Personal Computers and the Disabled

by

Peter A. McWilliams

Quantum Press
Doubleday & Company, Inc.
Garden City, New York
1984

First Edition, October 1984

Senior Editor: Christopher Meeks

Research Editors: Gregory Lee
                  Marko Sakren
                  Daniel Harris

Resources Editor: Ronald P. Gold

Paste-up: Robbie Uniacke

Copyright © 1984 by Prelude Press

Library of Congress Cataloging in Publication Data
McWilliams, Peter.
   Personal computers and the disabled.
   1. Self-help devices for the disabled. 2. Microcomputers. 3. Physically handicapped—Rehabilitation.
I. Title.
RD755.M38   1984   362.4'028'54   84-10309
ISBN 0-385-19685-7
Printed in the United States of America

OTHER BOOKS BY PETER A McWILLIAMS

The Personal Computer Book
The Personal Computer in Business Book
The Word Processing Book

Contents

Introduction 12
Chapter One
The Personal Computer 18
Chapter Two
Where Did They Come From and
    What Do They Do? 34
Chapter Three
The Right Stuff 42
Chapter Four
Personal Computers for the Deaf
    and Hearing Impaired 52
Chapter Five
Personal Computers for
    the Speech Impaired 62
Chapter Six
Personal Computers for People with
    Learning Disabilities 68
Chapter Seven
Personal Computers for People with
    Muscular, Motor, and Movement
    Disabilities 76
Chapter Eight
Personal Computers for the Blind
    and Visually Impaired 86
Chapter Nine
The Drawbacks of Personal Computers ... 92
Chapter Ten
Learning a Personal Computer
    Program 108

Chapter Eleven
Purchasing a Personal Computer *114*
Chapter Twelve
A Brand Name Buying Guide *128*
- Home Computers
  - Atari 800XL *132*
  - Coleco Adam *134*
  - Commodore VIC 20 .... *137*
  - Commodore 64 .... *138*
  - IBM PCjr *140*
  - Sinclair QL *142*
- Lap-Sized Computers
  - Epson Geneva/PX-8 .... *144*
  - Hewlett-Packard HP-110 .... *146*
  - Radio Shack Model 100 .... *148*
  - Teleram T-3000 .... *150*
- IBM and IBM-Compatibles
  - IBM PC *160*
  - IBM Portable PC *163*
  - Columbia MPC *164*
  - Compaq *166*
  - DEC Rainbow 100 .... *168*
  - Eagle PC PLUS-2 .... *170*
  - Eagle Spirit 2 .... *172*
  - Hewlett-Packard HP-150 .... *174*
  - NEC APC *176*
  - NorthStar Dimension *178*
  - Otrona 2001 .... *180*
  - Radio Shack Model 2000 .... *182*
  - Seequa Chameleon Plus *184*
  - TeleVideo Tele-PC *186*
  - Texas Instruments Portable
    Professional Computer *188*
  - Victor 9000 .... *190*
  - Xerox 16/8 .... *192*
  - Zenith Z-150 .... *194*
- Apple and Apple-Compatibles
  - Apple IIe *196*
  - Apple IIc *198*
  - Apple Lisa 2/5 .... *200*
  - Apple Macintosh *202*
  - Franklin Ace 1200 .... *205*

CP/M and Other Computers
   Cromemco C-10 207
   DECmate II 208
   Epson QX-10 210
   Jonos C2150 212
   Kaypro II 214
   Kaypro 4 216
   Kaypro 10 218
   Lanier TypeMaster 221
   Morrow MD-2 / MD-3 222
   Morrow MD-11 224
   NorthStar Advantage 226
   Radio Shack TRS-80 Model 4 228
   Radio Shack TRS-80 Model 12 230
   Radio Shack TRS-80 Model 16B 232
   Sanyo MBC-1150 / MBC-1250 233
   TeleVideo 802 234
   TeleVideo TS-803 236
   Toshiba T-300 238
   Zenith Z-100 240
Printers
   Epson FX-80 243
   Mannesmann Tally 160L 244
   Okidata 92 246
   Texas Instruments Model 855 248
   Hewlett Packard Think Jet Printer 250
   Bytewriter 252
   Diablo and Qume 252
   Daisywriter 253
   Comrex CR-II 254
   Brother HR-1/Comrex CR-1 255
   NEC 256
   Smith-Corona L-1000 258
   Transtar 130 260

HARDWARE, SOFTWARE AND
COMPUTER SERVICES 262
  Hardware and Software
    For the Deaf and Hearing
    Impaired 263
    For People with Learning
    Disabilities 265
    For People with Muscular,
    Motor and Movement Disabilities 267

  For the Speech Impaired, and
  for the Blind and Visually Impaired *287*
 Computer Appendix *311*
 Computer Services *313*

Chapter Thirteen
Resources 314
 I. Associations
  All Disabilities *316*
  Visual, Hearing,
  and Speech Impairments *319*
  Learning and Emotional
  Disabilities *321*
  Motor and Medical
  Impairments *323*
  Advocacy *326*
 II. Federal Government *327*
 III. Business: Training and Employment *334*
 IV. Higher Education *340*
 V. Information: Data Banks and Bases *345*
 VI. Media
  Magazines *349*
  Newsletters *352*
  General Computer Magazines *354*
  Major Newspapers *355*
  News Services and Syndicates *358*
 VII. Reading List
  Books *360*
  Directories *361*
  Book Clubs *362*
  Library Services *362*
 VIII. States *364*
  Addresses *395*

Introduction

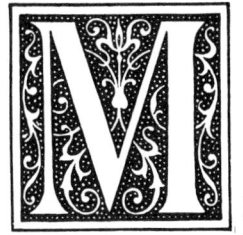y last computer book—at last. Were it not for the subject matter of this computer book, my last computer book would have been my last computer book.

My first computer book, *The Word Processing Book*, was a love letter to my fellow writers. Back then (1982), there were no books about word processing, most people didn't know what "word processing" meant, and many writers felt they were selling out if they used anything more electric than a pencil. In offices, people knew about word processing, but they thought it cost $20,000.

The message of *The Word Processing Book* was that word processing existed, that it was a creative tool more marvelous than any writer could imagine, and that it was far less expensive than most offices thought. Less than three years later, the rather radical message of *The Word Processing Book* is common knowledge. Every writer wants a word processor, and every office is planning to get one.

And so it is with personal computers and the disabled. (Yes, I remember the subject of this book. I may go off on autobiographical tangents now and again, but more often than not I return to the subject at hand.) Many people—including many disabled people—are not quite sure what a disabled person would *do* with a computer. Don't able-bodied people have enough trouble operating them? Aren't computers for the disabled terribly expensive? On the news, don't they show computers doing wonderful things for disabled people, but then don't they mention prices like $30,000, $50,000, $100,000?

In fact, personal computers for the disabled cost the same as personal computers for anybody else. The input devices, output devices and software might add to the price, but usually not that much. And, yes, sometimes disabled people have difficulty operating a computer—just as their able-bodied compatriots do.

And as to what personal computers can do for disabled people—well, personal computers can make the difference between communication and isolation, between productivity and non-productivity, between independence and dependence.

This may seem like a broadly sweeping statement, but consider:

• The deaf can now call anyone who has a computer and just "chat." Before computers, they could only call relatives and other deaf people who happen to have the same special communication devices.

• The blind, through synthesized voice output, have access to all the information available to personal computers—including news, research, correspondence, gossip, and thousands of other available services on data banks and bulletin boards. Before computers, the blind depended on the radio, talking books, Braille, and people who read to them.

• Computers allow people with muscular, motor and movement disabilities to work, create and communicate far more effectively than ever before. Disabled people who have control of only an eyelid, finger, toe, or eyebrow, can communicate, with unlimited vocabulary, and no outside help.

• People with learning disabilities find computers infinitely patient and thoroughly non-judgmental.

• Voice synthesizers give a voice to the voiceless.

All of the above, by the way, are available through off-the-shelf computers and currently available peripherals and software. Prices for complete systems range from $350 to $3,500, and prices are falling daily.

This is a book about what's available for the disabled person today, at reasonable prices. The $30,000 robotic arms, the $20,000 reading machines, the experimental computers that stimulate muscle groups allowing people to walk again—they're all wonderful, but they all remind me of the wonder drugs due on the market in "about five years."

Let's talk about what's here now, and in five years, as prices drop and as experiments become marketable products, we'll do a new edition and marvel at all the improvements.

A word about the words in this book: After much thought and long discussions with many disabled people, I chose the word "disabled" over "handicapped." Disabled simply means not able, and it's a word that applies to everyone about some area of life or another. (I have a disability when it comes to spelling and math. I am not able to spell most words longer than two syllables, and I still do not know my multiplication tables. Long division? Cringe. Fortunately, my computer and pocket calculator—a baby computer—are tools through which my disabilities become abilities.)

The word handicapped seems to have a greater stigma attached to it than simply "not able." Maybe it's just me and the way that I hear it, but handicapped has a slightly negative charge, and disabled is fairly neutral. "Crippled" is clearly negative, as James Watt found out the hard way.

Again, it's just me. I find the word disabled more comfortable to use than handicapped. I do not for a moment feel that most people who use the word handicapped mean to imply even the slightest negativity. The choice is a personal one, and I am not campaigning for the replacement of one for the other.

Those who do not suffer from the generally accepted disabilities will be referred to in the book as able-bodied. The condescension inherent in calling a non-disabled person "normal" is, I think, obvious. For the sake of variety, I will sometimes use "non-disabled," as I did in the previous sentence. It's a double negative of sorts, and my seventh grade English teacher will shriek. I will do my best to keep that usage to a minimum.

And a word about the humor (or, shall I say *attempts* at humor) in this book. When I told people I was going to write a book about personal computers and the disabled, they thought it was a grand idea, then they leaned over and said, conspiratorially, "But what about the *humor?*"

Well, I am here to state the obvious (I'm good at that—I make my living at it, in fact): the disabled have a sense of humor, too. The ability to occasionally laugh at oneself and the world is one of the most effective survival techniques I know, and disabled people know more about survival than anyone else. To leave humor out of the book would be the greatest insult of all.

It was all brought home to me one day a few years ago when a young woman, Marty Sheldon, stood in front of a room of about 200 people and told us, carefully forming her words syllable by syllable, "I do not have a speech impediment. I have a Cerebral Palsy accent."

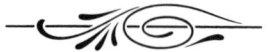

I hope that three years from now, everything in this introduction will be so much a part of the collective social consciousness that it will all seem silly.

I hope that publishers turn out as many books on personal computers for the disabled as they turned out books on word processing.

I hope that people will soon consider providing a personal computer for certain disabilities as automatic and as fundamental as providing a wheelchair or a leader dog or a pair of crutches.

I hope that there will be so much information on and action in getting personal computers to disabled people that this book will be but a minor footnote in a major campaign.

From a soothsayer's point of view, the signs are good. In 1982, between the time I wrote and the time I published *The Word Processing Book*, Sybex released a book on word processing. *The Word Processing Book* was second. Now, in 1984, Sybex is publishing a book on personal computers and the disabled between the writing and publishing of this book. Once again, I'm second.

Let's just hope that what happened to word processing from 1982 to 1984 is a forerunner of what will happen to personal computers for the disabled from 1984 to 1986.

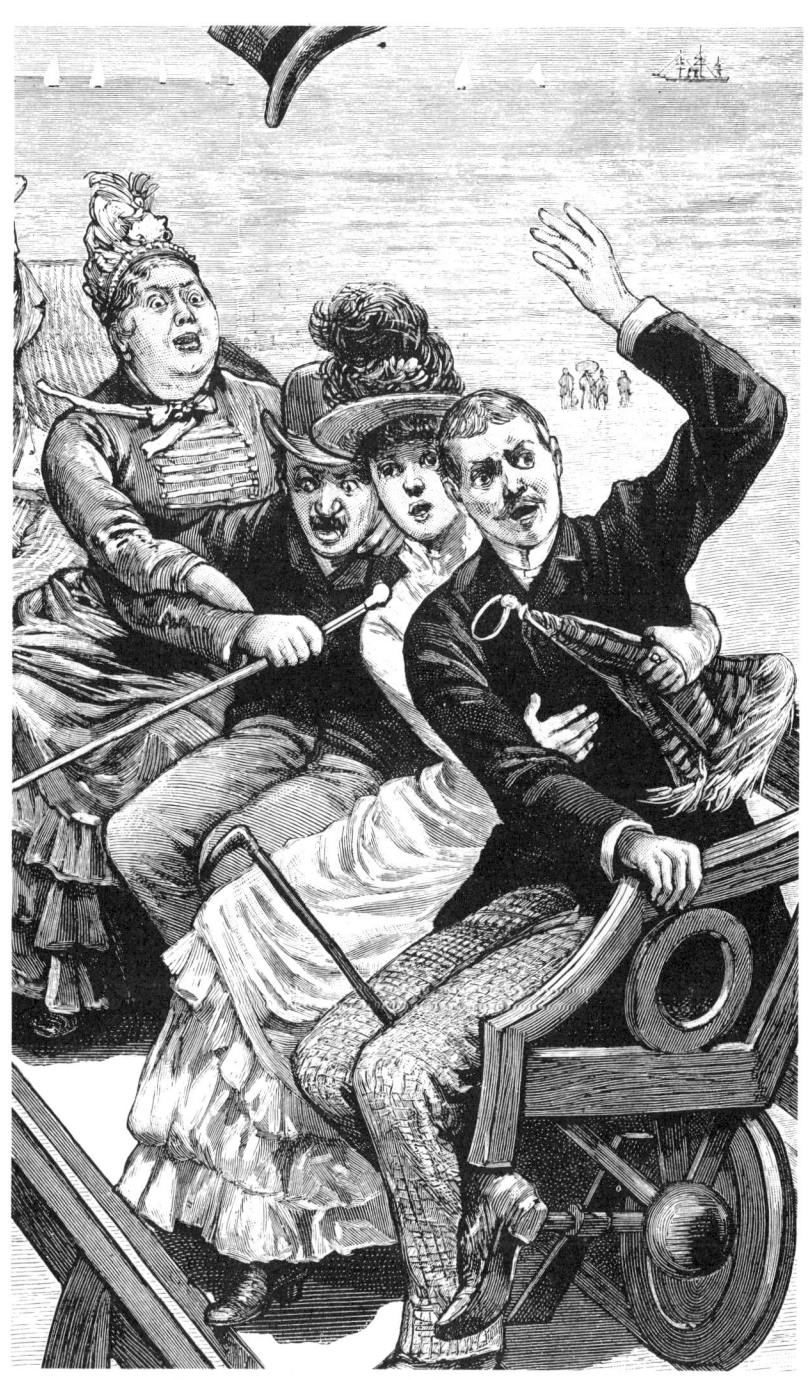
Hold tight everybody! Next stop, computers.

Chapter One

The Personal Computer

 o begin with, personal computers are just machines. The misconception that computers *think*, and that as they get smarter and smarter they will somehow take over our lives like HAL the computer took over the spaceship in *2001*, has caused some fear.

The fact is that computers no more think than tape recorders talk or phonographs sing. Personal computers are simply the latest technological goodie in a line of technological goodies (electric lights, telephones, phonographs, automobiles, airplanes, radios, movies, televisions, VegaMatics) that have, in the past 100 years, changed the face of the earth.

Let's take a look at the machine itself, the personal computer.

While exploring personal computers, I'll also provide you with a crash course in conversational Computerese. Computerese is intricate enough to qualify as the world's 297th language. The United Nations is currently providing translators fluent in Computerese to various delegations, and Berlitz is offering a basic course on cassette tape. There is even a book of Computerese sign language for the deaf. (I'm not kidding. It's called *Signs For Computer Terminology* and published by The National Association for the Deaf.)

After reading this chapter you'll be able to trade jargon with some of the best computer salespeople in town, and most of the time you'll even know what each other is talking about.

The heart of any computer is known as the **processor**. A processor sorts and re-sorts information at a very high speed. (It is the phenomenal speed of computers that gives the *illusion* of thought, just as the speed with which still pictures change on a movie screen gives the illusion of motion.) This repeated sorting is known as **processing**. Hence, the sorting of words is **word processing**, the sorting of data is **data processing**, and so on.

PERSONAL COMPUTERS AND THE DISABLED

In the old days (the 1940s), processors used vacuum tubes and filled entire rooms. Then transistors replaced tubes, and a **mini*processor** could fit in a single room. Then silicon chips replaced transistors, and soon you could hold a **micro*processor** in the palm of your hand. More importantly, you could build a computer around a microprocessor that could fit on a desk, and **microcomputers** were born. Microprocessors are also known as **CPUs**, for Central Processing Unit.

Microprocessors are fast, but stupid. They only know two things: on and off. Like all machines, computers are good at black/white, yes/no, open/closed. They are not good at shades of grey, "maybe," or "a little bit open but not quite closed." (Humans, on the other hand, tend to prefer the gradations of life, which is why many people feel uncomfortable in the presence of computers and religious fanatics.)

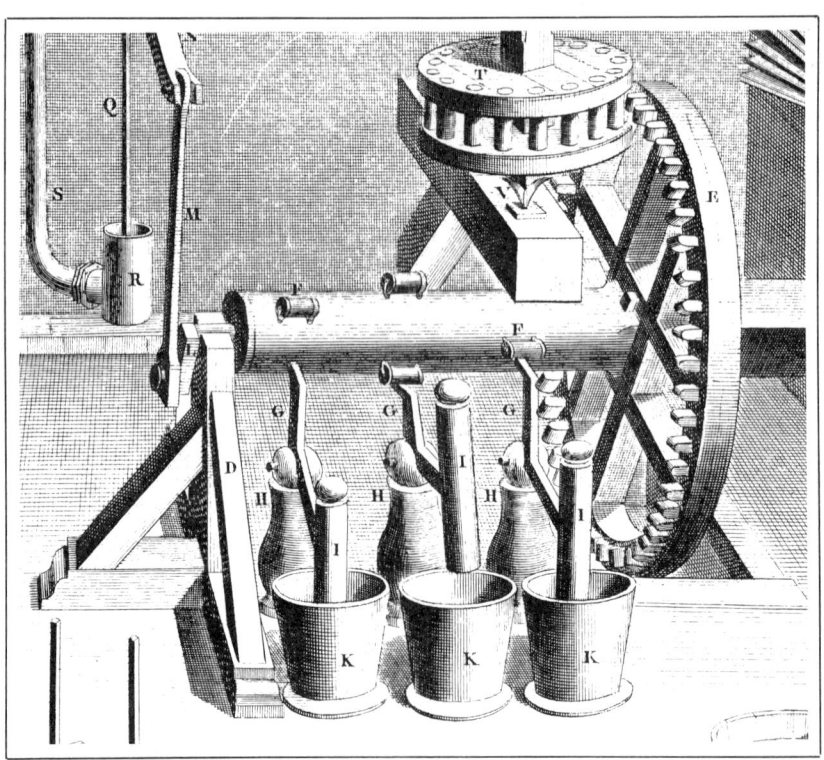

A microprocessor through the electron microscope. (Scale: 1 inch = 5 miles.)

The Personal Computer

This makes the **binary** system of numbers invaluable to computers. It's a system of counting that has only two symbols, 0 and 1. (The system we're used to is the decimal system, which has ten symbols: 0 through 9.) With the symbols 0 and 1, the binary system can represent any number, although binary takes up more room and is more cumbersome to work with than the decimal system. ("27 in binary is "11011," for example.)

Because processors are so fast, the cumbersomeness is not noticed. The computer translates from decimal to binary, does its work in binary, and translates the answer back to decimal so fast it seems instantaneous. (In working with a personal computer, by the way, you'll never know that this binaryness is going on.)

To process words, computers assign all the characters of language a number. To process music (for digital recordings), computers divide the audio spectrum into 50,000 slices, and the intensity of each slice is assigned a number from 0 to 65,000. This gives an accurate representation of the sound at a given moment in time. Play these moments back, one after another, and you have music. In this way, the computer reduces the masters of literature and music to 0 and 1.

This 0 or 1 choice is the smallest increment of computers. It is known as a **bit**. The more bits a processor can handle *simultaneously*, the more powerful the processor. Most small computers have 8-bit processors. Many have 16-bit. Some have 32-bit processors. (I'm not sure personal computers *need* 16 or 32-bit processors, but then some old fogies at the turn of the century didn't think that cars would ever need heaters or headlights.)

A **byte** is eight bits, which is enough to represent a single letter, number, or punctuation mark. A **kilobyte** is 1,024 bytes. Kilobyte is abbreviated simply **K**. Each generation has its measurements to brag about and to compare one's achievements against.

"My computer has 64K."
"What's a K?"
"I don't know, but my computer has 64 of them."

PERSONAL COMPUTERS AND THE DISABLED

To understand the amount of information in a K, imagine an 8½ x 11 sheet of paper, typewritten, double spaced, with generous margins. The amount of information on such a page is 2K. If you're blind, the 8½ x 11 analogy might not mean much to you. Put another way: a radio announcer, speaking at a moderate rate, reads about 1K of information per minute. Kilobytes are used to measure various forms of memory on personal computers. Bits are used to measure the power of microprocessors.

While some silicon chips ("silicon" is just a fancy word for glass, by the way) were designed for processing information, other chips were developed to remember what had been processed. (Microprocessors are fast, but they can't seem to remember what it was they did so fast.)

The two kinds of memory chips used in personal computers are **RAM** and **ROM**. RAM stands for Random Access Memory, and ROM for Read Only Memory.

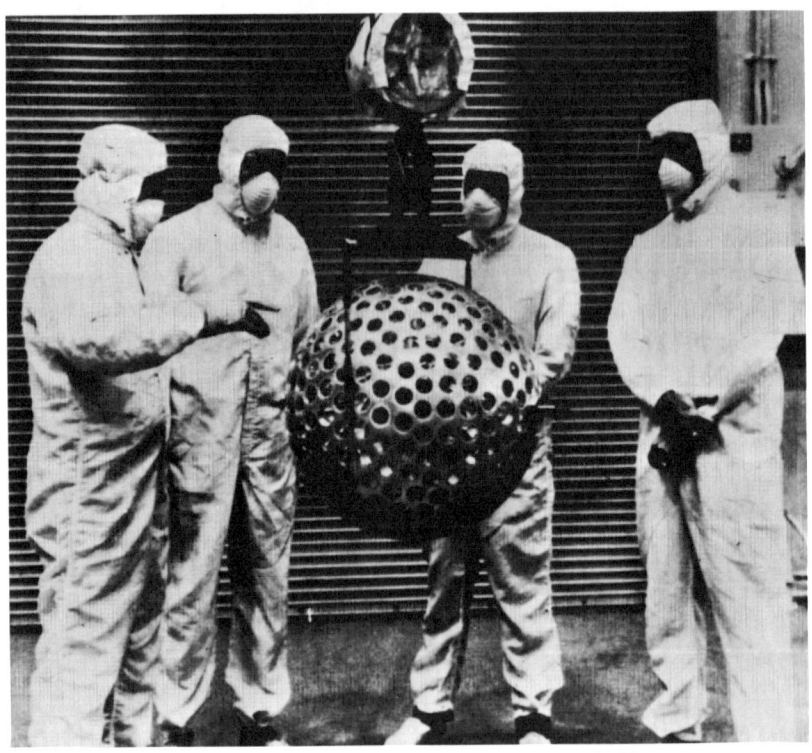

Bits must be handled very carefully.

The Personal Computer

ROM is a chip that contains information that cannot be changed. It's like a phonograph record. The CPU can play (or **read**) information from that chip as often as it wants. It cannot, however, record (or **write**) information onto that chip. (Hence "read only" memory.)

RAM is like a cassette tape. You can record information on it and play back information from it. You can erase, alter, take from or add to RAM any time you like. You have *random access* to this memory.

RAM is also known as **User Programmable Memory**. I have never seen this abbreviated UPM, nor have I ever heard of ROM referred to as Manufacturer Programmable Memory (MPM). The Noah Webster of Computerese is obviously asleep at the dipswitch. (A **dipswitch**, by the way, is one of many switches found inside a personal computer that is so small it requires the point of a pencil to flip it. Why this is called a dipswitch and not a microswitch, I will never know. I also do not know who put the dip in the dip-da-dip-da switch any more than I know who put the RAM in the rama-lama-ding-dong. My ignorance about computers is boundless.)

The amount of memory RAM can hold at any one time ranges from 1 kilobyte to 1,000 kilobytes, and larger memories are on the way. As you may have guessed, 1,000 kilobytes has a name of its own: one **megabyte**. Most personal computers have either 16K, 32K, 48K, 64K, 128K or 256K of RAM.

RAM, while more versatile than ROM, has a tragic flaw: Once electric current stops flowing through it, RAM forgets everything it ever knew. ROM, on the other hand, remembers everything, power or no power, indefinitely. This poses a problem if you want to store the processed information when it comes time to turn the computer off.

The solution? Most personal computers today use some form of **magnetic media**. These generally come in the form of tapes and disks.

Tapes used in personal computers are the standard cassette tapes that the record industry is blaming all its troubles on. When a cassette recorder is connected to a computer, it will record and play back computer impulses just as it records and plays back musical impulses when attached to a stereo.

PERSONAL COMPUTERS AND THE DISABLED

Cassette tapes, while inexpensive, are limited. The rewinding and fast forwarding necessary to read and write information to and from various portions of the tape is time consuming, and the number of "read/write" errors when using tapes is far greater than when using disks. Further, cassette tapes hold less information than disks.

Disks come either floppy or hard, and in sizes from 3½ to 8 inches. Disks are circles of plastic or metal, covered with the same brown garden-hoe variety rust (iron oxide) as tapes.

Disks spin like phonograph records, although much faster. The playback and record head (called a **read/write head**) moves across the disk like the arm on a turntable, and it can go quickly from one spot on the disk to another.

Floppy disks are circles of flexible plastic enclosed in a square, protective cardboard covering. The entire square goes into the computer's **disk drive**, and the computer has access to the disk through a hole in the center of the square and an oval slit on one or both sides.

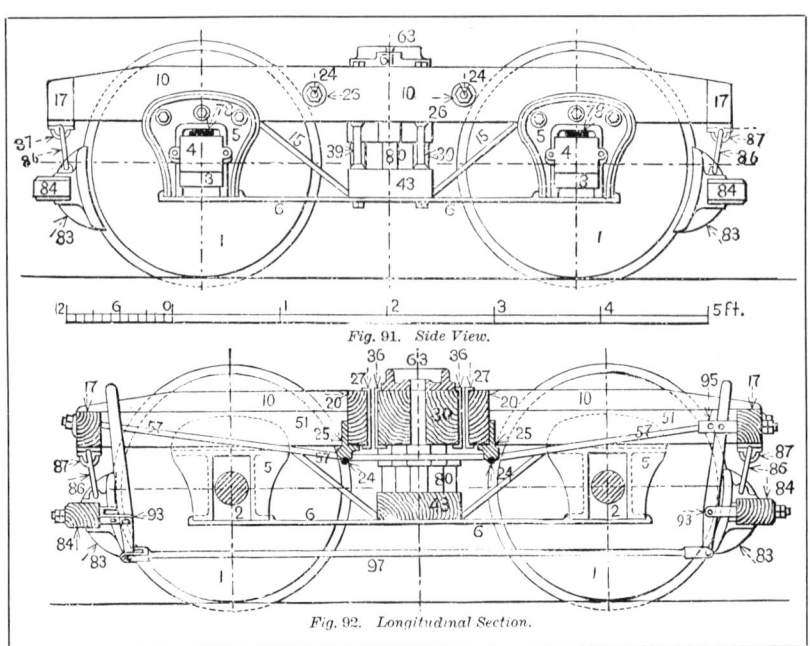

Fig. 91. Side View.

Fig. 92. Longitudinal Section.

Diagram of a dual disk drive. Please memorize all parts. There will be a quiz at the end of this chapter.

The Personal Computer

Information is recorded on floppy disks in circles known as **tracks**. Each track is divided into **sectors**. When twice as many tracks are squeezed onto one side of a disk, this is known as **double density**. When read/write heads are on both sides of a disk, this is **double sided**. When these two features are combined, it is, (logically, for once) called **double sided double density**.

Floppy disks on personal computers come in three sizes: 3½, 5¼, and 8-inch. The 5¼-inch disk is the most popular. Each disk holds from 71K to 2,400K (2.4 megabytes) of information. For greater storage, greater speed, or both, one usually needs a **hard disk**.

A hard disk is a platter of metal on which a layer of iron oxide has been bonded. The rapid spinning of these disks (about 30 revolutions per *second*) creates a breeze. The read/write head floats *above* the disk on this breeze. Because there is no head friction, and because the disk spins so quickly, hard disks store and retrieve information several times faster than floppy disks.

Hard disks also hold more information. The smallest holds 5 megabytes (5,000K) of information, and they go up from there. Naturally, they cost more than floppies.

Another form of magnetic media used in a few personal computers is **bubble memory**. This incorporates the best features of both ROM and RAM: You can manipulate the information as you please *and* it retains the manipulated information even after the computer has been turned off. Bubble memories have a flaw, too: at the moment, they are expensive. Broad exposure and popular acceptance should, like anything else, tend to cheapen them.

(The next mass storage device will be the laser disk. A standard video laser disk, the kind that shows movies and costs $25, will hold more than one gigabyte [one *billion* bytes] of information. That's roughly the amount of information in the Encyclopedia Britannica, including color photographs. These should be available within the next year or two.)

Magnetic media are not just used for remembering what absent-minded CPUs and fickle RAMs forget. Disks and tapes are also used for providing information and

PERSONAL COMPUTERS AND THE DISABLED

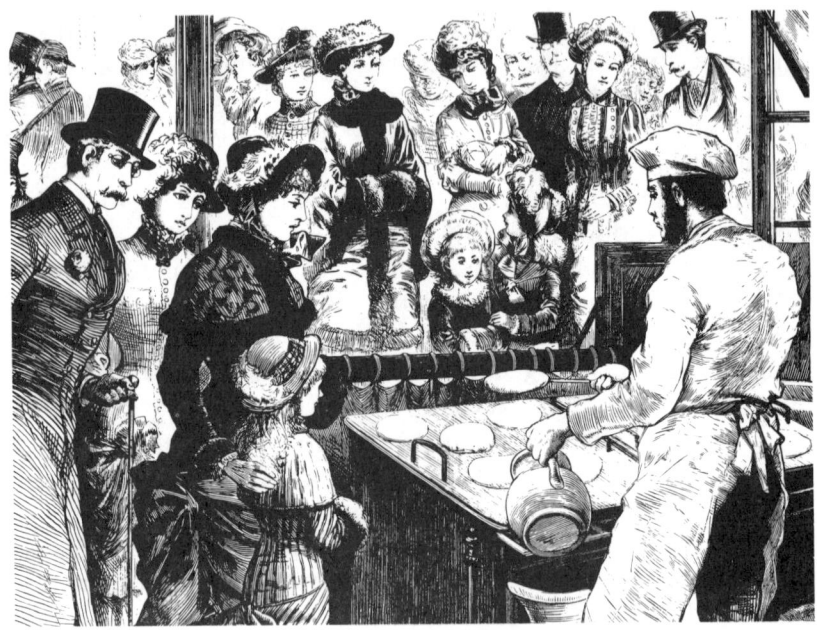

Some computer stores actually show disks being made, and the public is always intrigued.

instructions to the computer in the form of **programs**. Programs tell the computer what to do, how to do it, when to do it, when not to do it, and so on.

A program is to a computer as a record is to a phonograph. (Didn't you used to love those tests in school? "A rose is to a thorn as a ＿＿＿＿＿＿ is to an atomic bomb.") Phonographs play records. Computers **run** programs.

Programs (also known as **software**) are what give computers their enormous appeal. All the good things you hear about computers happen because programs tell the computer (the **hardware**) how to make it happen.

A computer running a word processing program is a word processing computer. (Word processing is the most significant advance in the manipulation of the written word since the advent of writing. I do not exaggerate. Every secretary, student and, certainly, professional writer will find their lives changed—dare I say transformed?—by the simple addition of a personal computer and a word processing program.)

The Personal Computer

The same computer running an accounting program becomes an accounting computer. (The incredible advantages large computers have given large companies are now available to small companies through small computers. Accounts receivable, accounts payable, cost projection, inventory control—all the repetitive numerical tasks that can make or break a small company—are manageable with ease, speed, and remarkable cost effectiveness.)

The same computer that runs a small business can, with a change of programs, help keep the wheels turning at big business too. (Although the company may have two or three large computers, an executive can have his or her own "personal" computer to help manage all the information that managers are paid to manage. In years to come, the small computer will become as familiar a desktop item in large corporations as an adding machine or typewriter.)

Remove the business program, insert a game program, and you have a game-playing computer. (Man does not live by information management alone, and computer games are not just for kids. Chess, backgammon, blackjack; you name it, computers will play it. Beyond the traditional games, there are action and adventure games that can only be played on computers. These are remarkably seductive, and may become your favorite waste of time.)

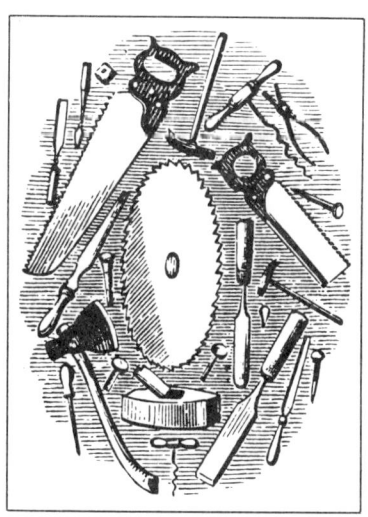

Hardware, circa 1957

PERSONAL COMPUTERS AND THE DISABLED

Most people buy prerecorded music, and most people buy prewritten programs. Some people record their own music, and some people write their own programs—but you need know nothing about programming to successfully use and enjoy a computer. (I know as much about writing computer programs as I know about writing music, which is as close to nothing as is metaphysically possible.)

Writing computer programs (**programming**) is, I am told, involving and occasionally delightful. (Anything some people find addictive is worth serious investigation.) Programming is a creative act, but one in which the creator has the dubious pleasure—shared only by film makers, Henry Higgins, Dr. Frankenstein, and God—of watching the creation take on a life of its own. Computer programs can be remarkably three dimensional. They interact. Randomness can be written in. And, maybe for the first time in your life, you can get a TV set to do what *you* want it to. Ah, power.

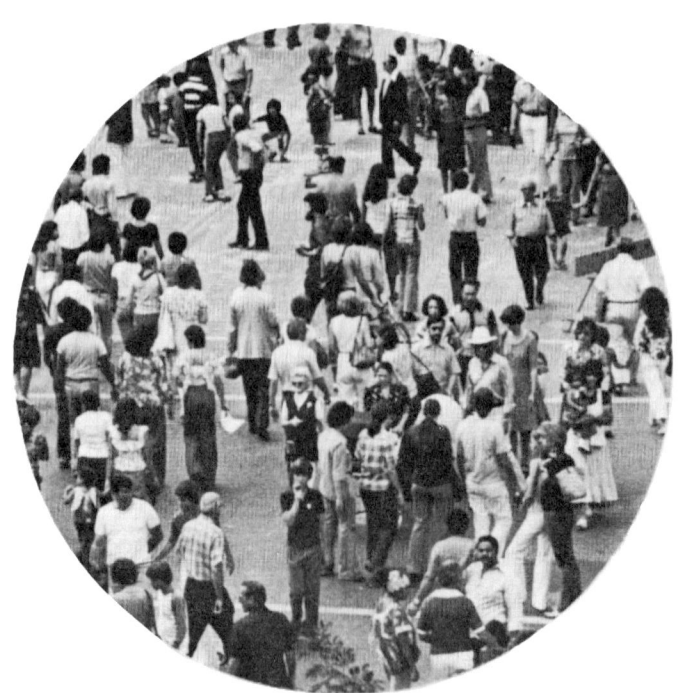

Here's the disk for a program called "Address Book." It holds about 300 people.

The Personal Computer

The enthusiasm of that last paragraph is second-hand. I have listened to the rapture of the converted, and believe it to be genuine. But, like jogging or marriage or backpacking across America, when it comes to the joys of writing computer programs, I have thus far resisted temptation.

When you write programs, or enter any other information into the computer, a **keyboard** comes in handy. This looks like an ordinary typewriter keyboard with a few extra keys added. (These keys are labeled CONTROL, ESCAPE, BREAK and other words taken from the dialogue of old Warner Brothers prison movies.) Some keyboards have a square with the numbers 0 through 9 in an adding machine arrangement. This is known as a **numeric keypad**.

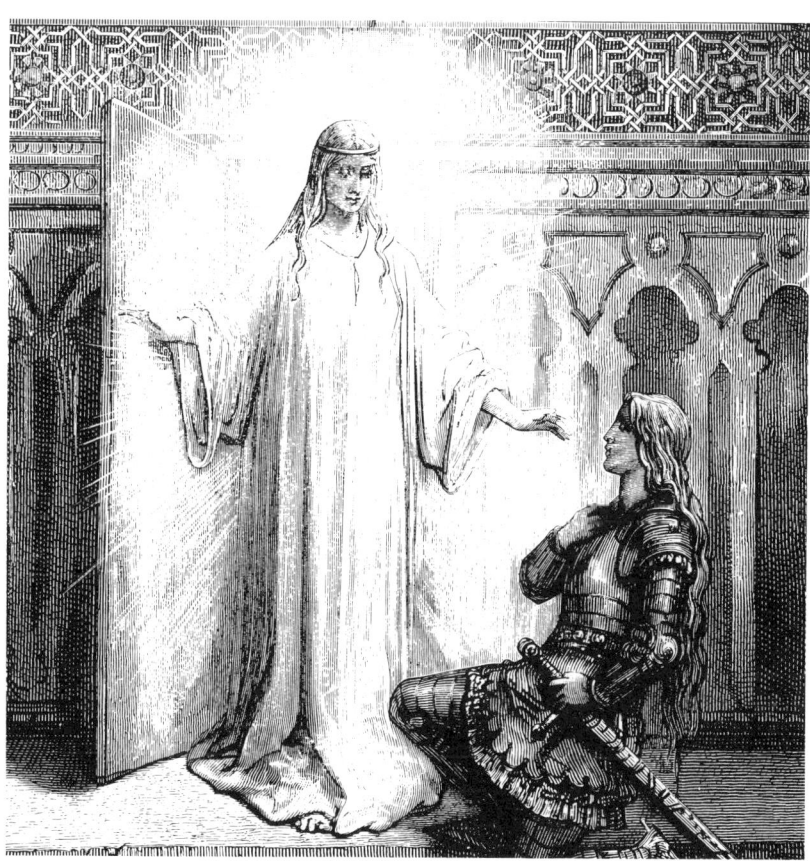

THE CURSOR. The cursor is a square of light that tells you where you are on the video screen.

PERSONAL COMPUTERS AND THE DISABLED

Another method of entering information is through a **joystick**. Joysticks are hand-held devices that move the space ship or submarine or Pac Person about. A **mouse** is a small, square device that is moved across the top of a desk. It's used to move a pointer around in business programs. (If you want to get rid of something, you move the pointer to a picture of a garbage can and push a button.) A mouse, then, is an executive joystick.

There are other **input devices** especially designed for the disabled. (An input device is any device used to put information into a computer. Clear?) We'll discuss these further along in the book.

It is helpful, of course, to see the information as it's being processed, stored, and manipulated. For this, computers use **video screens**. (We'll discuss the "viewing" options for the blind a bit later on.) Video screens in personal computers are the same video screens that have been showing "I Love Lucy" for the past several millennia. The fancy Computerese word for a video screen is **CRT**, which stands for Cathode Ray Tube, which is the kind of tube a TV picture tube really is.

Some computers, especially smaller home computers, use regular televisions for display. For business and word processing, most personal computers use **monitors**. Letters and numbers (known as **characters** in Computerese) are sharper and easier to read when displayed on a monitor.

Video displays can be either color or **monochrome**. (Monochrome means, literally, "one color.") Monochrome screens offer one color (usually white, green or amber) against a black background. Color screens, naturally, offer the full spectrum of colors. The best color screens are known as **RGB monitors**, so named because the three primary electronic colors are Red, Green, and Blue. (For some reason, in electronics, red and green, combined, produce yellow. Try telling *that* to your eighth grade art teacher.)

In general, color monitors are better for games and graphics; monochrome monitors are better for the display of characters.

When it comes time to print what one has processed, computers use **printers**. (Another rare example of logical

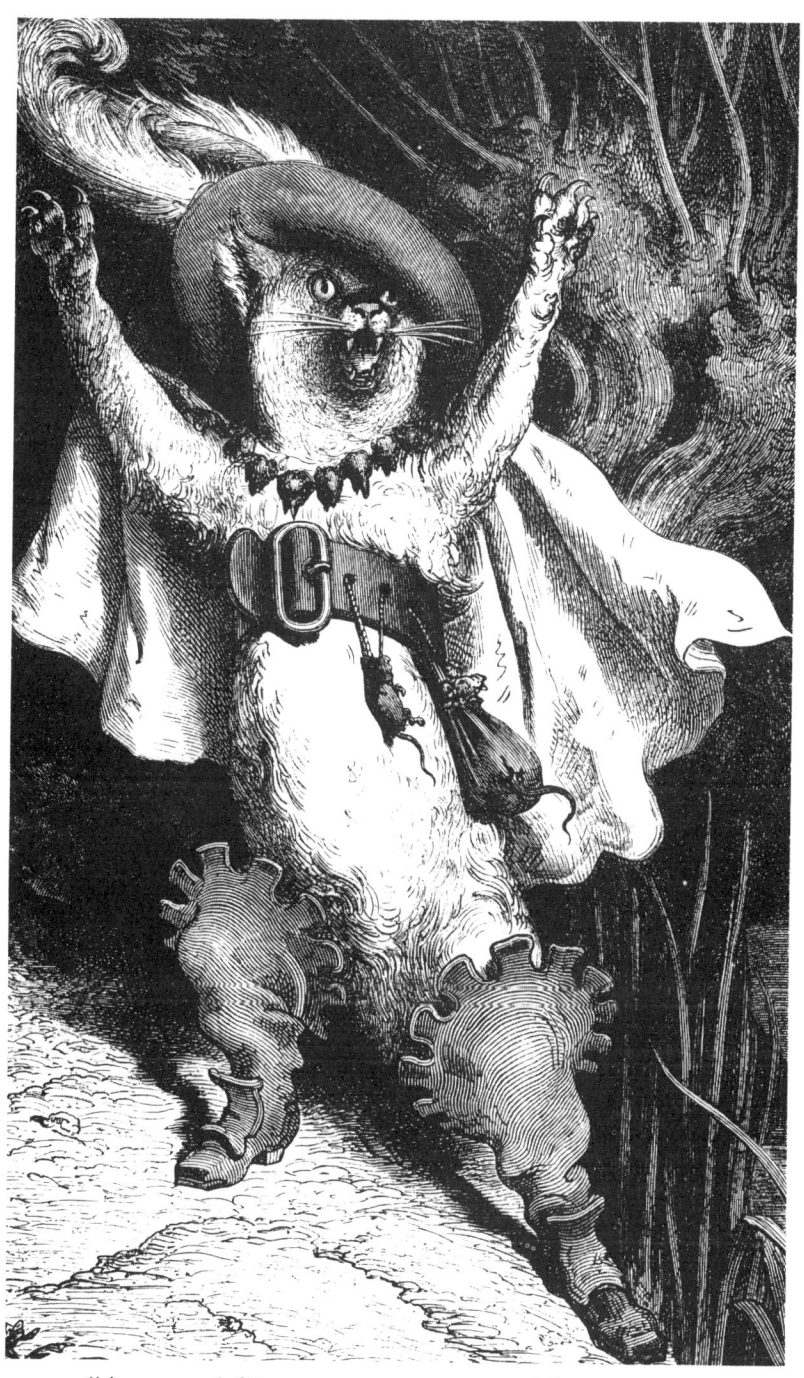
"A mouse! Give me a computer with a mouse!"

PERSONAL COMPUTERS AND THE DISABLED

labeling in Computerese.) Printers used with personal computers are generally of two types, **dot matrix** and **letter quality**.

Dot matrix printers form letters and numbers using little dots, like the signs on banks that display time, temperature, and current interest rates. Like these signs, dot matrix printers communicate information effectively, though not elegantly.

For elegance, one must turn to letter quality printers. Letter quality printers print one fully formed character at a time, like a typewriter. The term "letter quality" comes, I suppose, from the fact that it's hard to tell the difference between a letter typed on an electric typewriter and one printed on a letter quality printer.

Dot matrix printers cost less and print faster than their letter quality counterparts. Letter quality printers produce better copy. Dot matrix printers are necessary for graphics; letter quality printers are necessary for "serious" word processing. (Friends will be happy to get dot matrix letters, but writing bank presidents, asking for that million-dollar loan, requires letter quality.)

(Lasers, by the way, threaten to revolutionize printing as well as mass storage. Laser printers combine the best of both dot matrix and letter quality, at a speed that rivals offset printing. The cost, as you may have guessed, is high, but should be coming down in the next few years.)

To communicate with other computers over telephone lines, one requires a **modem**. Modem (pronounced mo-dem, as in Mo Dean) stands for MOdulate/DEModulate, which is what modems do to computer signals. Outgoing information is modulated (encoded), and incoming information is demodulated (decoded) by a little black box that plugs into your telephone line. (Not all modems are black any more. Many black boxes in the world of personal computers are now fashionably beige.)

The Personal Computer

So there we have it, the personal computer. But what do we have? Not much. It's not what personal computers *are* that's important (or even interesting, as you may have noticed). What's important is what personal computers *do*. And that is the subject of Chapter Two.

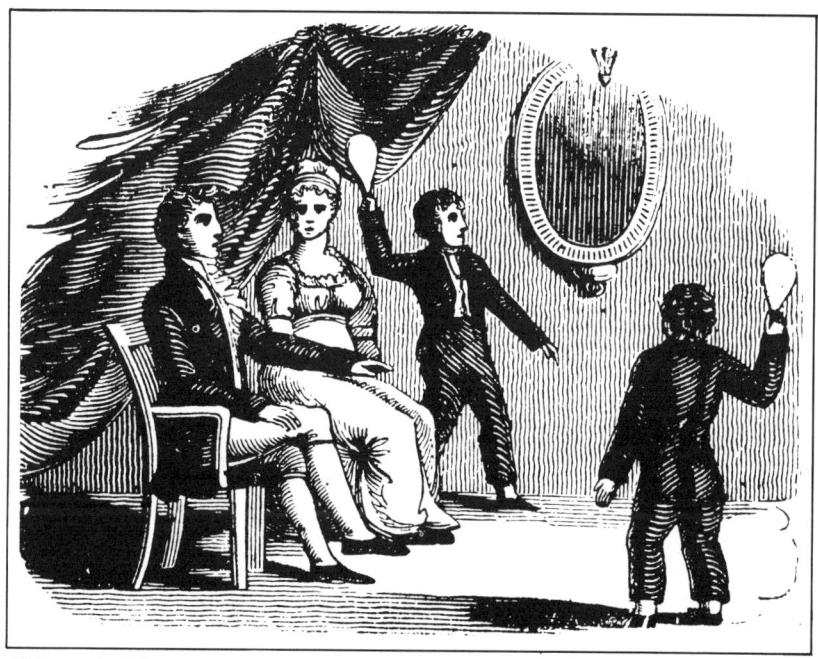

"The children seem to be enjoying the paddles quite a lot. Do you think we should get them a ball?"

PUBLISHERS NOTE: THIS DRAWING, AS FAR AS WE CAN TELL, HAS NOTHING WHATSOEVER TO DO WITH COMPUTERS FOR THE DISABLED. MR. MCWILLIAMS IS DRIFTING HOPELESSLY, AND WE OFFER OUR SINCERE APOLOGIES.

Chapter Two

Where Did They Come From and What Do They Do?

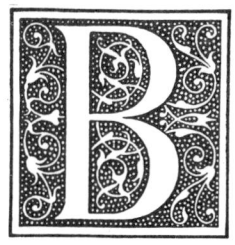efore we look at how computers can help individuals with specific disabilities, let's take a broad view of what computers generally do well, and why they have become so popular in such a short time. Let's begin with a bit of history.

One hundred years ago, the population of the United States was growing so fast that the 1880 census took eight years to count. It was estimated that the 1890 census would take twelve years. At this rate, we would know by 1985 what the population was in 1930. A better way of counting people had to be found, and it was: The 1890 Census Machine.

This was the brainchild of John Shaw Billings and Herman Hollerith. Hollerith distributed to the census takers dollar bill holders and preprinted punch cards. (The dollar bill holders were already invented, hence the size and shape of computer punch cards for generations to come was determined by the dimensions of the 1890 dollar bill. There's an irony in there somewhere.)

The census taker would put a punch card in the holder, punch holes in the appropriate locations while conducting the census, and send the completed cards to Washington. There they were fed into a machine that read the holes and tabulated the results. The 1890 census took three years to complete, and Hollerith was a hero.

To market his invention (now called the Tabulating Machine), Hollerith turned to big business. The consumer public was, after all, having trouble accepting such recent inventions as the lightbulb, the phonograph, the automobile, the telephone and indoor plumbing. Hollerith joined a company that eventually called itself International Business Machines.

In 1938, IBM joined with Harvard and created the first electronic computer, the Mark I. This machine was the size of a 7-Eleven and had 46,000 vacuum tubes. (One

PERSONAL COMPUTERS AND THE DISABLED

tube burned out, on the average, every six minutes.) This behemoth could add, subtract, multiply, divide and, most importantly, make mathematical tables for the forthcoming world war.

By the mid 1950s there were Univacs and IBMs all over the big business landscape. Digital came along with its cheaper computers in 1960 (a mere $120,000 per), and, while most of America was deciding whether to invest $500 in a color TV, thousands of big and pretty-big businesses were buying computers.

The late 1970s brought personal computers. Some small business people started using personal computers for accounting or word processing or cost projection. The big computer companies said it couldn't be done. Then Radio Shack and Apple and a few others made a lot of money, and the big computer companies said, well, maybe. Then IBM introduced a small computer, and the other big computer companies said, but, of course, we have one, too.

And so personal computers were firmly established in business, and they all lived happily ever after. End of history lesson.

But what is it about personal computers that makes them so irresistible to businesses, both large and small? Well, they're cheap for one thing. Sure, two, three, four, five thousand dollars is expensive for you and me, but to a business it's not much, especially when you consider what a business gets for its money.

In these days of increasing labor costs, and decreasing labor skills, personal computers have become the Mighty Mouse of business. ("Here I come to save the day...") Computers do their work, reliably, uncomplainingly, 24 hours a day if necessary, with no vacations, sick leaves, unemployment benefits, unions, salary, or coffee breaks.

Besides, computers are best at the kind of work human beings hate: mechanical, repetitive manipulation of words and numbers. A personal computer, for example, can sort a mailing list of 10,000 into zip code order in about ten minutes. Can you imagine how long that would take a human? And how painfully dull that process would be? (To give you some idea, this chapter has about 2,000

Where Did They Come From

words. Imagine five times as many words, and each word a five-digit number. Then imagine trying to sort them into numerical order. Ugh.)

But the computer does not care. You can tell it to re-sort the list in alphabetical order by last name, and ten minutes later a new list of 10,000 alphabetized names is ready. Want to find the name of the person who lives on Elizabeth Court? Ask it to find "Elizabeth Court" and it will, within minutes. (In a mailing list of 10,000, that's roughly equivalent to skimming through every page of this book, looking for a single word.)

These are extreme examples, showing how a single personal computer can eliminate hours, if not days, of tedious work. Not everything the computer does telescopes two days into ten minutes. Even if, on the average, a personal computer only doubled the efficiency of the person using it, it would pay for itself in six months (and that's including two months of training and transition time).

Here are a few of the tasks that have made personal computers the darlings of the business world:

Word processing. I cannot spell and I'm a terrible typist, so when I heard about this marvelous machine that would correct my spelling and never make me retype anything ever again, I knew I had to have one. That was my introduction to personal computers.

Four years later, I can't imagine writing, or running a business, without one. Letters, articles, or reports can be revised and "retyped" (reprinted, actually) in a matter of minutes, not hours. Personally "typed," personally addressed form letters can be churned out at the rate of one per minute. Labels for our mythical 10,000-person mailing list can be printed in less than a day. Over and over, time is saved and tedium reduced with word processing.

Word processing is a boon to the creative process. Word processing, in fact, goes on in the human mind. The various tools of word processing—pens, pencils, type-writers—are simply there to remind one what has already been processed. A personal computer, outfitted with a word processing program, is the best tool for assisting the word processing mind to date.

PERSONAL COMPUTERS AND THE DISABLED

Accounting. Accounts payable, accounts receivable, invoicing, payroll, general ledger, inventory control—all those things that are handled by the dp (data processing) department of large companies, can now be moved from piles of books to piles of disks in small companies.

Computers love manipulating numbers. A bookkeeper may not, at first, enjoy becoming a computer keeper, but once he or she writes his or her first invoice with only twelve keystrokes, and marvels as the information is automatically posted to accounts receivable, general ledger, and the invoiced items are automatically removed from inventory, resistance will melt.

Cost projection. On a computer this is known as electronic spreadsheeting or electronic worksheeting. It's putting information in rows and columns, and then playing the game of "What If?" What if the cost of goods goes up 5%, how much will we have to raise the retail price? What if the cost of goods goes up 5%, but sales go up 7%? What if we charged $1.95, how many widgets would we have to sell before showing a profit?

These questions once took paper-and-hand-held-calculator spreadsheeters hours to answer. A personal computer does it in seconds. Electronic spreadsheeting allows one to be creative with numbers. You can play What If for an hour, and have considered more options than could have been considered in a week.

Data banks. Data banks are like money banks, except they hold data instead of money. You contact a data bank by using a personal computer, a modem, and a telephone. You can get up-to-the-minute stock market quotations, financial histories of any traded stock, read AP and UPI stories before Dan Rather, make travel arrangements, do research, and on and on.

The three most popular data banks are The Source, CompuServe, and The Dow Jones Information Service. There are many, many others.

Electronic mail. Electronic mail allows information to get across the country in seven seconds, not seven days. ("And on the seventh day, the Postmaster said, 'It will do,' and he rested.") Letters, memos, reports, charts—anything that can be displayed on a video screen can be sent to any other connected computer (again, through modems and phone lines) almost instantly.

This costs more than a first-class letter, but less than Federal Express. Many computers and modems have auto-send and auto-receive capabilities. A letter can be sent and received at 3 AM, when phone rates are cheap and when the computer is not likely to be in use. No one needs to be at either end; the computers will take care of it all. An average letter takes only a few seconds to transmit, and the information is stored on a disk.

MCI Mail will give you, free, your own electronic mailbox. Anyone with a computer can send you a letter to your mailbox, and it will be waiting for you when you check in. The box is free, checking your box is free, but sending a letter to your box, naturally, costs something.

Another version of electronic mail is teleconferencing. This allows several computers in various parts of the world to be connected for a conference. This can happen in "real time," that is, everyone can be "online" at the same time, or it can happen over time, with the various conference participants checking in from time to time, reading what's been said, making comments, and checking out.

Graphs. Some companies have whole art departments that do nothing but prepare bar graphs and pie charts. Computers can make graphs and pie charts in minutes, not hours, and in color if necessary.

This gives the small business its own art department. And, while the large business will no doubt retain its art department to produce bars and pies for corporate reports, the daily flow of graphs from screen to screen and (when printed) from hand to hand should increase dramatically in boardrooms across this great land of ours. (Someone might even do a bar graph charting the increase.)

Games. There are uses for computers that have little to do with business, the favorite of which is games. Computers play games very well, from chess to backgammon to a new genre of recreational activity called, appropriately enough, computer games. Computers provide worthy opponents for solo play, or impartial refereeing and accurate scorekeeping for paired combat.

There are mental games, strategy games, and action games. Computer games are marvelous recreation. Far from viewing them as a waste of time, I tend to go along with Professor Harold Hill, who said in defense of billiards long, long ago: "I consider that the hours I spend with a cue in my hand are golden. Helps you cultivate a horse sense, and a cool head, and a keen eye." The same could be said of joysticks today.

Education. And finally, computers are great for education. If there lived a person as patient as a computer, that patience and three miracles would qualify him or her for sainthood. Computers will present information over and over, without judgment, until it is grasped by the student. Ten times or ten thousand times, the computer does not care.

Knowing the pressure is off, the student is free to actually learn something, not just *pretend* to be learning, fearing the disapproval of an impatient authority figure. Most people have experienced a situation in which the pressure to perform was the one thing that made performance impossible. Computers remove the pressure, and let education take place.

Computers allow students to go as fast as they want or as slow as they need—the speed always dictated by the student and by what was learned, not by what the "class average" is ready for. Computers release the student from the Tyranny of the Average.

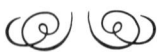

Now that we have a basic understanding of what computers are and what they do, let's explore various disibilities and see how, and under what circumstances, personal computers might help.

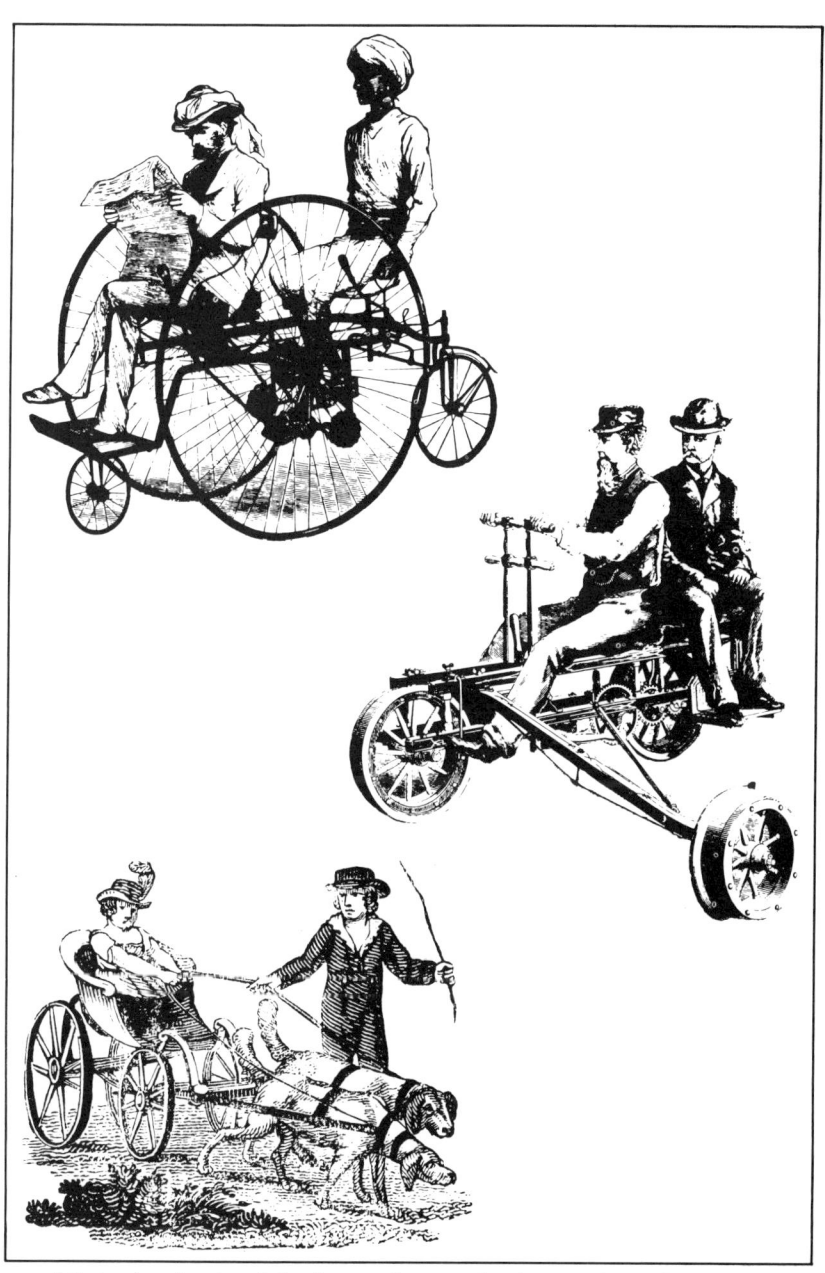

Motorized wheelchairs, prior to the invention of motors.

Chapter Three

The Right Stuff

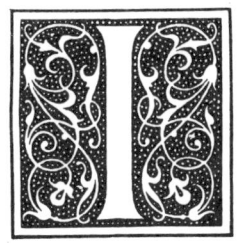 spent most of this evening talking with an aerospace engineer from Rockwell International. He worked seven years on the space shuttle program and was Launch Director of the first five flights. He designed 43 of the 47 control panels inside the cockpit. ("When you push a button in a weightless environment," he asks, "how do you know if the button will be pushed in, or if you will be pushed away?" I'm going to sell that to the local Zen Center for their book of Space Age Koans.) He has won four Astronaut's Awards (the coveted "Silver Snoopy") for professional excellence.

His name is Gerry Schwartz. Although his list of NASA and other aeronautic achievements goes beyond impressive and approaches staggering, we spent very little time discussing manned flight. (We did, however, discuss the movie "The Right Stuff." I couldn't resist.)

What we talked about was our mutual passion: computers for the disabled. The admonition to beat one's swords into ploughshares is being faithfully followed by Mr. Schwartz. "They're working on a bomber that will fly at nine Gs, and will deliver a nuclear missile with zero inaccuracy by voice command alone." Evidently, at nine Gs, a pilot can move very little but his mouth, so the mouth becomes the tool for control. Gerry is applying the bomber voice technology to people here on earth who are as immobilized as a nine G pilot.

"I'm trying to make my life help-oriented," Gerry says in his characteristically straightforward style that lacks both conceit or pretension, "rather than develop killing systems." To that end he founded the HOPE Center (Hands Off Program Experience) in Huntington Beach, California (714-962-8689). If he keeps this up, he might just qualify for a Nobel Peace Prize.

Gerry can make any computer do almost anything with voice commands alone. The number of words his

PERSONAL COMPUTERS AND THE DISABLED

system can recognize is limited only by the amount of available RAM. A 64K computer can recognize about 80 words. Word processing, for example, can be done with the basic commands ("OPEN FILE," "DELETE WORD"), a primitive vocabulary ("IT," "AND," "THE," and so on), and the alphabet. Most words are spelled out one letter at a time, just as on a keyboard. The same could apply to accounting programs, spreadsheet programs, or to the writing of programs themselves.

There are several voice recognition devices on the market. Gerry Schwartz's gift is one of software, and matching the computer to the user. He has three goals when helping a disabled person select a computer, and all three must be met for Gerry to consider the job well done.

First, the machine must be usable at once. (The computer will grow more useful as time goes on, but it should be able to do *something* right away.) Second, the purchase of it shouldn't destroy the disabled person's budget. Third, the system must have room for growth.

One of the most interesting uses is a computer program he wrote for a young man with cerebral palsy. At first, the computer accepted a broad range of pronunciations for the command words, but as the weeks went by, the acceptable range was narrowed, and, consequently, the young man's speech considerably improved. Improving the young man's pronunciation was not the primary goal, but it was an added benefit that can come when computers are used creatively to serve the disabled.

When speech is not possible, Gerry arranges for the disabled person to communicate with the computer using Morse Code. "Morse Code seems to be the standard for certain disabled applications," I said.

"Yes," said Gerry, "but is it right? Is it the best, the most useful? It's what we tell the disabled to use, but I hope they'll use it for a few months and come back and say, 'You idiot: why did you stick us with Morse Code when this or that would work so much better?'"

The Right Stuff

Gerry looks forward to the day when the disabled people he works with will tell him not only what they need but also how to best fulfill their need. "What's right for them is what's right."

And it is that attitude—the joy of being wrong if a better answer can be found—that is known, I suppose, as the right stuff.

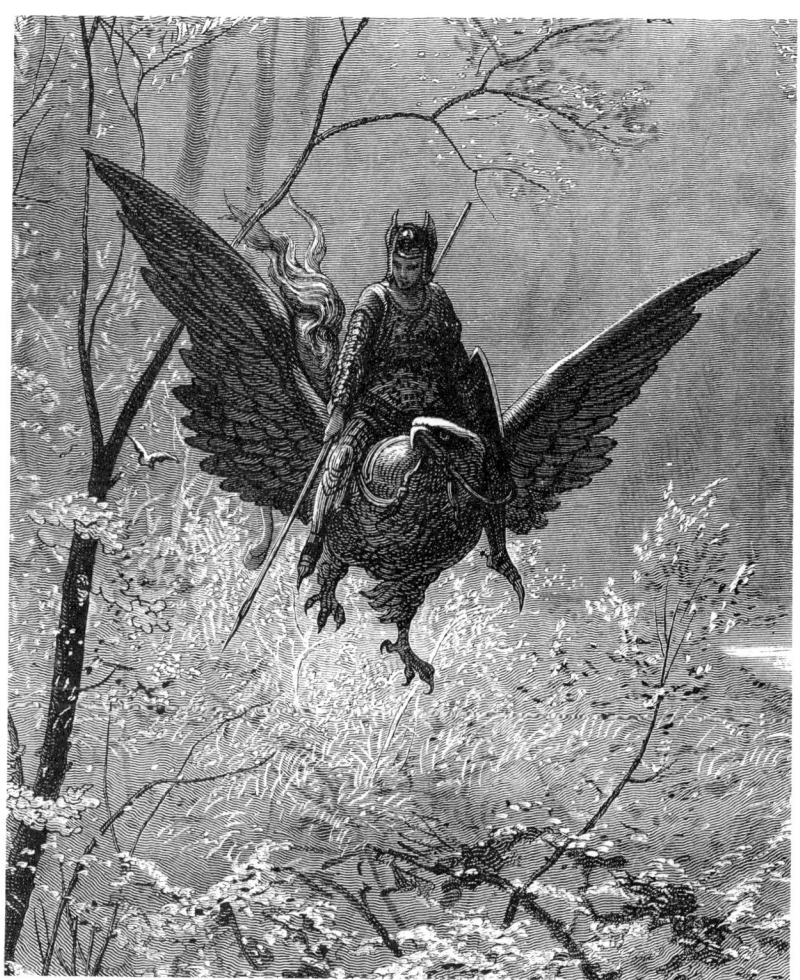

Some disabled people are finding leader birds helpful in getting around.

PERSONAL COMPUTERS AND THE DISABLED

Walt Woltosz began his work with computers and the disabled in 1980 when his mother-in-law was diagnosed as having amyotrophic lateral sclerosis—ALS, or Lou Gerhig's Disease. She unfortunately died before the software and input devices could be fully developed, but the event had a profound effect on Walt Woltosz's life, and the work continued.

Walt left his job as Aerospace Engineer for United Technologies Corporation and started Words+, Inc. in Sunnyvale, California (408-730-9588). (Words+ does not, by the way, market The WORD Plus spelling checker; that's Oasis Systems in San Diego.)

Walt Woltosz developed a computer/software package called the Words+ Living Center. This sounds like a planned environmental community for writers, but is in fact a Radio Shack Model 4 computer, with special software, and input and output devices. It is designed so that even the most severely disabled person can communicate—slowly, albeit, but fully.

It works something like this: A sensor is placed on or near the muscle group over which the disabled person has the most control. The only movement necessary for successful applications need be the tapping of teeth, the twitch of a thumb, the raising of an eyebrow, or the wink of an eye. When activated by the tap, twitch, raise or wink, the switch gives a single command, roughly translated as "This One."

I tried the Living Center with an eye switch, an infrared device developed by Mr. Woltosz's father. The switch fits over the head and in front of the eyes, like a pair of racing goggles. When an invisible beam of light, reflecting off the eyeball, is broken by a wink or a squint, a "This One" signal is sent to the computer.

On the screen is the alphabet, along with numbers and some punctuation, laid out in a grid, five across and ten down.

A pointer starts at the top and, traveling down, stops for a moment at the first letter of each row. After all ten rows are visited, the pointer returns to the top and makes the trip down again. A wink at any row causes the pointer to travel horizontally across the selected row. A second wink selects a specific letter, and a new screen appears.

The new screen has fifty words on it, all starting with the letter chosen, and arranged in the same five-across-ten-down format. The pointer continues its vertical search, and a wink causes the pointer to travel horizontally across the chosen row. A second wink selects a specific word. The word is added to the work area at the bottom of the screen, and the top of the screen returns to the alphabet.

In this way, sentences are built, word upon word. It's slow—five to ten words per minute (about as fast as I type)—but considering the fact that complete thoughts and ideas can be expressed by someone who has control over the movement of just one *eyelid*, it's remarkable. One of the tragedies of ALS is that the mind remains clear and alert while all the methods of communication, including speech, are taken away. The Words+ Living Center will allow people with ALS or other severe disabilities to communicate with friends and loved ones longer than ever before possible.

The Words+ Living Center costs $2,200 without printer or voice output, or $2,900 to $3,500 complete, depending upon input device. The software, switches, or any component of the system can be purchased separately at reasonable prices.

The "+" part of "Words+" includes games, the ability to draw, a voice synthesizer, and the on/off control for electrical appliances and environmental control.

Also in Walt Woltosz's arsenal is the Words+ Portable Voice. This is an Epson HX-20 computer with a speech synthesizer and a portable power supply. Type in a message, and the Portable Voice will pronounce it. The Portable Voice can also store sentences and say them on command. Fourteen-year-old Pam Adams, who has cerebral palsy, writes and gives speeches using the Portable Voice.

The Words+ Portable Voice costs $1,675.

Anything Words+ makes can be adapted by Walt Woltosz and his associates for specific needs. He is a man

PERSONAL COMPUTERS AND THE DISABLED

dedicated to serving the disabled. Why did he give up an outrageously high paying job in aerospace for the non-paying (thus far) job of developing computer systems for the disabled? "You only go through life once, and you've got to do what feels best. Unlocking people's minds gives me the most satisfaction of all."

The concept of unlocking is one that carries through in his company logo, a key, and the company motto, "Unlocking the Person."

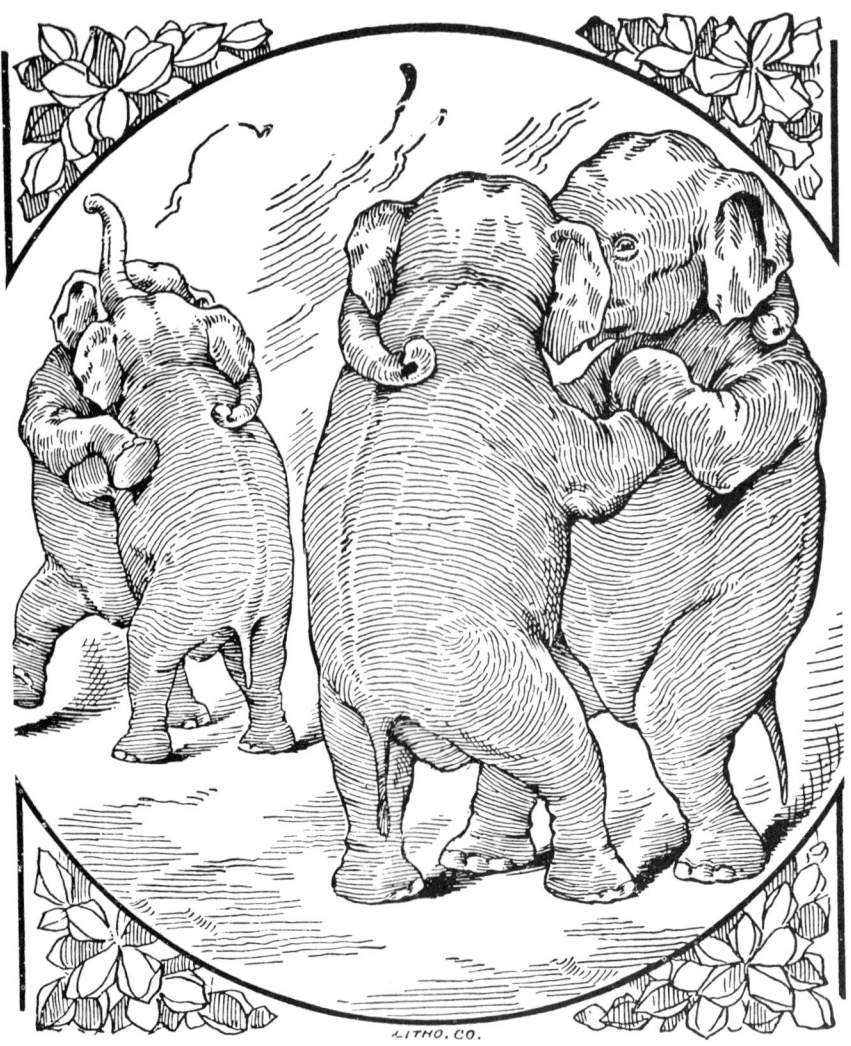

Elephants have disabilities when it comes to, say, dancing.

The Right Stuff

Ken Yankelevitz is a flight simulation engineer for McDonnell Douglas. In his spare time he makes joysticks for the disabled. But aren't joysticks for playing *games*? Do disabled people want to use computers to play games? As Ken explains, "Disabled people are just like everybody else—especially kids."

And kids seem to be Ken's specialty. Although disabled adults appreciate the opportunity to play Pac Man or chess or Decathlon, Ken seems to take special delight in helping disabled children control the hopping about of Qbert, or walking with Big Bird down Sesame Street.

Ken works regularly with the younger members of the Rancho Las Amigos rehabilitation center in Downey, California. "Some of them use the same type device as the game controller to operate their wheelchairs," Ken explains. "Playing games teaches them accuracy and coordination, which they can use in steering the chairs. It can also be good exercise." So, there are practical benefits to game playing. "Sure," says Ken, "but mostly it's just fun." It's also fun to watch disabled youngsters trounce ablebodied friends at video games.

Ken's controllers are designed for use with movements of either the hand, head, mouth, foot or tongue. They attach to Atari, Sears, and ColecoVision video games, and to Atari 400/800 and Commodore VIC-20 computers.

Trying to get game controller devices for his quadriplegic friends proved impossible, so Ken invented some. He demonstated them to Atari. They were not interested in marketing them, but anytime a disabled person called Atari looking for a special joystick, Atari gave them Ken's name.

He formed KY (Ken Yankelevitz) Enterprises in Long Beach, California (213-433-5244). Yet to show a profit (Ken's special controllers are generally less expensive than regular mass-produced joysticks), Ken refers to the entire activity as, "An expensive hobby." His wife, Diane, takes part in the family hobby, too.

The controllers can, of course, be used for more than playing games. ("More" implies that game playing is lowly

PERSONAL COMPUTERS AND THE DISABLED

and other computer activities are not. This is not my intent. Recreation, it seems to me, is as valuable as creation. Let's say that controllers can be used for purposes *other* than playing games.)

Many educational programs use the joystick as an interactive device—selecting letters, numbers, pictures and so on. The controller can be used as a cursor movement device. The keyboard can be used—perhaps with a mouth stick—to enter information, and the mouth-activated controller for zipping about the file while editing. The controller becomes a sort of mouth mouse.

One of the exciting things about the mouth controllers is how inexpensively an education/communication/game system can be assembled for a disabled person. Video games or VIC-20 computers cost about $100, and the less expensive Atari runs $200 or so. Add one of Ken's controllers ($20 to $65), buy a few cartridges, hook it up to any television, and it's set to go. $120 to $265 may seem like a lot to some budgets—especially considering the other financial obligations disabilities bring—but such a configuration offers a great deal of fun and learning for a price much lower than most people think a computer especially adapted for a disabled person might cost.

Were I writing this as a feature piece for a local newscast, I might end it with something syrupy like: "Ken Yankelevitz helps simulate flight for grown-ups during the day, so that he can stimulate flights of fancy for young people at night."

Fortunately for us all, this is not a TV news feature. I can close this piece by simply saying, Good work, Ken. Film at eleven.

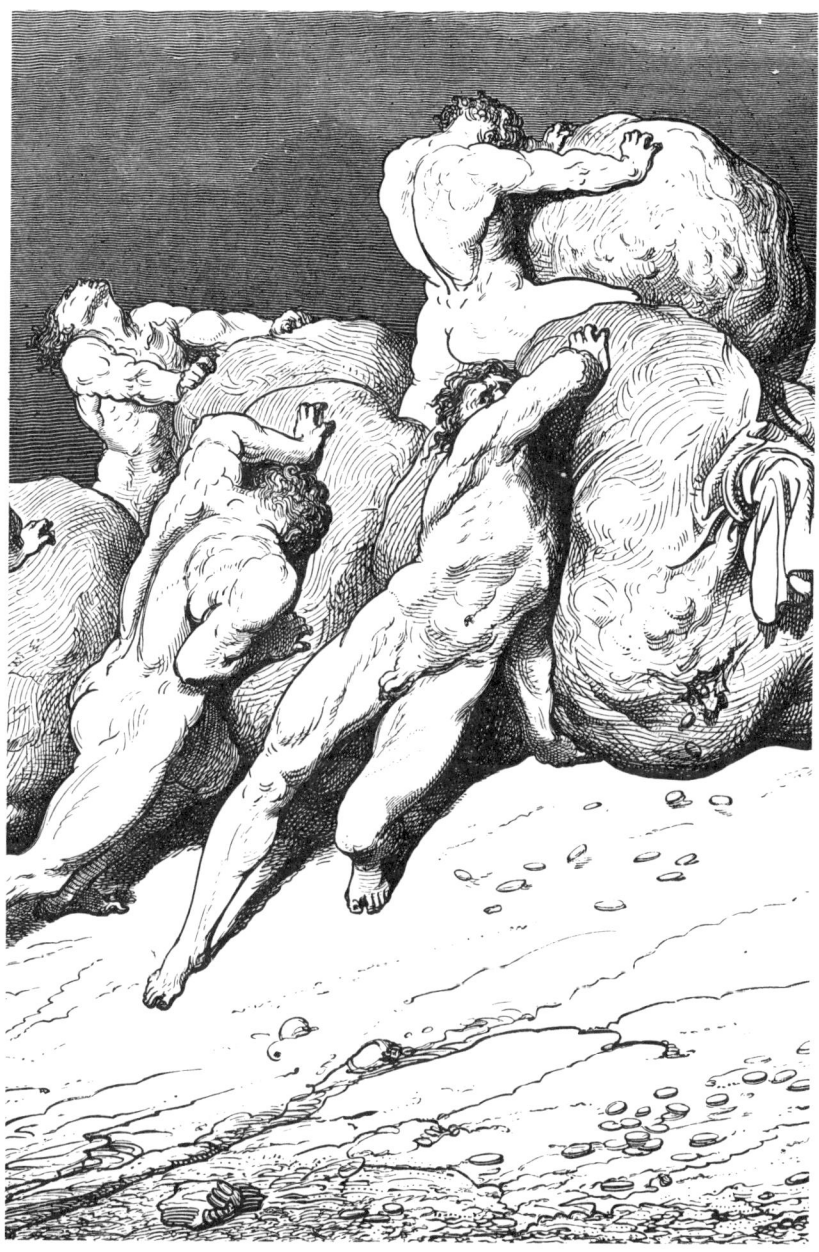

The accountants of certain big computer companies roll the profits to the banks.

Chapter Four

Personal Computers for the Deaf and Hearing Impaired

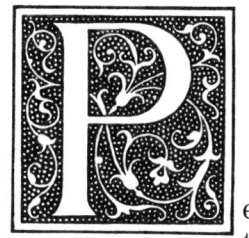ersonal computers are easily adapted for the deaf. All the necessary elements can be found in any computer store—or computer department of any K-Mart, for that matter.

And yet, although the implementation is easy, the results are profound. For the deaf, it is as though the telephone has just been invented. They can call anyone with a computer, and, for the first time, using screen and keyboard, *chat.*

It seems altogether fitting that the telephone should finally be available to the deaf. One hundred years ago, the telephone was invented by Alexander Graham Bell while researching hearing aids for the deaf. For the better part of a century, everyone *but* the deaf got to enjoy the fruits of Mr. Bell's labor. (Bell Labs invented the transistor, and other components which led to personal computers, so it seems that Mr. Bell's company did have something to do with getting the telephone to the deaf—in a painfully roundabout way.)

It's easy to see why computers are so usable for the deaf and hearing impaired. The primary output device is the screen (or printed text) and the primary input device is a keyboard. Both of these are *visual,* and require no hearing. (In fact, with the racket some printers make, deafness might prove a minor advantage.)

The only time a computer uses sound to communicate is for the explosions, laser rocket fire and Pac Man munching of video games, and an occasional beep with some programs when an error in entering has been made. In neither case is hearing what the computer's saying essential to appreciating and using the program.

I "talked" with Henry Kisor, book editor for the *Chicago Sun-Times,* and rival syndicated computer columnist. (The *Los Angeles Herald-Examiner* dropped my column and replaced it with his—demonstrating, once

PERSONAL COMPUTERS AND THE DISABLED

again, their infinite good taste.) We hooked our computers together over phone lines and I, the supposed expert, could not figure out how to save—either on disk or in print—what we were typing back and forth. After much fiddling, Henry kindly offered to save it on *his* end and mail me a copy. Although this is like asking someone for an interview and then asking them to take notes for you, I gratefully accepted.

In it we discuss, among other things (including sex! Stay tuned), Telecommunication Devices for the Deaf, or TDDs. These are basic keyboards with one line of text display and, sometimes, a printer that prints on adding machine paper. Unfortunately, TDDs are not compatible with most computers, although translation programs for computers are becoming available. The problem is, most computer owners will not buy this program unless they have a deaf friend or relative.

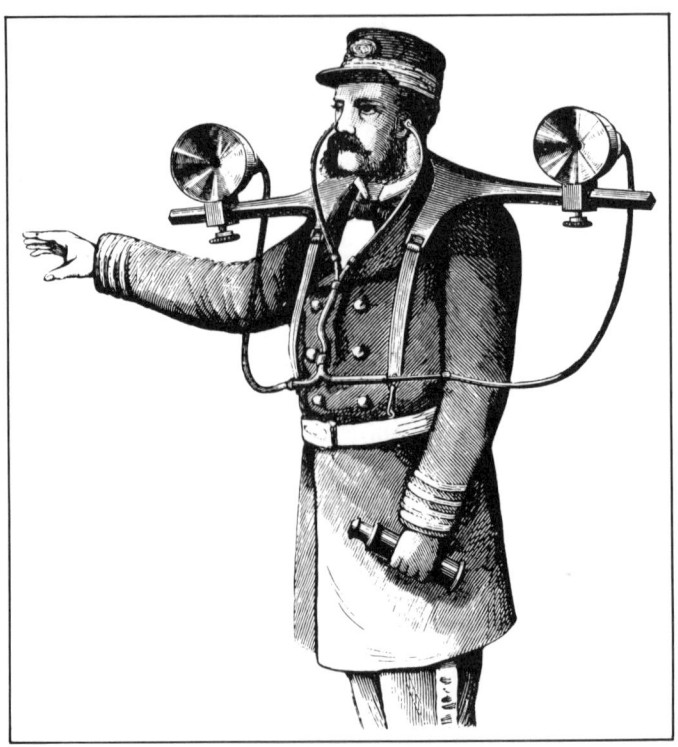

An early hearing aid.

Deaf and Hearing Impaired

Computers communicate using a code called ASCII (pronounced "ASK KEY"). TDDs communicate using Baudot code. Some TDDs come with both ASCII and Baudot capability. As the world of computers is clearly ASCII, this is a trend in TDDs that should be encouraged.

Here's a mildly edited transcript of our conversation. (I only took out the parts that made me look unbearably stupid.)

Please tell me about your own deafness. You were not always deaf, I understand. More like Beethoven.

I lost my hearing postlingually, at age 3. (That's shrink-speak for losing hearing after acccquiring language.) Meningitis. Learned to read print right away, so never lost the ability to use language.

In your interview (the one in *Infoworld*) you mentioned that deaf people have trouble acquiring reading and writing skills. Why?

Those are the deaf-born. Unlike hearing children, they aren't born into a world of language, experiencing it from the moment of birth. Deaf people can only see and feel things. Hearing babies learn simple abstractions quite early. Deaf people take a lot longer ... and some never achieve enough language to score in the "normal" range of IQ tests though they might be otherwise extremely bright.

Do you think computers will help them with the learning of English?

Yes. I don't know what is being done in this field, but logically a computer can be used as an interactive teaching tool with the deaf. A child presses a key; the computer reacts instantly. A computer is a lot easier to read than the lips of another person.

This saddens me. For some time now, I've thought that all a deaf person would have to have is a computer and they'd be able to communicate with anyone else who had a computer. But you are suggesting that there may be a greater problem of literacy here.

That's true. If you called the average deaf-born person on the computer, most likely you would be struck

PERSONAL COMPUTERS AND THE DISABLED

by the bare-bones grammar. It would be very like sign language ... subject, verb, object, with few frills. Almost broken English. But I think the computer would *add* to the literacy of the deaf-born. After enough time passed, perhaps this general literacy level could be close to that of the hearing. It really depends on individual cases—general intelligence, residual hearing if any, and so on.

Doesn't reading increase the vocabulary and teach sentence structure, or is reading difficult for people born deaf?

I'd better be careful here: I don't know. Reading is a passive, not an interactive activity. Some people might get a lot out of it, some might get little. The inability to manipulate abstractions easily could make reading difficult.

Born-deaf people have trouble handling abstractions, more so than other people, that is?

Here again, I am speaking from hearsay. One, I think, needs language to deal with abstractions ... not necessarily mathematical ones (those are easy to grasp) but linguistic ones.

Easy? I don't even know my multiplication tables. Thanks a lot.

Ho, ho. But I'll reiterate my conviction that computers, being an interactive tool, will help the deaf a great deal.

How have computers changed your life, if indeed they have?

1. For the first time, I am able to roll up as large a phone bill as my wife does.

2. For the first time, I am able to communicate with hearing people without having to look at their lips or write them letters and wait days for them to be delivered.

3. I am able to interview writers on the phone, as you are doing (though this is still a matter of potential ... most writers still use the goose quill, not word processors, and you can forget about modems, so far as they are concerned).

Have you had much experience with TDDs?

I have three ... one at home, one at work, and a portable. I call my wife every day for the domestic news. I have used it to make motel and train reservations. But it isn't as large a part of my life, since TDDs are generally limited to the world of the deaf. I don't mean to criticize them. They were the first big step out of the electronic isolation of the deaf; the microcomputer is the second.

Do you think TDDs are necessary for deaf people who own computers?

At present, it is difficult to make computers communicate with TDDs. Special hardware and software is necessary. TDDs will be around for quite some time simply because enough people have them to make the changeover slow ... they're reluctant to spend more on a micro. TDDs are also cheaper ... $200 or even less.

What specific suggestions do you have for a deaf person exploring computers?

Get a modem! One can get a Commodore 64, a modem, a terminal program and a cassette recorder for under $400. That opens up an enormous new world one never knew existed.

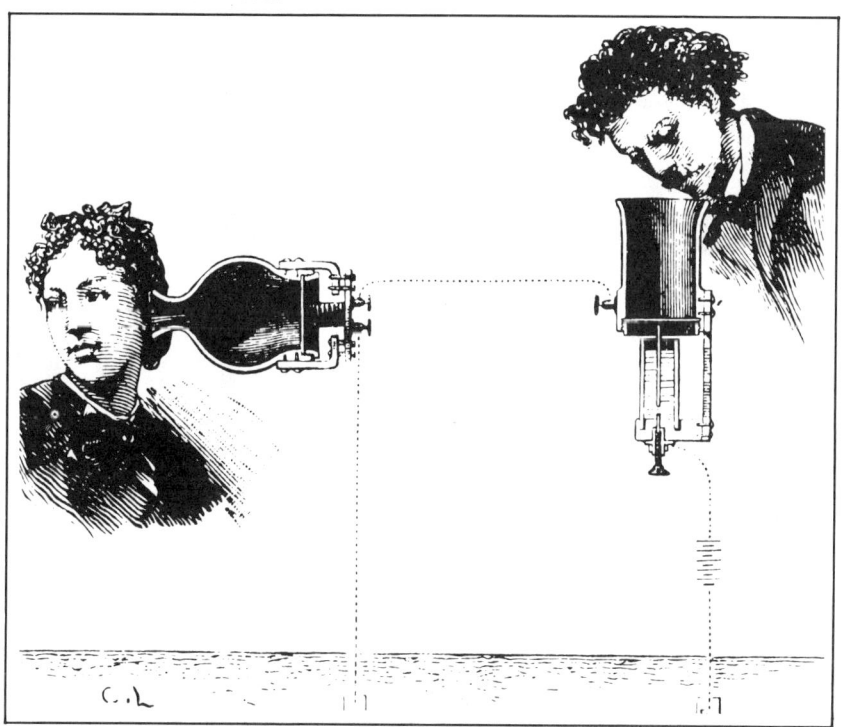

PERSONAL COMPUTERS AND THE DISABLED

What should the deaf look for in computers? Any special requirement?

I can't think of anything ... beyond what it takes for a hearing person to go online.

Tell me about your experience with bulletin boards. What are they and what do you use them for?

I use them for three reasons:

1. To get my technical questions answered about my Osborne and Radio Shack Model 100 computers, and to download free software.

2. To pass on questions my readers ask about their computers—in 24 hours you'll have answers from 50 hackers.

3. To communicate for the joy of it with electronic "penpals."

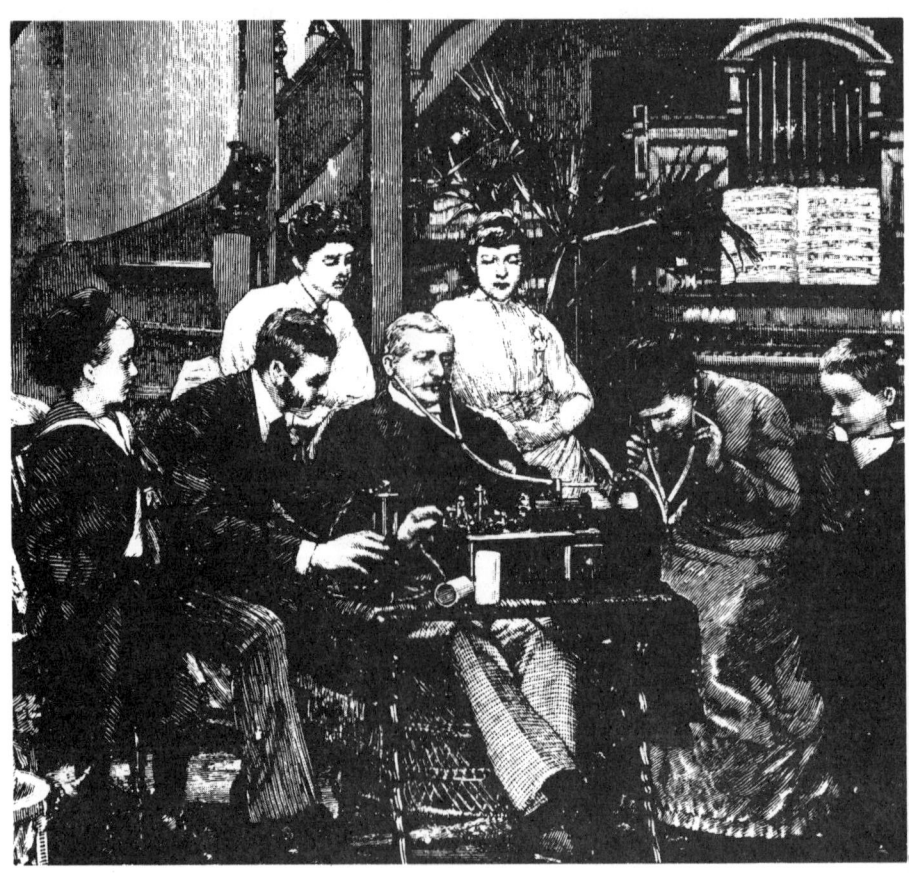

Deaf and Hearing Impaired

Do you use the "Chat" feature of The Source or CB on CompuServe?

Yes ... I've been on CB a lot lately (but at 6 bucks an hour I will be on a lot less in the future). The slow turnaround time is a pain. Especially in the evenings when CompuServe and The Source are slow in general. But given the alternatives, I should not complain.

Is there any message about computers you'd like to give to the deaf readers ... or friends of deaf readers ... who will be reading my book?

Just to make a modem the first peripheral they buy, even before a printer. And I suggest also they look into a lap computer, such as the Radio Shack Model 100 or whatever seems most affordable, as their first or even only computer. The 100 is so portable that it can accompany them everywhere (I take mine in my briefcase most places).

In an emergency, they could call CB and ask someone to make a voice call for them (this is theoretical ... it would take some convincing of other CBers that it was no joke). More practically, I have heard of a new network of bulletin boards called Deaf-Net being set up in various cities as an experiment. It will bridge the gap between computers and TDDs and serve as a clearinghouse of information as well as an emergency phone center.

I have heard of lap computers attached to speech synthesizers, but know very little about them. That's one possibility ... especially if the synthesizer could be attached to a phone (but how's the deaf person going to know if anyone answers, and how to get a reply?)

Yes. We're into the chapter on the blind. Have I forgotten to ask you anything?

No...but I have an interesting observation. You are aware of CompuSex on CB, aren't you?

Yes, but my Bible prohibits me to explore anything but missionary electronics.

Har de har har ... I was talking to a psychologist who is also a CBer and made horrified noises about CompuSex to her. She replied that a lot of CBers are people with severe physical disabilities who have no means

PERSONAL COMPUTERS AND THE DISABLED

of finding sexual partners. She contends that a lot of them find sexual fulfillment with erotic conversation on CB. Makes sense, I guess...

Oh. I think I'll put that in the book. I think that people take to CompuSex (and PhoneSex for the hearing) who have the most basic (sexual) disability of all: they're not attractive enough for the "market" and can pretend to be anything they want. Funny, though: they're getting off with someone who is likewise saying, er ... exaggerated things.

I guess so. Maybe most "normal" people would look askance at CompuSex, but I think it serves a good purpose for those who have no other outlet.

We should point out that people use CB for more than sex. I am told by a psychologist that CB has proven very useful to people recovering from disabling accidents. Some of the first reaching out they do has been to other CB users.

I enjoyed our "talk." There's only one problem with this form of communication: I *still* don't know how to pronounce "Kisor."

Kaiser! (As in "Frazer.")

Thank you. Over and out.

Right. Goodbye.

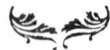

Because computers require skills that most deaf people have (the ability to see) and can acquire (typing), the job market for deaf people working with computers is large, and growing larger every day. Jobs that require inputing data (programming, data processing, word processing) and no telephone interaction would be ideally suited for a deaf or hearing impaired person.

And, if you want to be truly independent, you can always start your own computer column. Maybe the *Los Angeles Herald-Examiner* will bump Henry's column for yours.

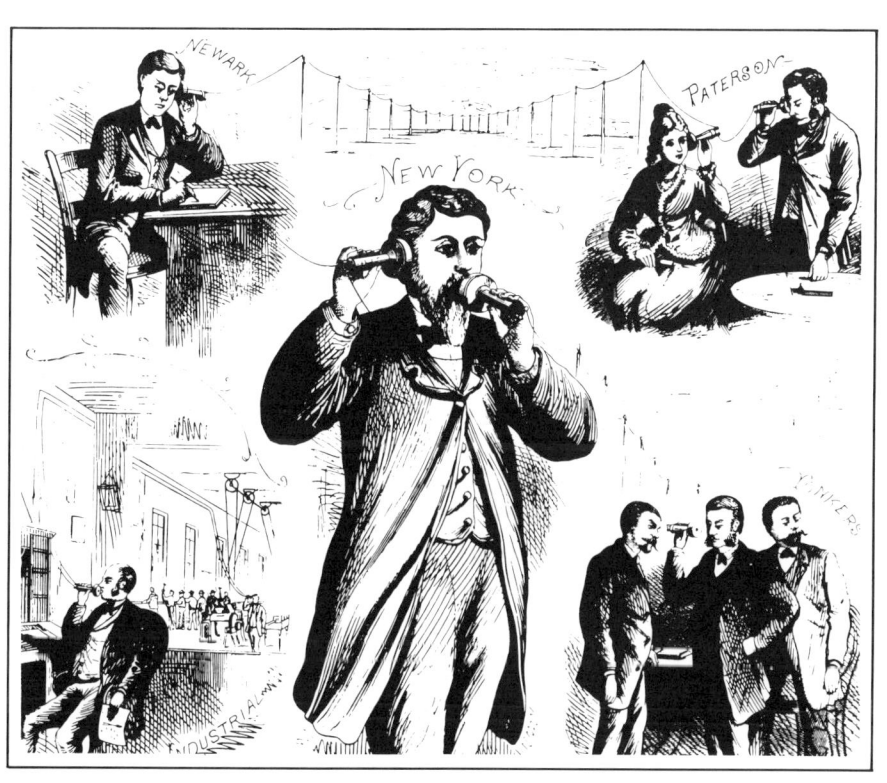

Chapter Five

Personal Computers for the Speech Impaired

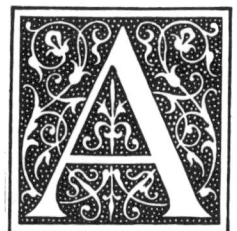great many people have speech impairments, for a great many reasons. People born deaf often have trouble speaking because they've never heard what understandable speech should sound like. Cerebral Palsy sometimes causes speech that is difficult to understand. Strokes, tracheotomies, and laryngectomies frequently cause speech loss of varying durations. Cancer, MS, ALS and other diseases silence tens of thousands every year.

The causes are many, but the result is the same: no voice, or an inability to pronounce words that are easily understood.

Until now, those who were unable to speak communicated with written messages or a point board. A point board (or lap board) is a flat surface with the alphabet and a series of frequently used words, symbols and phrases on it. ("I'm hungry," "I love you," "I don't think Sartre had precisely that in mind," etc.) The user points to the words and letters, and the observer gets the message. Point boards are especially helpful to those who have insufficient motor control to write.

While written messages and point boards work, they have their limitations. Neither notes nor point boards are of any use on the telephone. Summoning aid in an emergency without the ability to speak is a considerable task. Point boards require someone to look over the pointer's shoulder, or sit next to them, and do nothing else but watch while the message is constructed, letter by letter.

Voice synthesizers to the rescue!

Voice synthesizers are relatively inexpensive ($200 or so) and connect to almost any computer. Most plug into the printer port and, rather than printing what is said, it speaks it. The speed and pitch can usually be adjusted.

PERSONAL COMPUTERS AND THE DISABLED

External audio speakers can be added for more volume or better fidelity.

The voice it synthesizes, alas, sounds unmistakably like a computer. Even the most expensive (the DECtalk, at about $4,000) sounds like no human from this planet. But voice synthesizers are nonetheless understandable, are quickly adjusted to, and many find them a valuable alternative to message writing and point boarding.

Disabled people who go from point board to voice output find the pressure is off to point quickly and accurately. The message can be worked on—while others are talking or reading or fixing dinner—and when it's ready, the synthesizer speaks it out. Interaction is slower, but is more casual and conversational than with a point board. Also, with a voice synthesizer, several people can hear at the same time. Very important when telling a joke.

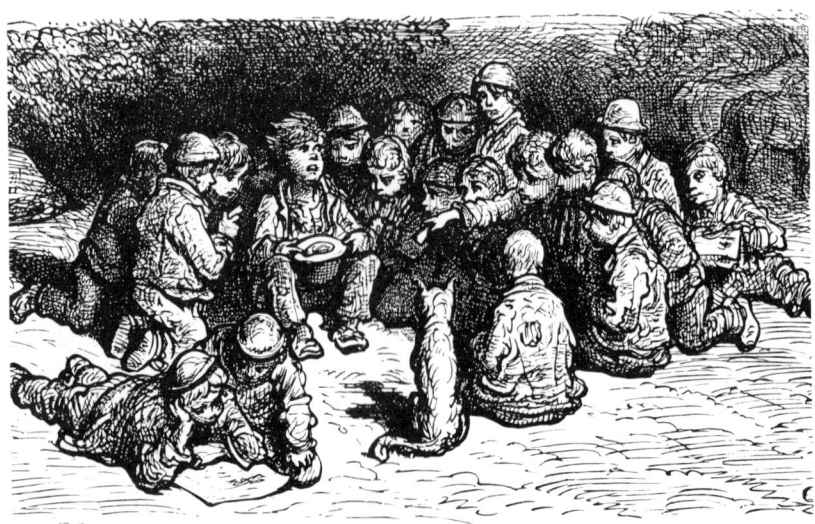

A road company of "Oliver," sung completely with synthesized voices.

Speech Impaired

Almost all the information in the chapter on computers for the deaf applies to those without a voice as well. Computers do not require that one either hear *or* speak to operate them. Any job using a computer can be held by a voice-impaired person. The only limitation would be the amount of verbal interaction necessary. (Word processing, data entry or computer programming would be easier than, say, phone reservations.) And the ability to call anyone with a computer and "chat" opens new worlds of communication.

Telephone communication with people and companies who do not have computers or any special equipment (such as TDDs) is possible with a voice synthesizer. For example, to find out if tickets are available for a given concert, you can type in the message, "Hello. I am not able to speak, but I can hear, and my computer is doing the talking for me. Could you please tell me if you have any tickets for the Beethoven (or Van Halen, or whomever) concert on Friday the 14th? If so, could you tell me in what locations and at what prices?"

You dial the ticket information number, wait until someone answers, and push the "speak" button (it's different for different computers), and the message goes out over the phone. The person on the other end gives the information, you write it down, push another button, and have your computer say "Thank you. Goodbye."

If you want the tickets, you can program in the information, such as your credit card number, address, price of tickets, number of tickets, and so on. Another call, and the tickets are on the way.

The same system can be used for ordering groceries, sending telegrams, checking bank balances, getting phone numbers, and arranging with friends when to next have a genuine computer-to-computer chat.

Most computers have a way of programming in a given number of frequently used sentences—whole paragraphs, sometimes. In this way, "Hello, I'm glad to see you. How have you been?" or "I bid hearts" or "This is just an ordinary personal computer with a speech synthesizer added" need not be typed each time.

PERSONAL COMPUTERS AND THE DISABLED

For portable use, there's Walt Woltosz's Words+ Portable Voice. (Please see the chapter *The Right Stuff*.) Less expensive, but of more limited use, is the Texas Instruments Vocaid. This has a series of preprogrammed words and phrases that are activated by the push of a button. (For a further review of both products, please see the buying guide at the end of this book.)

Elaine Marlowe, who lost her speech because of ALS, continues her work as a children's librarian, using a computer to tell stories—complete with music, sound effects, different voices and even graphics. According to Ms. Marlowe, "If children can relate to Star Wars and computers, they certainly can relate to their librarian talking through a speech synthesizer."

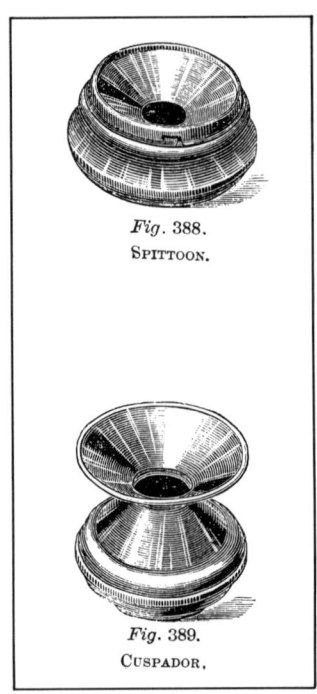

Fig. 388.
SPITTOON.

Fig. 389.
CUSPADOR.

These two illustrations should clear up the difference between a spittoon and a cuspador once and for all.

PUBLISHER'S NOTE: WHAT CAN WE SAY?

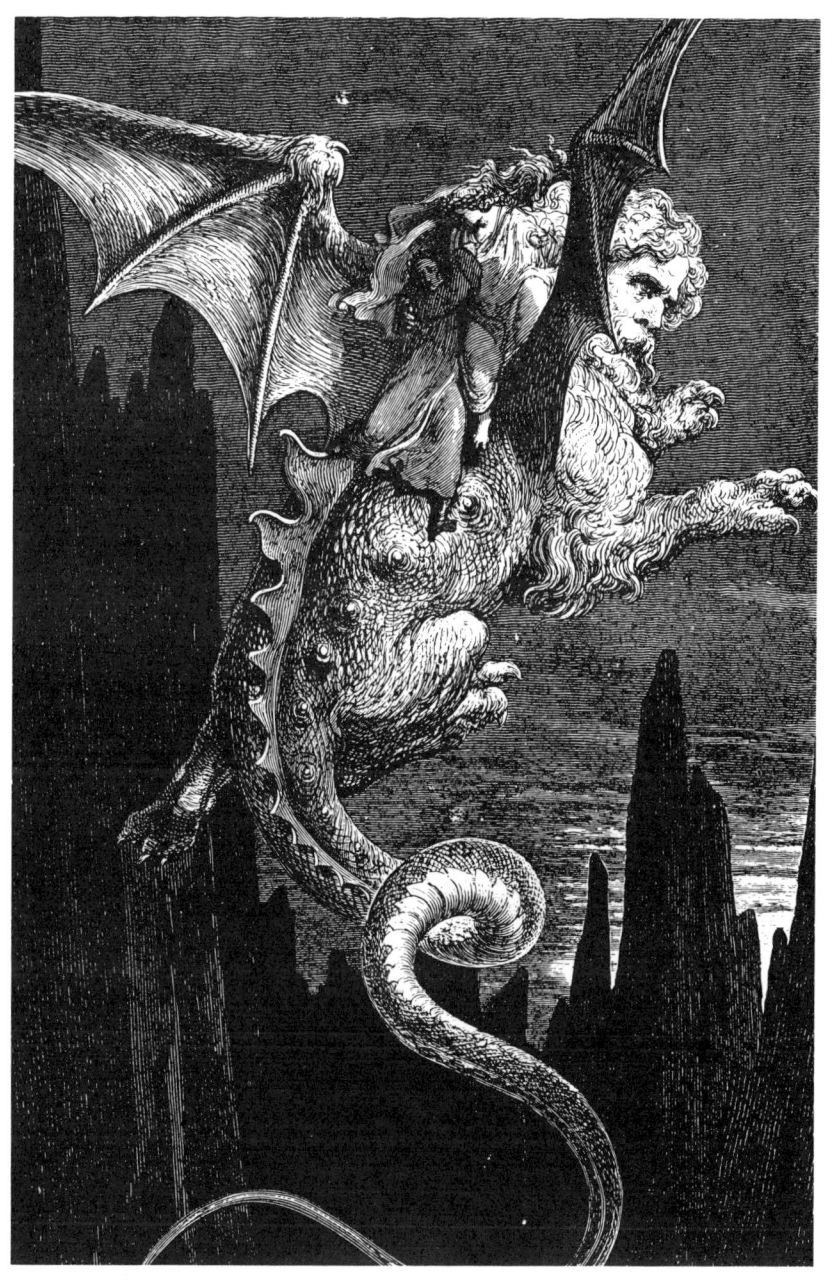

One of the new breed of disabled transport animals.

PHOTO COURTESY OF GENCO—BETTER LIVING THROUGH GENETIC ENGINEERING

Chapter Six

Personal Computers for People with Learning Disabilities

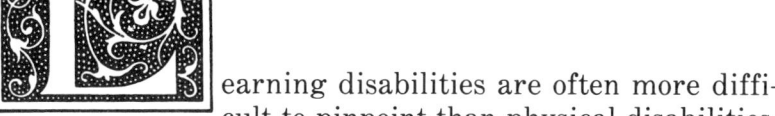earning disabilities are often more difficult to pinpoint than physical disabilities, but they are just as real and can be just as limiting. In many cases, personal computers can help overcome these limitations.

Before we begin, let us explore for a moment a myth. This myth goes something like this: Computers are cold, impersonal, aloof, distant machines, devoid of a single positive human emotion. Believing this, one wonders what good computers could possibly be to anyone, let alone to people with learning disabilities.

This myth grew up in the black and white 1950s and flowered in the anti-establishment 1960s. During that time, the only "people" who could afford computers were big business and the government. Computers were programmed to be cold, impersonal, aloof and distant. Considering their owners, this is not surprising.

The only interaction the average person had with computers was the DO NOT FOLD, SPINDLE OR MUTILATE enclosed with every bill. (If a bill was past due, there were two cards.) Businesses started to blame everything that went wrong on "computer errors." Science fiction movies increasingly portrayed the computer as an arch villain. And if we ever met someone who actually knew something about computers, these people seemed cold, impersonal, aloof and distant, too. They must have gotten it, we thought, from too much contact with the computer.

In fact, the computer got it from too much contact with *them*. These were the Computer Programmers. They spoke a special language even the owners of the million-dollar computers couldn't understand. They had a closed club. They created the computer in their own image. Not that all computer programmers were like that—just the ones hired by the people who owned the computers.

PERSONAL COMPUTERS AND THE DISABLED

A computer, in fact, is neutral—like a phonograph. Just as you can play either Mahler or Midler on a phonograph, you can program a computer to be either cold and aloof or warm and cuddly.

The concept of warm and cuddly programming is new, but it's catching on. It's the next step after "user friendly." A warm and cuddly program would probably spoil a big businessperson's lunch, but it's just the thing for people with learning disabilities. (See? I got back to the subject. I don't know how, but I got back.)

When one imagines the ideal situation for teaching people with learning disabilities, a series of human qualities comes to mind: Love, understanding, compassion, caring, support and encouragement. But there are some super-human qualities that come to mind as well: infinite patience, inexhaustible energy and unlimited availability.

Given that the first six can only be provided by another person, it's nice to know that the last three can be provided by personal computers.

Patience. If it takes a student 10,000 tries before learning that six times six is thirty-six, that's how many times the computer will present the problem. At no point will the computer get angry, upset, frustrated or in any way human. (Some programs offer encouragements such as, "That's closer! Let's try again.")

This infinite patience takes the pressure off the student. It is frequently the pressure that people with learning disabilities have difficulty with. In an effort to make fewer mistakes, they make more. This causes more pressure, leading to more mistakes. A thoroughly non-judgmental "partner" in learning breaks this cycle of expectation and failed performance, allowing the student to learn at his or her own pace.

Energy. A computer will never say, "I'm too tired, we'll do it later." If it's on, it's ready to go; any time, all the time, 24 hours a day. Barring a power failure or a breakdown, the alertness of a computer never varies. The lesson is presented with the same "enthusiasm" at 8 AM as at 10:30 PM. Answers are given or checked as quickly at noon as at midnight. Hyperactive children have finally found their match.

Availability. The best special education teachers in the world seldom have the time to give each student all the attention he or she may need. They have other responsibilities, other students, a family of their own, social and personal needs.

Computers, on the other hand, are simply *there*, to be used or not used, as the student desires. The computer adapts to the student's personal timetable. People with learning disabilities frequently respond poorly to the "We've done enough science; it's ten o'clock, time for geography" system of education. And who can blame them? Just as the light of cognition is about to glow, some idiot pulls the plug because "it's time."

Computers also make available the next lesson precisely when the student is ready for it. This is how computers could have helped me in elementary school. In half my subjects I was ahead of the class; in half my subjects, I was behind. I spent my days alternating between boredom ("When will these people ever catch up?") and frustration ("They got all that so soon? I don't get it at all"). I consequently became a "behavior problem," known in non-technical circles as the class clown.

Who says that one hour is the correct amount of time for each subject? And who says how much should be covered in that hour? That monster known as The Class Average decides. Never mind that the best students will be bored and check out, and that the worst students will fall hopelessly behind. The average student has been served, and what more can we hope for?

This is a problem in traditional classroom education, and is even a greater problem when working with the learning disabled. Special education classes frequently mix not only students with varying disabilities, but also various grade levels.

Computers provide personal instruction, at the speed the student is ready to learn, the distance the student is ready to travel.

PERSONAL COMPUTERS AND THE DISABLED

Unfortunately, this chapter is the most theoretical and speculative in the whole book. All I've been able to do is discuss the *potential* computers have in teaching people with learning disabilities. The computers are there, the software is not—but it's on the way. Just about every major educational publisher is developing a line of educational software—and they've got the money to do it, too.

There are good programs that teach the alphabet, spelling, or basic math, and these are a good start, but the *continuing* programs are missing. Until that vacuum is filled, computers will only be selectively useful in educating people with learning disabilities—being invaluable to some students, peripheral to others, intermittently helpful to most.

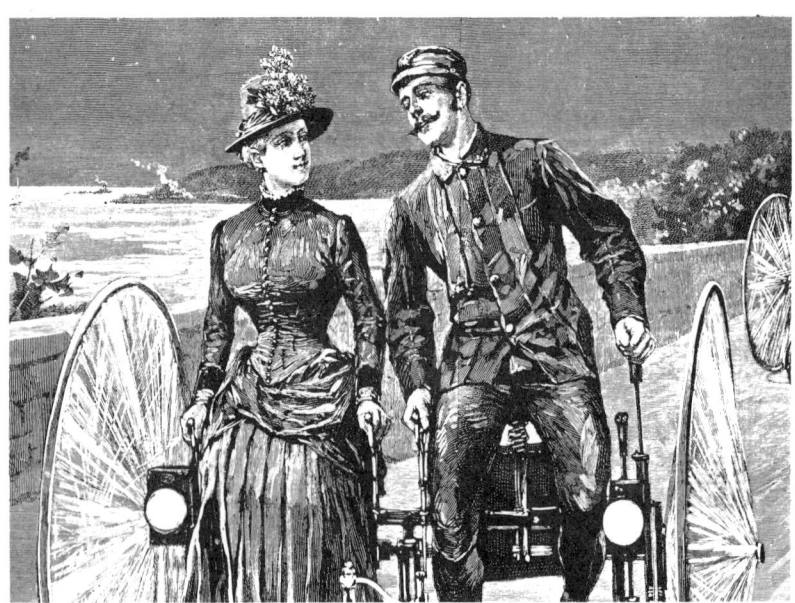

Wheelchairs built for two were very popular around the turn of the century.

Learning Disabilities

One of the most successful tools in teaching people with learning disabilities is Logo. Logo is a computer language that uses a turtle (cursor) to draw graphics designed by the student. Here's a report by educator Susan Jo Russell.

Logo in Special Education

By Susan Jo Russell

The word "slow," when used to describe children with special needs, is a literal description of how we teachers see them—it takes them longer to get where they are going. That is why the solution at first appears to be to pack more time into the school day. But the child with special needs, like all other children in our classrooms, is an individual who thinks, learns and communicates in an individual way. Instead of more time for learning, we need more worlds—more environments that allow individual styles and paces, that offer engaging content, and that provide new opportunities for teachers to observe and interact with children's thinking. That is where the computer can help us.

During the last two years, I have been working on a project using the Logo program with six-to-ten-year-olds who were physically handicapped and/or learning disabled. Two facts have impressed me: first, how readily many children, even those who have experienced much failure in school, make Logo their own; second, how much of their work with Logo tells us about their thinking.

Therese first came to school—a school for physically handicapped children—at age ten. She had a severe hearing loss but had never worn a hearing aid. She used few words, relying on sounds to express her feelings. She had a rare syndrome that resulted in immature growth and made her need braces on her legs and lower body. She looked as if she were five and communicated as if she were two. The school staff knew little about what Therese knew or how she learned.

We began using the turtle robot that functions with Logo, and a button box (a plastic box with widely spaced buttons used as a substitute for the keyboard). Therese showed immediate delight at the movement of the turtle on

PERSONAL COMPUTERS AND THE DISABLED

the floor. After a few sessions, she clearly distinguished the functions of the button labeled F (for forward) and T (for turn). Later we introduced her to the same commands using the computer keyboard and screen in a version of single-key Logo. She had difficulty coordinating the actions of watching the screen and finding the right key on the keyboard: moving her eyes to the screen, she would lose her place on the keys. Despite this difficulty, as well as the barriers of hearing and speaking, she persevered.

One day she outlined a large square on the screen with her finger. Then she outlined something in the bottom center of the square. "Open the door," she said. After making the door, she said, "and a window" and outlined several windows within the square. I imitated her movements: "A window here? A window here?" She pointed again and said, "One, two, three, four, five," showing me five positions for windows. This conversation was the longest and clearest I had ever had with her. It may not sound monumental, but to have shared an experience with Therese in which she was directing, in which words and ideas were understandable, was a rare experience.

Willie is almost nine years old. He repeated first grade and is now completing second in a public school classroom. His skills in mathematics and reading are well below what would be expected for his age. When he entered school, Willie cried for hours daily and almost never talked. Now, three years later, he still talks infrequently and often does not answer even when addressed directly. Despite a supportive classroom environment and popularity among his peers, tears come to his eyes when he is confronted by new material.

One of Willie's first Logo pictures was a car. While he made it he spoke little, but when he was ready to make the wheels, he asked me how to make a circle. It was the first time he had addressed me directly. In his fifth and sixth sessions he made a picture called "the plane in space." For this picture he chose his numbers unerringly, showing a strong sense of proportion and design. His working style was consistent: he worked silently and steadily on his own, asking me questions when he needed a new tool for what he wanted to do.

Willie's language skills are poor, but Logo provides a world in which he excels. Willie draws as well on paper as on the screen. But what is interesting about his work in Logo is that he can translate what he knows about shape and proportion into Logo commands, which require him to estimate, compare, sequence, visualize, plan and use numbers. He chooses his own problems and solves them, communicating his ideas in a mode that is comfortable for him. Although his schoolwork with two-digit numbers is shaky, in this context he uses them confidently.

For Therese and Willie, Logo provided compelling motivation in a world that is both structured and open—structured because the child has to work with particular commands that produce particular effects; open because an unlimited number of ideas can be implemented with it. Both Therese and Willie were limited in their spoken and written communication. The context of Logo encouraged the expression and sharing of ideas. Unlike drawing, for which they could guide the crayon directly, Logo required them to translate their intentions into a series of commands understood by the turtle. To do that they had to analyze and plan—in effect, to think about their own thought.

Therese can now handle only the simplest single-key commands. It is a manageable environment for her, yet one in which she can direct the action. Willie, who can use most of the regular Logo commands, manages a more complex environment. Because Logo is accessible yet powerful, both of these children can gradually expand their knowledge of the tools Logo offers them. If we do not limit children's access to new worlds because of our expectations about their abilities, then they will show us unexpected strengths.

Chapter Seven

Personal Computers for People with Muscular, Motor, and Movement Disabilities

his is, understandably, the longest chapter in this book (next to the buying guide) because it covers people with disabilities involving movement, the largest population of disabled people in this country. This includes severe arthritis, amputees, spinal cord injuries, degenerative nerve and muscle diseases, cerebral palsy, strokes, accidents and many other causes. Whatever the cause, the result is the same: impaired movement of some portion of the body.

When I was in the fourth grade, we received an insurance policy for young folks (of which I was one at the time). It had a list of what our parents would be paid for which injuries to our little bodies. "Loss of one arm, $5,000. Loss of one leg, $5,000. Loss of two arms, $10,000. Loss of two legs, $10,000. Loss of one arm and one leg, $10,000. Loss of one arm and two legs, $15,000. Loss of two arms and two legs, $20,000. Loss of one eye, $5,000. Loss of two eyes, $10,000. Loss of one arm and one eye, $10,000."

And so went the seemingly endless list, combining body parts at $5,000 per, until the "Maximum Payable Benefit" of $25,000 was reached.

I have a fear that this chapter might at times start sounding like that insurance list. I'm going to have to go through various combinations of motor disabilities—both partial and complete—in order to examine how computers might prove useful to people with those disabilities.

Those who have limited or no use of their legs might find themselves agreeing with Gary Figelski: "As far as computers go, my disability makes no difference whatsoever." Gary lost movement from the waist down in a military accident ten months ago. "I used computers

PERSONAL COMPUTERS AND THE DISABLED

before the accident, and I use computers after the accident. The only difference is that now I sit in a wheelchair."

Gary is 23 and writes graphics programs for his Atari 800. He is the recipient of a new Kaypro 4, which he hopes will improve his typing skills. "I hate to type," he says. "I wish they'd perfect voice input—not because I need it, but because I'm lazy." He may work for his brother's computer store, "But first I'm going to learn how to drive my hand-operated van and travel around the country for a while." He plans to take his computers with him.

Because computers use the hands and eyes for input and output, those who have use of hands, arms, head, and eyes have no reason to read this book. ("Why did he wait this long to tell me?") Any computer book applies to you without alteration, as does any computer. No special software or input/output devices are required.

This is what makes people with full upper-body ability such good employees for companies who use computers. Disabled employees traditionally have far less turnover than able-bodied workers. (The turnover rate for able-bodied computer operators—data processors, programmers, word processors—is enormous.) Companies frequently get tax breaks for hiring the disabled, and, quite frankly, it's good PR.

All this bodes well for those with able upper bodies. Personal computers are turning up everywhere in business, both large and small. This is opening up job opportunities for the disabled faster than anything before.

In addition, at-home businesses—accounting services, word processing, writing, programming, consulting, and dozens more—can be started with and supported by personal computers. As your business grows, soon you'll be giving able-bodied people what they say they really want in life—a chance.

Muscular, Motor, and Movement Disabilities

Ed Loundey finds himself in precisely the reverse situation of Gary Figelski. Although he has full use of his legs, an illness left him without the use of his hands and arms. Ed, working with Scott Arnold, developed several methods of input for his computer.

All involve the use of that ancient art, Morse Code. The dots and dashes that make up the letters, numbers and computer commands are communicated to the computer through a series of devices.

The first is a foot switch. Operated by the big toe of each foot, one toe is dots and the other toe is dashes. Ed is quite proficient in this form of entry, and could no doubt beat me in a typing contest.

A second method is the sip and puff switch. This is a tube, rather like a straw, that responds to slight changes in pressure as the operator sips in or puffs out small quantities of air. The computer translates the sips and puffs into dots and dashes. This method obviously requires no use of muscles below the neck, making it a valuable input device for quadriplegics.

The third device is a head switch. The rocking of the head left and right sends dots and dashes to the computer. This method requires the use of neck muscles alone.

Ed is able to change disks and turn his computer on and off with his feet. Other people with use of their legs and feet but limited use of their arms use computer keyboards and type with their toes. Ed feels the use of his foot switch with Morse Code is faster. (Adapt-A-Computer: 818-906-0349)

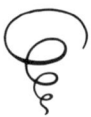

David Geffen broke his neck in a diving accident two years ago. It left him with no use of his legs and only partial use of his hands and arms. He's attending law school, and uses his Kaypro 4 primarily for word processing.

PERSONAL COMPUTERS AND THE DISABLED

Before getting his computer, he was using an electric typewriter. He had a device designed that attached to his wrist and held various objects. Strapping a pencil in the holder, he used the eraser end to hit the keys one at a time. Entering text on the typewriter was slow but tolerable; making changes and correcting mistakes he found exasperating.

Now, on his computer, he simply moves the cursor to the spot he wants to change, makes the change, and goes on. When the document is perfected to his satisfaction, he prints out a final copy. This ease of alteration is one of the primary reasons word processing is so beloved by writers, secretaries and students—disabled or not.

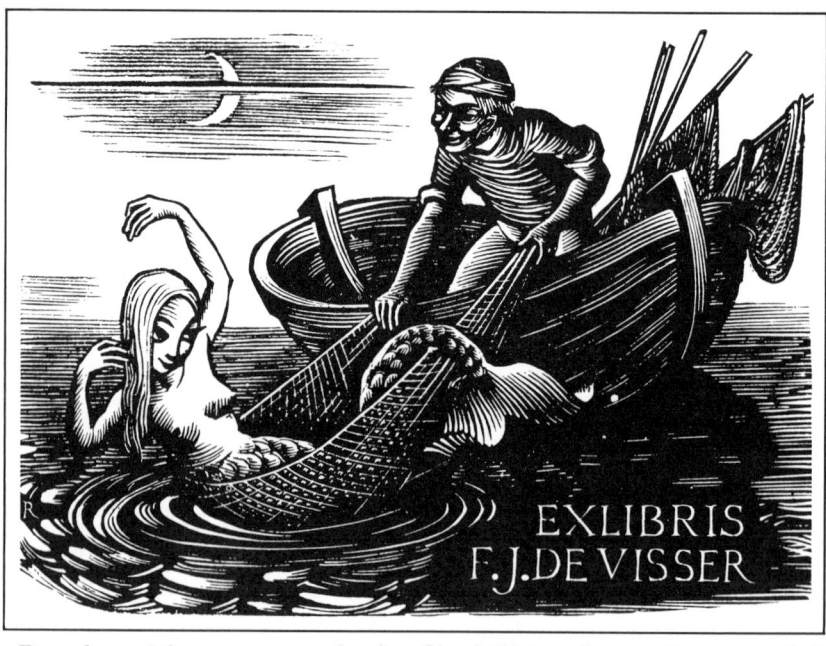

People with no upper-body disabilities have few special needs when it comes to operating computers.

Muscular, Motor, and Movement Disabilities

Money Luckett was born at the end of the Depression. "I was named Money because my parents said I was the only money they'd ever get," laughs Miss Luckett. (" 'Ms.' is a manuscript," she says.) Polio at the age of twelve left her with the use of only her lower left arm. (She calls herself a Born Again Southpaw.) Money sleeps in an iron lung at night and must use a portable respirator during the day.

She "auditioned," as she puts it, for a special government program for "the severely disabled." "They did all these tests, Money says, "and they determined I was too severely disabled for the severely disabled program."
She finds this rather amusing, as do the hundreds of people she corresponds with regularly. She writes more than a thousand letters each year.

Professionally, she is an investor and military analyst, describing herself as "slightly to the right of William F. Buckley, Jr." ("Is there *room* to the right of William F. Buckley, Jr.?" I asked. "Oh yes," she answered, "I can even take my wheelchair.") Does she mind her lack of of mobility? "Oh, no. I've got too much to do to get around."

Having the use of only one hand presents a problem at times in computing. Computers have something called a **control key**. When pushed, it gives every key on the keyboard a different value. Holding down the control key while hitting the letter "G" would, in some programs, send a command to the computer. (In the word processing program Money uses, WordStar, "control-G" tells the computer, "Delete the letter under the cursor.")

Now all this control stuff is fine if you have two hands, or even the use of one finger on each hand. But with only one hand, hitting "control-P" can be impossible—unless you have awfully large hands. (The same is true for people using mouth sticks, which we'll discuss shortly.)

The solution is to have the keyboard adapted (by software or hardware, depending on the computer) so that the control key, when pressed, is activated and remains activated until it is pressed again. In this way, the control key works like a shift-lock on a typewriter: once you hit it,

PERSONAL COMPUTERS AND THE DISABLED

everything is typed in capitals until you hit it again. The method for hitting "control-P", for example, would be CONTROL KEY (turning it on), then "P", then CONTROL KEY (turning it off). "The Kaypro people did this for me, and they never even cashed my check," says Money.

An additional aid is SmartKey. This program turns any key on a computer keyboard into any other key. With SmartKey, hitting a single key can add *pages* of text to your documents. Frequently used commands, such as "control-KSQP" ("save to disk what I've written thus far, and return the cursor to the spot I'm at now"), can be assigned to any unused key. (How often would you use the "|" key for example?)

Many computers come with numeric keypads. This gives two sets of numbers on each keyboard—the set above the letter keys and the set on the keypad. One set of numbers could be turned into SmartKeys, and, with a single keystroke, you could add your name and address, or today's date, or character names in a story, or the formal name of your condition (it's usually long and Latin), or frequently used words or phrases or sentences or paragraphs.

People with the use of neither arms nor legs—but who have full use of head and neck—have several options for computer input. One is the sip and puff straw or the head switch discussed earlier in this chapter. Another is the spoken input described in the chapter *The Right Stuff.* Also mentioned in that chapter were joysticks that operate by tongue or head movement.

Some people with only head movement use a mouth stick. As its name describes, this is a mouthpiece with a pointer attached, used for hitting keys on a regular computer keyboard.

Special plates are available that fit over regular keyboards. These provide a hole for each key, and a physical separation between keys. These plates are valuable if the movement of the head is shaky or uncertain. A plate makes it more difficult to hit the wrong key. These plates

Muscular, Motor, and Movement Disabilities

are also good for people with cerebral palsy or other disabilities in which the hands are available for use, but control over the hands is trembling or erratic.

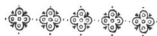

The more severely disabled who have use of enough groups to make two distinct movements—no matter where on the body these movements take place—can communicate with the computer using Morse Code. If someone has use, say, of his right toe and left thumb, devices would be connected to toe and thumb that sensed motion. The motion of one would be dots; the movement of the other dashes.

The most severely disabled, who have use of only one muscle group, can use the Words+ Living Center (described in the chapter *The Right Stuff*). Dr. David Rabin is a professor of obstetrics and gynecology at Vanderbilt University's School of Medicine. He wrote the following on the Words+ Living Center.

Trapped in My Body, I Electronically Escape

By David Rabin

Among the catalog of terrifying diseases one learns of at medical school, none frightened me more than amyotrophic lateral sclerosis. I have often asked myself why during the four years since I developed the illness.

Was it the picture of that first patient etched indelibly in my memory? We had gathered in one of those awful, gloomy basement lecture rooms that used to be an indispensable part of the architecture of teaching hospitals—rows of stark benches rising steeply from the "well", more appropriately the pit, which sported a blackboard, a lectern and one medieval chair. That chair was occupied by a seemingly elderly man stripped to the waist. Perhaps it would be more accurate to say that the chair occupied the man, so small, so cachectic, so vulnerable, so insignificant. He was reduced to flesh and bone, and what remained of his muscle was engaged in a macabre dance of death—the dreaded fasciculations of ALS.

His voice was all but gone, and to this day, I wonder what private hell he silently endured during that hour as

PERSONAL COMPUTERS AND THE DISABLED

the neurologist detailed the myriad physical signs on his broken body. The booming voice of the neurologist rendered the prognosis: "Hopeless! This is creeping paralysis! He will be demeaned, isolated, frustrated, unable to communicate, and probably will be dead in six months."

Today, I am the man in the wheelchair. However, I do not feel demeaned. I have combated isolation by speaking out to those of my colleagues who still retain the obsolete views of my neurologist "teacher" and as a family we have tried to divert our frustrations into creative energy—all of which require the ability to communicate. I lost the use of my hands more than two years ago, and as I faced a tracheotomy, my worst nightmare was whether this would finally turn me into a nonperson—every sensory perception intact but strictly one-way traffic.

Fortunately, miraculously, none of this would prove correct. On the day after my tracheotomy, I received a letter from a fellow physician who also has ALS telling me what countless prior inquiries had failed to elicit, that a computer was available that could be operated with a single switch. Not "on the drawing board," not "just around the corner," but with specifications on hardware and software, a purchase price and a delivery date.

The significance of the single switch is that it can be operated by anyone, however physically handicapped, who retains the function on one muscle group. For me, my eyebrow muscle is strong enough to depress a very light switch and thereby gives me access to the full power of the computer. Other patients have a functioning finger or toe. The first person to use a similar computer program had a switch fitted to her mouth and bit down.

The screen presents the alphabet to me. A pointer ("cursor") moves at a speed that I select, and I press the switch when the pointer is next to the letter I want. This opens an electronic dictionary to a page of words beginning with the desired letter. The process is repeated, and with the aid of the pointer, a word is selected. It takes longer to explain than to do!

What has the computer, in conjunction with a printer and voice synthesizer, afforded me? I talk to my family—that is most wonderful. I can make conversation with friends—the jokes take a little longer, but they don't seem to mind. I can work independently again—write papers, review manuscripts, cooperate by mail with other scientists—and I am able to interact with the persons in my laboratory. I write out my ideas before we meet and sum up afterward. Because of the loyalty and devotion of this group—and for me the indispensable ability to communicate—our research continues to be original and productive.

After 27 years of marriage and total sharing, Pauline and I have discovered the joy and satisfaction of writing together. Topics come from the news, from books we read, from our own experiences and from the human comedy all around. Ideas seem to be generated simultaneously, one of us prepares a draft—I, of course, use the computer—and then we enjoy a dialogue whereby we attempt without haste to use the rich textures of the English language.

A computer program such as mine, operating from a diskette no bigger than a 45-rpm record, can change the lives of hundreds of patients who retain cognitive function but are unable to communicate. While it was originally developed for a patient with ALS, its application in selected patients with stroke and other neurologic-syndromes, and in individuals who have lost their vocal cords, should be equally helpful. The main problem appears to be a dearth of information among health-care professionals about the medical applications of the computer. Advertisements for a variety of communication programs designed to meet the needs of the handicapped have appeared in the Summer 1983 issue of *Communication Outlook*, a publication of the International Society for Augmentation and Alternative Communication. However, this publication is not likely to reach the desk of many physicians.

Coping with ALS is a grim ordeal—but it is not hopeless. Every patient needs an infrastructure of love and support. Now, for those of us who could no longer communicate, the computer provides ALS patients with an Alternative Life Style.

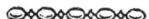

That thoughtful and beautifully composed piece was written with the movement of *a single eyebrow*. Dr. Rabin illustrates that courage and determination are the driving force behind the use of personal computers for the disabled; the force that will ultimately decide how practical and useful personal computers will be for each individual disabled person.

Chapter Eight

Personal Computers for the Blind and Visually Impaired

s the advertisement reads, "Close your eyes. Now have someone read you this page." That explains as well as anything the difficulty blind people have using computers. So much of computing is visual—video screens, printouts, instruction manuals, computer books and magazines. Adapting personal computers for the blind can prove to be one of the greatest challenges in computing.

(Autobiographical aside: My grandfather rented Ivy Green, Helen Keller's birthplace, from Captain Keller after the Keller family moved on. My father was raised there, and while I was growing up, I was told stories about Helen Keller. When we watched *The Miracle Worker* on television, my father gave us a running commentary on which bits of architecture were accurate and which were not. Later, when we went to visit Ivy Green, now a national shrine, my father said, "I never thought I'd pay two dollars to get back into *this* place." End of autobiographical aside.)

Fortunately, most blind people know touch typing and numeric keypads. Putting information into a computer is not much of a problem. (Have you noticed, by the way, that the arrangement of numbers on a computer or adding machine keypad is different from the arrangement on a telephone keypad? We seem to have a national disability when it comes to creating and accepting standards for things.)

Input being no problem, the question for blind people is, How do I get the information out? There are basically two methods, speech synthesizers and Braille.

Programs are available that instruct speech synthesizers to read all or selected parts of the computer screen. Capitals are indicated by either a beep or a higher pitch. Commas are indicated by a pause, periods by a longer

PERSONAL COMPUTERS AND THE DISABLED

pause. In the proofreading mode, words are spelled out letter by letter, commas become "comma" and periods become "period," and so on.

This system is obviously more useful with some programs than with others. It seems to work well with word processing and writing programs. Both involve a fairly linear progression of ideas and numbers. Electronic spreadsheeting and accounting are more difficult. Spreadsheets have rows and columns of numbers that are identifiable to sighted people by quickly checking the top and sides of the screen. Blind users must travel to the top, side, and back to where they were to find out the value of a single number.

Accounting programs tend to change screen formats frequently. Sighted people can quickly scan the screen and find the desired figures. Blind people must frequently have the entire screen read out (taking several minutes) to find the one piece of information a sighted person could have found almost at once.

These scenarios are of blind people using off-the-shelf software. Adapting popular and powerful programs for the blind is not a high priority for most software houses. They're more interested in adapting programs for various computers. It's one of those vicious circles: because the market for blind computer software isn't there, blind people do not buy computers. Because blind people do not buy computers, the market for blind computer software isn't there. Neither, for that matter, do instruction manuals on cassette tape or in Braille exist.

Another problem with some off-the-shelf software is that it imbeds control codes in the text. These codes tell the programs what to do with certain words or numbers. They are never displayed on the screen, but *are* sent out to voice synthesizers. These codes can send synthesizers into a tizzy. Beyond that, programs that rely heavily on graphics are obviously of little use.

As time goes on, more and more blind people will discover the value of computers, and more software will be written for the blind user. As it stands, good programs are available for the blind, especially for word processing.

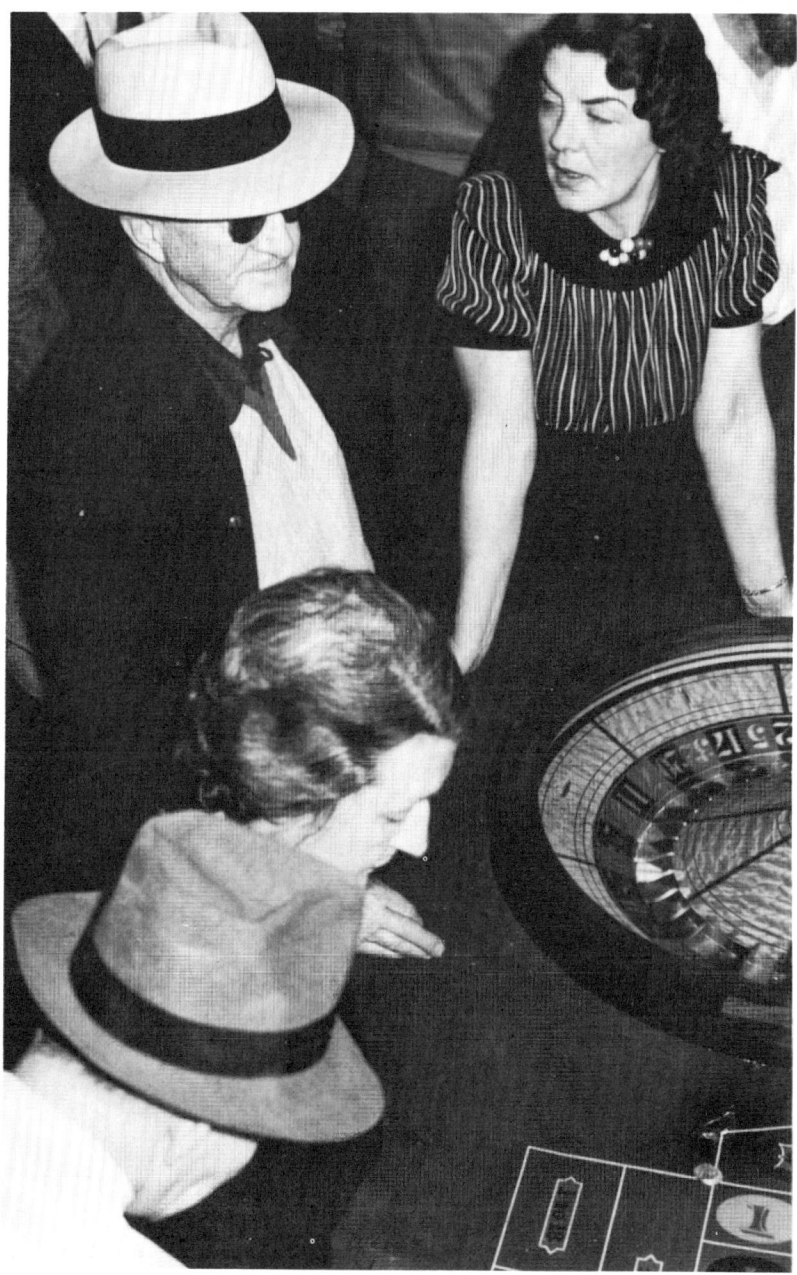

"No, this isn't a computer store, but you just won $10,000."

PERSONAL COMPUTERS AND THE DISABLED

Using a computer, a voice synthesizer and available software, the blind person can create, edit, review and print text without an expensive Braille reader or the help of a sighted person. Some programs will even print out in Grade II Braille using a standard letter quality printer. (The platen is replaced by a softer rubber one and the "period" prints the text, backwards, in Braille. When removed from the printer, the reverse side of the sheet is in Grade II Braille.) This allows for written communication to both blind and sighted friends and associates.

Computers with voice synthesizers also allow for access to the thousands of services available on data banks. These range from at-home shopping to daily newspapers and on-line encyclopedias. (The best book on data banks and what they have to offer is Alfred Glossbrenner's *The Complete Handbook of Personal Computer Communications—Everything You Need to Go Online with the World;* St. Martin's Press, 175 Fifth Avenue, New York, NY 10010—212-674-5151). A modem added to the computer, and a subscription to the service, are all that's needed.

(Whenever possible, put the information from the data bank on disk, exit the data bank, and then "read" the information. This saves the hook-up charge to the data bank, which is usually billed by the hour.)

For the visually impaired who are not completely blind, the above uses of computers can be valuable, as well as a few others. Many visually impaired people find that reading from a video screen is easier than reading from paper. The light is coming *from* the letters on the screen, not reflected *off* them, as is the case with type on paper. The contrast and brightness can be adjusted for maximum ease of reading. One program is available that enlarges the type on the screen several times. Another idea is to use a 25-inch video monitor rather than a 12-inch one. This gives a full-sized screen display in large letters.

Many blind people find that connecting their VersaBrailler to a computer speeds the editing process. (The VersaBrailler is a $6,700 machine that allows editing and printing in Braille. It has proven very useful to blind people, but, considering its price, is beyond the range of

Blind and Visually Impaired

this book. Information can be obtained from Telesensory Systems, Inc., 455 North Bernardo Avenue, Mountain View, CA 90443.) While we're on the subject of "useful to the blind but beyond the range of this book," there's the Kurzweil Reading Machine. It reads aloud, in a synthesized voice, and prints from almost any book. The major drawback is the price, around $30,000. Information is available from Kurzweil Computer Products, 185 Albany Street, Cambridge, MA 02139 (617-864-4700).

Prior to computers, the blind had basically two forms of written communication: Braille typewriters and regular typewriters. Braille typewriters allowed for no editing, correcting or inserting. Once the paper was punched, that was it. (Some blind people, I understand, got good at flattening down unwanted dots with their fingernails and adding desired dots with a pin.) Regular typewriters allowed for input, but no way to check what was written without sighted assistance.

Computerized word processing for the blind is as wonderful as it is for everyone else—if not more so. I highly recommend a book put out by the National Braille Press, entitled *A Beginners Guide to Personal Computers for the Blind and Visually Impaired.* (National Braille Press, 88 St. Stephen Street, Boston, MA 02115—617-266-6160.) In our excitement about what personal computers can do, however, we should remember that there is a lot of work to do in making available other computer programs to the blind and visually impaired.

Chapter Nine

The Drawbacks
of Personal Computers

(*Pilfered from* The Personal Computer Book.)

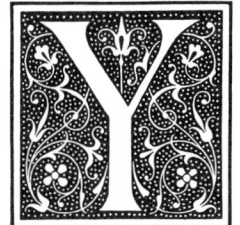Yes, there are drawbacks to personal computers, and I'll tell you what they are. You won't have to hear it first from Geraldo Rivera on a *20/20* expose.

There are drawbacks to everything, of course, and drawbacks must be weighed in proportion to benefits. Further, most drawbacks can be reduced or eliminated if approached creatively. So, in this chapter, we will be looking not only at problems, but also at solutions.

Here they are then, the several drawbacks (and suggested remedies) to personal computers I have encountered.

1. Computers are expensive. Personal computers cost a lot in terms of both time and money. Some people I know have enough money, but they don't have much time. Some people I know have enough time, but don't have much money. Most people I know have neither enough time nor enough money. Personal computers require a sizable investment of both.

Will this investment pay off? Will it be worth it? Like installing a swimming pool, it's hard to know until you take the plunge. Health clubs could not exist without the remarkably high drop-out rate of their members. Fully 80% of the people who join, signing up for several years at several hundred dollars, never go near the place after the first month. If everyone who joined made use of the facilities, health clubs would be five times more crowded than they are now, a burden they would be unable to bear.

A personal computer is something that you will buy, use a few times, and then abandon, a monument to your impulsiveness and lack of determination—like a Cuisinart. Or, you will buy a personal computer, wonder how you ever got along without it, and use it daily for a variety of tasks you would never dream of doing again by hand, a

PERSONAL COMPUTERS AND THE DISABLED

living example of your good taste and practical nature—like a Cuisinart.

Recommending that you "start small" doesn't help much. As those who bought a discounted version of a Cuisinart will tell you, most of the knock-offs were no bargain—they butchered meat rather than sliced it, and mangled vegetables rather than chopped them. The very people who might have been happy with a *genuine* Cuisinart, found the imitator unacceptable, assumed the praise heaped upon food processors was grossly overstated, and returned to the processing of food by more traditional methods.

If you want, for example, to do word processing, and attempt it on a $300 machine, you might find it unsatisfactory; whereas, if you were to attempt it on an $1,800 machine, you might be thrilled; and if you were to try word processing on a $5,000 machine, you might find yourself unable to write even a shopping list without it.

If you don't process words (or do bookkeeping, or have a passion for electronic games, or one of the other things that personal computers do remarkably well), it's hard to know if the many things that personal computers do marginally well will appeal to you enough to cause a change in habit.

If you are in the habit of calling your broker or waiting for the daily newspaper to see how the stock market is going, you might not find the allure of an updated-only-fifteen-minutes-ago stock price worth turning on your computer. In some areas, personal computers might offer more power than you'll ever need—and in other areas, they may offer much less.

I wish I could give the rather pat advice, "Try before you buy." Unfortunately, personal computing is rather like flying a plane or visiting Europe or sailing a boat—you'll never know if *you* will like it unless you try it, and trying it is expensive.

If you're uncertain, continue your investigation. If any of the "drawbacks" in this chapter seem like sound, logical, clear-headed arguments for not buying a personal computer, then you probably shouldn't get one—yet. If these drawbacks seem like intolerable nit-picking that no reasonable person would consider for more than a few moments at most, then you're ready.

How long that readiness will last is anybody's guess, and if you guess wrong, it could be a costly error.

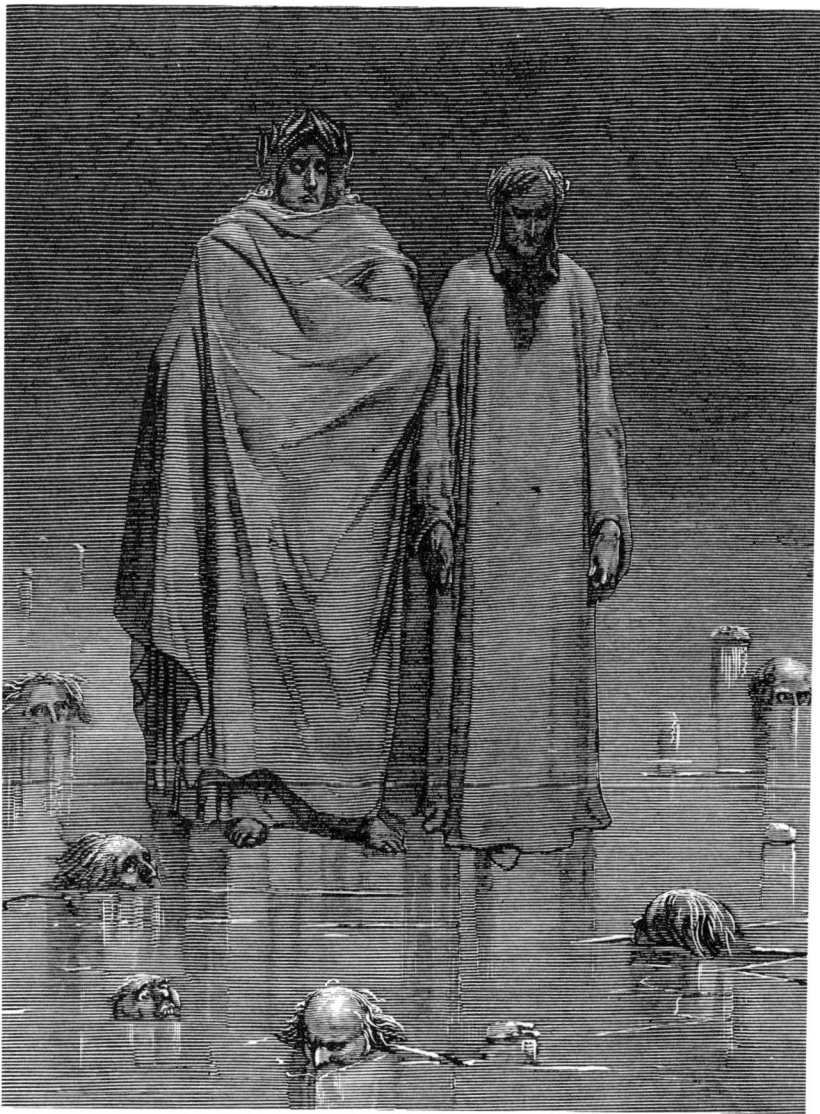

"They paid too much for their computers and got in over their heads. What can I say? Let's move on."

PERSONAL COMPUTERS AND THE DISABLED

You can minimize the chances of disappointment by lowering your expectations. Personal computers do many things well, many things not-so-well, and a broad spectrum of things somewhere between "well" and "not-so-well."

Don't expect a personal computer to change your life, unless you are a professional writer who already knows how to use a typewriter; a small businessperson who has fairly standard small business needs (word processing, accounts receivable, accounts payable, etc.); or someone who devotes a large portion of their time doing something personal computers do well (electronic spread-sheeting, stock marketing, cross-index filing, and the like).

If you don't fall into one of those three categories, it might be best if you lower your expectations to a workable minimum. By "workable minimum" I mean, don't lower them so much that you don't get the computer, but lower them enough so that disappointment will not be one of your peripherals.

Another way to help insure that you'll use your personal computer more often than your Norman Rockwell Thanksgiving Turkey Platter is to choose carefully. As much as possible, select the computer and programs that meet your current needs and fit comfortably into your lifestyle.

If you want to play computer games, buy the best game-playing computer you can afford—and make sure you like the games that are available for it.

If you are running a small business, there is no need to buy a computer and software designed for a ten-million dollar corporation. (Yes, the salesperson might say, you can grow into it. When you're grossing ten million, however, you can *buy* into it.) If you get more program than you need, you'll have to learn about the complexities of a program that you might use only 25% of, and those complexities—besides being expensive—might one day cause the computer to be turned off for good.

If you're just curious about computers and want to get your feet wet, a fish pond will do—there's no need to install an Olympic-sized pool.

As pointed out before, however, if you need word

Drawbacks of Personal Computers

processing, plan on spending enough for a decent personal computer, a letter quality printer, and the best word processing program you can find. The same is true of business: buying too much computer can be a bother; buying too little, disastrous.

There's a quote about suiting the action to the word and the word to the action, but we've already quoted once from *Hamlet* in this book, and one profound Shakespearean reference per computer book is sufficient, I think.

2. Computers are powerful and, therefore, capable of powerful mistakes. It is hard to duplicate, using ordinary methods, the efficiency and effectiveness of a computer. It is equally hard to duplicate, using ordinary methods, the degree of devastation and disaster possible on a computer—unless you consider fire, flood, and nuclear fission "ordinary methods."

Let's assume, for example, that you run a company and have all of your accounting information on a single hard disk. A hard disk is a platter of metal, usually aluminum, spinning at something like 1,800 revolutions per minute, which is equal to 30 revolutions per second. Pretty fast. Let's say that one day, the hard disk decided it was tired of being a hard disk and wanted to become a frisbee.

The disk exercises a remarkable amount of free will for a disk, releases itself from its normally secure housing, and flies out the window, landing in the *Guinness Book of World Records* for The Greatest Distance Traveled by a Personal Computer Hard Disk.

Television news crews are dispatched to interview your disk, while Tom Brokaw and Roger Mudd argue over which one of them will handle the story. (Neither one wants to, but they hear that Dan Rather is opening his broadcast with it, so they feel *somebody* has to interview the damn thing, Tom Snyder and Rona Barret having both refused.) Roone Arledge can't decide if the story should be on *The ABC Evening News* or *ABC Wide World of Sports*. He decides both.

The MacNeil Lehrer Report cancels its planned satellite interview with Fidel Castro and devotes a special, expanded 90-minute version of the show to your disk.

PERSONAL COMPUTERS AND THE DISABLED

Also at PBS, both William F. Buckley, Jr. and Dick Cavett are trying to get the disk on their respective shows. "The disk is a celebrity, not a politician," says Cavett. "It belongs on my show."

"The disk is a projectile, and therefore belongs on *Firing Line*," counters Buckley.

In a ceremony on the White House Lawn, your former hard disk is made an honorary frisbee. "This is one small step for disk," the hard disk says as you flip off your TV and mutter something about ungrateful hardware. You try to figure out a way to recover months of priceless financial data, and decide there is no way.

A company once, in a less colorful way, lost all of its accounts receivable information. The company sent out polite form letters asking how much money, if any, each customer owed. Not surprisingly, the company was soon out of business.

Even a single floppy disk, holding 170 pages of information, can be a tragic loss. The entire text of this book fits comfortably on three 5¼-inch floppy disks. If I were to lose one of these prior to the publication of the book, and I had failed to make back-up copies (which I almost always fail to do), it would surely go beyond tragedy and deep into soap opera. O, the gnashing of teeth and the pulling of hair. Cecil B. DeMille never directed *angst* on a grander scale than I would emote.

There are two possible causes for such unthinkable, but possible, occurrences: computer error and operator error. As much as I hate to admit it, the latter far exceeds the former. By "computer error," I mean both hardware and software. Once again, the latter is the cause of far more difficulty than the former.

The causes of costly mistakes, in order, are:

A. Operator error.
B. Software error.
C. Computer error.

Using software that's been around for a while and a computer that's a relative newcomer, the last two categories might trade places. Almost without a doubt, though,

Drawbacks of Personal Computers

operator error will be responsible for more "computer errors" than anything else.

Suggestions for minimizing this drawback are:

First, make sure you know what you're doing. It's fine to experiment with a computer—there is almost nothing you can do from the keyboard of a personal computer that will cause any permanent damage to the machine—but don't experiment while you're working on something important or irreplaceable.

Before trying anything new, try a test first, or *at least* save whatever is in memory on a diskette. If, for any reason, the computer "crashes," (shuts down, freezes up, or turns off), whatever was in the memory is lost. If it is put on a disk (a simple, swift procedure), then the chance of retrieving the information is greatly enhanced.

Second, buy quality, time-tested software. This may not always be possible. You may need a program that is one-of-a-kind and newly introduced. In that case, watch for bugs and be very careful. If you are using the program to process information that is important to you, call the software manufacturer periodically and ask if any bugs have been reported that you should be aware of.

On the whole, however, most of the major categories of software—word processing, spell-checking, accounting, electronic spreadsheeting, filing—have products in each category that have been around at least a year, have sold thousands of copies, and have had most of the bugs removed.

Third, take good care of your machine. It doesn't require much. It is estimated that the majority of electronic parts that do not fail within the first twelve months will last for 500 years. How they make such calculations—the transistor being less than thirty years old and the silicon chip less than twenty—I shall never know.

It's a comfort, though, to think that, unless Life Extension Science takes the same dramatic leaps as Computer Science, and soon, our personal computers will be giving pleasure to generations yet unborn. Well, maybe it won't last *that* long, but a computer should hold up until you buy your next computer.

PERSONAL COMPUTERS AND THE DISABLED

The only parts of the computer that need periodic servicing and attention are the moving parts, and then only the disk drive and the printer. (A good keyboard seems to go on forever, and a joystick, well, use it for twenty years and buy a new one.)

Disk drives should be cleaned periodically. It takes about two minutes: all you do is put a special disk-cleaning disk in the drive and turn on the computer. Most "read/write" (disk) errors are caused by dirty heads, which two minutes of cleaning would have prevented.

Even if the computer misbehaves totally and eats a disk, the failure of the operator to make a back-up disk—again, about a two-minute procedure—can cause the problem to be much larger than necessary.

Power failures, too, cause the computer to lose its memory. Power failures happen with varying degrees of frequency in various locales. While living in Detroit, I don't recall any, except during electrical storms. In New York there were only two, although they lasted several days each. In Los Angeles, the power company named in honor of Mr. Edison seems to fail, on the average, once every other month.

Murphy's Law #253A states, "The power will fail only when you are about to find out 'whodunit' in a television mystery, have a souffle in the electric oven, or put something irreplaceable into the memory of your computer and have been too lazy to save it on a disk." Law #253B reads, "This will only happen when you are dangerously behind schedule, exhausted, and in a bad mood."

A good slogan to adopt while working with a computer is that of the compulsive bargain shopper: "Save, save, save." I am very bad at this sort of thing, but I do make it a habit to save whatever I am working on whenever I get up. Given that I get up at least every fifteen minutes, it's a rather good plan. Other people less antsy than I might want to save at the end of every page, or every ten minutes (set a timer), or at some predetermined interval or place in their work.

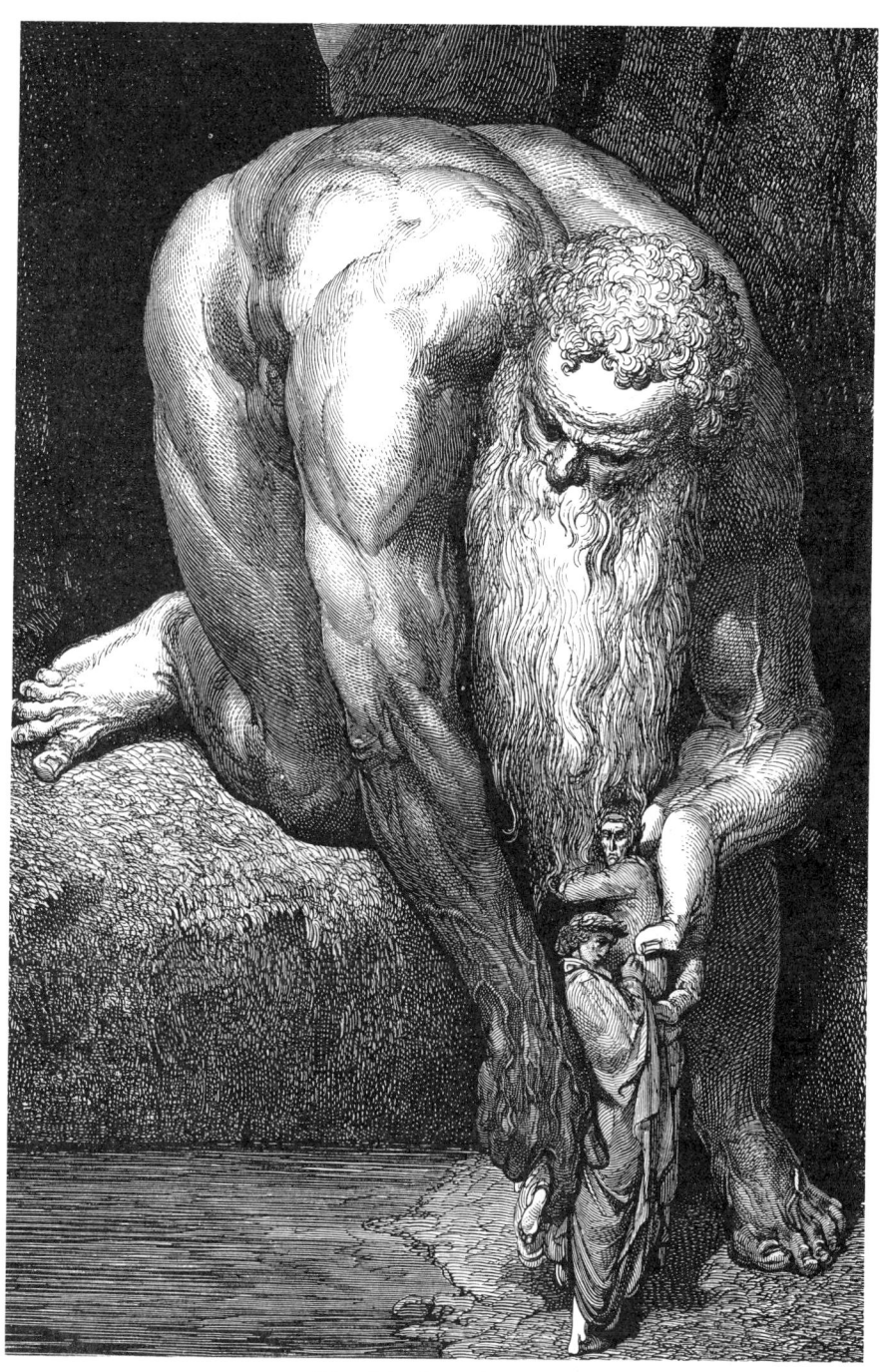

"Is this the IBM?"

PERSONAL COMPUTERS AND THE DISABLED

3. Eyestrain. Some people find that peering into a video screen causes eyestrain, and some do not. For those who do, here are some suggestions.

First, try using a monochrome video display rather than color. The images on color screens are not as sharp as images on monochrome screens. The fuzziness might be causing the problem.

Second, a monitor (a video display that plugs directly into the computer) rather than a recycled TV set, gives a sharper image. Again, fuzziness may be the problem. (When a screen display is fuzzy, the eyes strain to sharpen the focus. This constant straining can cause headaches.)

Third, green phosphor is supposed to be easier on the eyes than white. Try a green phosphor screen for a while.

Fourth, the glare of room lights off the glass of the video screen can cause eyestrain. Get a filter (Polaroid makes a good one) that reduces the reflected light. (The Polaroid filter also improves the contrast of the characters on the video screen, making them easier to read and further reducing eyestrain.)

Fifth, try a "slow phosphor" video display. The image on a video screen changes thirty times per second. This rapid changing is what gives the illusion of motion when Laverne hits Shirley in the face with a pie or a pizza or something. Ordinary video screens are designed to display the one-thirtieth-of-a-second-image, and then to fade quickly to make way for the next flash.

Slow phosphor holds the image for a longer period of time. Before the last image fades, another has already taken its place, and before that one fades, another has taken its place, and so on. This delivers a video display that is rock-steady.

The disadvantage of slow phosphor is that, because it holds onto a light image so long, when you change something on the screen, "ghosts" of what were formerly there will momentarily remain. These poltergeists remain for less than a second, but for someone used to quick-fade phosphor, it can be annoying. It is, however, far less annoying than eyestrain.

Drawbacks of Personal Computers

Sixth, read the solutions to disadvantages 4 and 5 below.

Eyestrain does not affect the vast majority of people who use video screens. These suggestions were offered for those who do have trouble.

4. Neck and back strain. Most back and neck strain experienced in front of a personal computer comes from maintaining the same posture, hour after hour.

If the keyboard and video display are all in one piece, your options for shifting positions are limited. You must reach the keys which, attached as they are to the screen, are not easily moved. This makes varying your position difficult. Not surprisingly, this sameness of position is a pain in the neck, a pain in the back, and a pain in any other portion of your anatomy you care to name.

The solution is a simple one: a detachable keyboard. A detachable keyboard allows you to place the video screen where it's most comfortable for viewing, and the keyboard where it's most comfortable for typing.

We have grown accustomed to looking *down* at a page when we type. This is because those of us who learned typing on a typewriter found that, invariably, that's where the paper was. The paper was where the typing was, and that's what we wanted to see.

Video screens can be placed a bit higher—closer to eye-level—and not having to look down for hours at a time can, in terms of neck and back strain, make quite a difference.

Also, the video screen need not be as close as the keyboard. As I write this, the video screen is at least four feet away. To read the entire screen, I only have to move my *eyes*, not my head. (The closer I get to the screen, the more my head would have to move—some law of physics at work there, no doubt.) This causes less strain on my neck and back. Further, the field of my vision encompassed by the video screen is small compared to the amount that would be involved if I were up close. I don't know if it's true or not, but my mother always told me it was bad for my eyes to sit too near the TV screen.

PERSONAL COMPUTERS AND THE DISABLED

I will, mom's advice notwithstanding, move closer to the video screen when I edit this piece. I will be looking at the text in a critical character-by-character way. Now I'm just looking at words, sentences, and ideas. For those, four feet is close enough.

But even when I move up close, I will never be as close as I would have to be if the keyboard were permanently glued to some spot directly under the video screen.

A detachable keyboard also allows for an infinite variety of positions. Some of this chapter I have written with the keyboard on my desk, some of it with the keyboard on my lap. Were I so inclined, I could have stood up, lain down, or assumed any of a dozen other positions.

Maybe it's true that the straight-backed rigid posture is the best for long-term typing, but I never learned to sit like that, and I doubt if I ever will. There is too much else to learn before and after getting a computer. Who wants to have to worry about learning a new way to *sit?*

I would rather have a computer that adapts its shape to my posture, not one that demands I adapt my posture to its shape, especially when that shape is dictated by an 1874 invention. Personal computers with attached keyboards were modeled after computer terminals, and computer terminals were modeled after typewriters. This was because computer terminals were designed for secretaries who were already familiar with typewriters.

Besides, if there's any validity to the next point, the further away the video screen, the better I feel.

5. Radiation. *All* TV screens, including the one in your bedroom and the one in your living room, give off radiation. The electron gun shoots electrons, "radiating" the phosphorus until it glows. Some of this radiation leaks out.

How much leaks out is not known. How much is safe to be exposed to is not known. What the effects of this are over time are not known.

Drawbacks of Personal Computers

A few things are known:

A. The farther you are from the video screen the less radiation you are exposed to. Radiation levels drop quickly with distance. A few inches from a video screen, a measurable amount of radiation is given off; several feet away, the amount is no longer measurable.

B. Color monitors give off more radiation—as much as five times more—than monochrome.

C. Radiation is not good for you.

I remember looking at a sign in front of a building on my first trip to Los Angeles in the early 1970s. It said, "UCLA CENTER FOR UNCLEAR MEDICINE."

I thought, only in Southern California would a medical center admit that there were any areas of medicine that were unclear; and to put it on a sign, and to devote a whole center to it—well, I was impressed.

A friend had to point out to me that the sign read UCLA CENTER FOR NUCLEAR MEDICINE. Since that time, I have been unable to look at the word NUCLEAR without seeing the word UNCLEAR.

The reports that have surfaced over the past ten years have only made it more unclear. Atomic bombs, meltdowns, nuclear energy, annihilation—did this perplexing subject have to pop out of Pandora's Box *on television*, too? Do we have to face major moral, social, and medical issues every time we turn on the TV or switch on the computer? I mean, can't they leave us *SCTV* and Space Invaders? Is nothing sacred?

A polling of the scientific community only heightens the dilemma. Some say radiation from video screens causes cataracts, miscarriages, leukemia, and arthritis, especially in the fingers because, on computers without detachable keyboards, the fingers are closest to the video screen for the longest periods of time.

Other scientists say that the chance a radioactive electron has of passing through the glass of a video screen is about the chance you or I would have of driving through Nevada with four feet of beachballs on the ground and a gallon of gas in the car. (I did not make that up. A nuclear scientist made that up. A man with credentials.) They say

PERSONAL COMPUTERS AND THE DISABLED

that even the sun gives off radioactivity, and that there is as much danger being exposed to daylight as there is to video light.

The more intricate the arguments, the more persuasive each side became. The only advice I could offer concerned computer users: use a monochrome video screen, and put it as far away from you as possible. (Yet another argument for the detachable keyboard.)

But then I wondered: should I be giving this advice at all? Maybe there's no danger to begin with. What's the point in scaring people? *The China Syndrome* was bad enough. No point in starting *The Computa Syndrome.* I was in the midst of deepening confusion when, suddenly, a solution appeared.

The Langley-St. Clair Company began marketing lead-impregnated acrylic screens that fit over regular video screens and block, according to Langley-St. Clair, 100% of all x-rays and most ultraviolet radiation. The acrylic, it turns out, was originally designed for windows in nuclear power plants.

I ordered one. It arrived, a sturdy piece of plastic, about a quarter of an inch thick; transparent, with a slight tint. It attached easily to my video screen with velcro tape. I felt safe from radiation, like Lex Luthor felt safe from Superman when wearing his Kryptonite-impregnated leisure suit. It was the magic shield of Gardol from my youth.

The only problem is that the acrylic screen reflects light almost like a mirror. Who wants to trade safety for annoying glare? (It's trade-off time again.) The Langley-St. Clair people readily admit the problem and have solved the problem by covering their acrylic with a mesh antiglare screen. The whole package lists for $129.

Well, those are all the drawbacks I've discovered about personal computers, except for unknowledgeable salespeople, lack of product support, and manufacturers' arrogance and incompetence. But I'll discuss those in the chapters ahead. Besides, I never let those things stop me from having something I want. If I did, I wouldn't have a telephone.

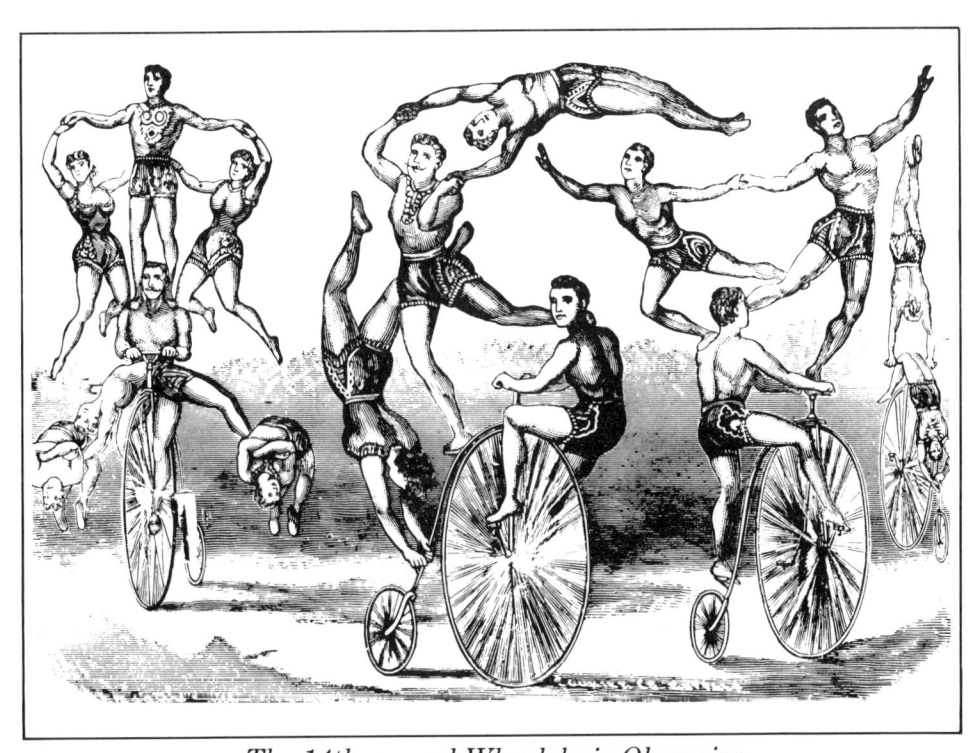

The 14th annual Wheelchair Olympics.

Chapter Ten

Learning a Personal Computer Program
(*Pilfered from*
The Personal Computer in Business Book.)

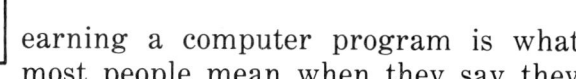earning a computer program is what most people mean when they say they want to learn "how to use a computer." After turning the computer on, anything you do, from copying a disk to writing a novel to running a business, involves programs. They can be simple programs that involve only one instruction (**command**), or more complex programs that baffle the uninitiated user with hundreds.

Generally speaking, the more commands a program offers, the more powerful and flexible the program is. A word processing program, for example, *requires* only six commands: a way to create a file, a way to insert text, a way to move the cursor around, a way to delete text, a way to save the file, and a way to print what you have saved.

But most sophisticated word processing programs have a hundred or more commands. These extra commands add extra features, but also add to the amount of time it will take to learn the program.

If you plan to frequently use your computer for a given task, accounting say, it pays to choose an accounting program with all the features you need, or might reasonably need in the future, and then invest the time and attention necessary to learn it properly.

On the other hand, occasional and infrequent tasks performed on your computer might require a program that is not as "powerful," but is easier to learn and use: A simple mailing list program, for example, rather than a full-scale data base management system.

What follows are some hints on making the process of learning a program as painless as possible.

1. Take your time. Learning a program takes time, so set the time aside.

2. Don't plan to do anything with the program until you have mastered it. The time to learn a few basic phrases in German is before you arrive in Berlin. Don't try to learn an accounts receivable program on Thursday if you need a trial balance on Friday, and you're expecting the computer to provide that balance. All it will provide is frustration and anger at everything and everyone connected with computing.

(You should see some of the letters I get from people in the throes of learning a complicated program under pressure. Tokyo Rose didn't get such hate mail.) Use replaceable, unnecessary information until the program is fully learned, *then* begin work on the company books or the great American novel or whatever you bought your computer for in the first place.

3. Read the manual from cover to cover. You would think the instructions for your program would be called the "instruction manual." No. Too simple. In Computerese it's known as **documentation**. ("Never use a simple word if a complex word will do." Rule #2.3a of The Computerese Manual of Style.)

Before even turning the computer on, read the documentation from cover to cover, quickly, without attempting to grasp anything. Don't stop to study intricate passages or make sense out of technical data; just read everything, lightly.

Some might say this lets all the information seep into your subconscious mind so that at least *some* part of your being has access to all the information. Others might say that a quick reading ("skimming" they call it in academia) gives an overview of the material to be learned. I say it lets you know what you're up against. (See next point.)

4. Don't expect manuals to be clear, simple, easy to understand, or contain all information necessary to learn the program. The personal computer industry is in its infancy. In any industry less than eight years old, there are bound to be some weak links. The weakest link in the world of small computers is documentation.

Where else can you spend $500 to $1,000 on a program, and find the manual so incomprehensible that you'd have to spend from $15 to $50 more on a book that

Learning a Personal Computer Program

will tell you how to use the program? In computerdom, it happens all the time.

Manuals are frequently written by the same people who write the programs. These dear souls, while they can communicate with computers eloquently, have not yet learned the joys of communicating with their fellow human beings using the written word.

Extracting information from some of these dense packs of prose can be difficult at best. The only way to survive some of the passages with your humor intact is to pretend you're playing a computer game.

The game is one of the many variants of *Raiders of the Lost Ark*. You have discovered a box containing some more Dead Sea Scrolls, which you refer to as Not-So-Well Sea Scrolls. A passage has been translated into a form of English. Your task: Figure out what some doomed Egyptian *really meant* by this collection of words.

You have a Rosetta Stone (your computer). You try it this way and that way and another way until, lo, one command suddenly works. You make a notation as to what was really meant, reward yourself with a date, and move onto the next passage.

At certain points, the information will simply not be there. You may need to visit the Scholars (the dealer who sold you the program) or, if the Scholars don't know, you may have to contact the Oracle (manufacturer of the program) directly.

5. Find a friend or colleague who uses the program. The phrase "A colleague in need is a colleague indeed" could be coined for just this situation.

6. Look for other information. Several popular programs have books written on how to use them. You might want to have a look at these. But remember: Just because they're books doesn't mean they're going to be any clearer or more informative than the documentation.

Computer magazines will often have articles written by users about the pitfalls of learning specific programs. A library with a first-rate periodical section should be able to help.

PERSONAL COMPUTERS AND THE DISABLED

7. Join a user group. There is no doubt *some kind* of user group in your area. Even though the group may be formed around a specific *machine* (Apple, IBM, Kaypro, etc.), and even if you don't have that machine, you may find someone there who uses the *program* you're trying to learn. Most programs operate almost the same from machine to machine.

8. Hire a consultant. Someone who knows and uses the program you are trying to learn can be well worth the $10 to $50 per hour consultants charge. To find a consultant, you might call the computer stores in town and ask for the salesperson who knows the most about your program. Tempt them with cash. Lead them astray.

Some computer stores have bulletin boards. A notice posted there might prove valuable. Another method is to call temporary help agencies. Some of these agencies specialize in small computers and in providing personnel familiar with certain programs. When the temp arrives, ask him or her to *teach* the program rather than *run* the program. They may have a full-day or half-day minimum, so be prepared to work.

9. Make notes. After deciphering the documentation, rewrite difficult passages in your own words. Also, get some highlighting pens, and mark in different colors the sections you think you'll use frequently, often, sometimes, seldom, and never.

10. Don't be afraid to experiment. You can't hurt the computer (unless you throw it out a window in frustration), and the worst you can do to a program is erase it. (At which point you go to your back-up disk—you *did* make a back-up disk, didn't you?) If you wonder as you go along, "What would happen if I did this?", do it and find out. You may discover a use for the program even the programmer didn't consider.

11. Congratulate yourself. Learning a powerful computer program is no easy matter. Pat yourself on the back frequently.

12. Have fun. If you've removed the time and task pressures, learning a program, like exploring any new territory, is an adventure, and adventures, so I'm told, can be fun.

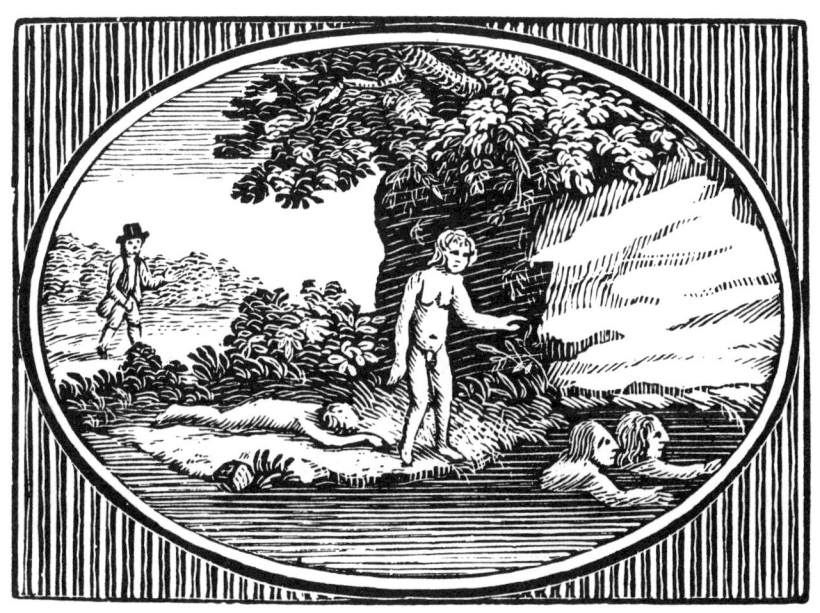

CAN YOU FIGURE OUT WHAT'S GOING ON IN THIS PICTURE? If you can, you'll probably have no trouble figuring out computers from available documentation.

Chapter Eleven

Purchasing a Personal Computer

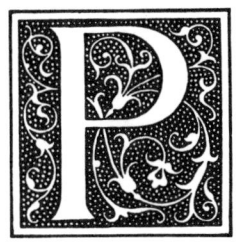urchasing a personal computer will, for most people, require visiting a new kind of retail outlet: The computer store. Seven years ago there were no computer stores. Today, they're everywhere.

Please keep in mind that personal computing is in its pioneer days. You'll get along a lot better at computer stores if you treat them like trading posts on the frontier rather than modern and sophisticated retail outlets.

When spending several thousand dollars on a consumer item, it is reasonable to expect some expert guidance, some personalized attention, and, yes, even a bit of pampering. At a computer store, you're lucky if they open on time.

A couple of years ago, there were only a few computer stores, owned and operated by knowledgeable, well-intentioned computer addicts who knew how to build, fix, operate, and program any computer in the store. There was only one problem with these people: they could not speak English. They had spent so long in the land of RAM that they were unable to describe life in anything but bytes.

All a prospective computer buyer had to do was take a Berlitz crash course in Conversational Computerese and he or she was set. Once you learned how to communicate with the people in the computer store, in their language, you could find out anything you wanted to know.

Then the gold rush came. Someone took a look at the sales curve of personal computers and decided there was gold in them there hills. A great many someones did. Personal computers became the domain of entrepreneurs and investment bankers and venture capitalists and Wall Street. These people were in it for the buck, not for the love of computing.

And so the marketing was turned over to the advertising agencies, store designs to architectural firms,

PERSONAL COMPUTERS AND THE DISABLED

and sales to professional salespeople. These people knew how to speak English, but they didn't know beans about computers. Selling was selling, or so the theory goes, and if these people were good at selling widgets, they'd be good at selling computers.

Selling is a skill, just as knowing how to operate a computer is a skill, and I'm afraid there are precious few people in the world of computer retailing who know both. Computer merchandising is growing at such a rapid rate that if a person *did* know both, he or she would wind up as sales manager of the company within six months, and you'd never see him or her on the selling floor again.

The fact that you will get neither stellar service nor sage advice from computer stores is nobody's fault, really. It would be nice to blame it on corporate greed or laziness or some recognizable evil, but I can't seem to find one.

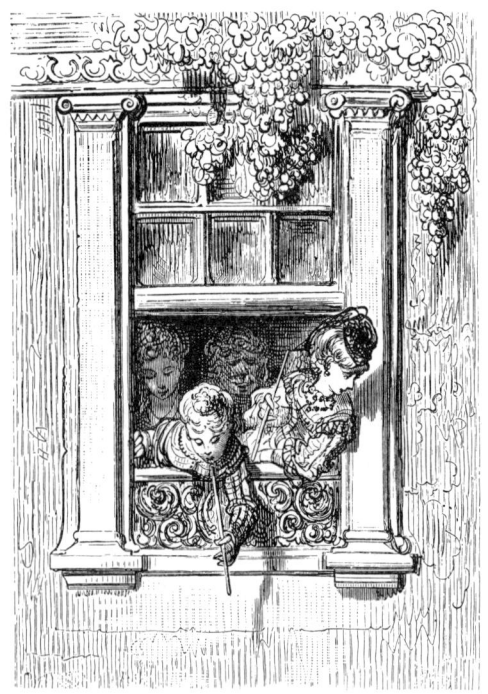

Computer salespeople, using pea shooters to attract the attention of customers in the street below.

Purchasing a Personal Computer

The computer salespeople I have met are well-meaning and willing to help, they just don't have enough information *to* help.

Look at what they're up against:

1. Computers are changing all the time. If a store sells two or three different kinds of computers, one must know what's currently available, what's planned for in the near future, what peripherals are available, how each of these works, and what they do.

2. Further, one must know what the competition is doing, planning, marketing, and so on. A customer may come in and say, "I saw an ad for The Super Computer in *Time*. Why is your machine better?" A good salesperson should have a good answer.

3. Software is a jungle unto itself. Imagine being asked to know, in even a cursory way, something about every program in a given computer store, much less on the market.

Someone shopping for games might ask, "Do you have the game that's like *Dungeons and Dragons*, except that it has the Red Baron in cell number seven and the green tiger? I played it at a friend's house last week."

Someone shopping for word processing might say, "I need to do script formats, indexing, and footnoting, but proportional spacing is not necessary."

An accountant might ask, "Will this process receivables on a year-to-date or periodic basis?"

And so it would go for every software category. Computer people are not the only ones who have jargon.

4. It would help if the salesperson were a master of psychology. (Ph.D., with a minimum of three years' clinical experience, well-grounded in crisis intervention.) People have the strangest reactions when confronted with a world as unusual and different as computers. For some, the defenses rise to battlestation proportions. Others become so defenseless that they believe anything. Terror, disorientation, hostility. Sometimes it's hard to tell the difference between the waiting room at an out-patient clinic and a computer store.

5. Most people come to computer stores looking not

PERSONAL COMPUTERS AND THE DISABLED

for computers but *solutions*. This and this and this is wrong with my business, my children, and my life. Which machine will fix it, how will it fix it, and what will it cost? For a computer salesperson, the wisdom of Solomon seems to be another prerequisite.

6. Computers appeals to a broad spectrum of people, from prepubescents to post-doctoral candidates. A salesperson must be able to discuss programming with ten-year-olds and video games with Nobel Laureates. If you're opening a computer store, you might check on the availability of Henry Kissinger.

7. After people spend $5,000 (or $2,000 or $3,000) on something, they expect *service*. "I didn't spend $5,000 on a machine to have it..." People can be awfully demanding.

Naturally, the person who must carry the brunt of whatever dissatisfaction the customer might have is the salesperson. He or she must be, in other words, an expert troubleshooter, a crackerjack repair person, and a diplomat extraordinaire.

8. A salesperson also has to deal with the demands of his or her boss and the many manufacturers of software and hardware sold in the store. This takes the patience of Job and the integrity of Serpico.

9. Thus far I've only discussed the problem salespeople have keeping up with regular computers for able-bodied people. To serve the disabled, the salesperson would have to have a vast amount of information about various disabilities, know what's available in special input devices, output devices, software and support.

One could begin to construct a picture, then, of the ideal computer salesperson. If you were to find such a person, you could easily get him or her elected President—or Pope. It is doubtful that, unless you came upon a Saint slumming it for a lifetime or two, this person would be selling computers.

The problem is that it's all so intricate and all so new, and it's getting more intricate and newer everyday. I don't know anyone who has successfully kept up with it all. I certainly don't pretend that I have. People pick an area and specialize: hardware, languages, games. I'm rather fond of word processing myself. You may have to talk to a lot of people in order to capture the gestalt of the whole thing.

There are ways of getting the most out of what computer stores have to offer. Here are some that I have found useful:

1. Do your homework. Contact the companies, organizations and individuals who might have information on the best hardware/software configurations for your specific needs. The information from these sources will narrow the range of computers that will best serve your needs. The input device or output device or software you'll want might only run on a limited number of computers. Those are, obviously, the computers to look at.

2. Make an appointment. Call the store and ask to speak to the expert in the field you are most interested in: accounting, games, word processing, electronic spreadsheeting. All you have to say is, "Which one of your salespeople knows the most about accounting?"

It might not be a bad idea to call (or write, or have a friend call) all the computer stores in your area, describe your disability—being quite specific as to what you can and cannot do with regard to operating a computer—and ask if they have any experience in helping someone with your particular needs.

Of ten stores you contact, you may find one or two that have that experience. These would be the stores to start with. If possible, contact the person (or people) who have similar disabilities and have been supplied by a particular store with a computer. They'll be an invaluable source of information.

When you contact the store, make a specific appointment. They may try to get off the hook with, "I'm here every day from nine to five. Drop by anytime." Counter with, "Fine, how about Tuesday at three?" Call in the morning to confirm (i.e., remind them).

With an appointment, you are more likely to speak with the person who knows the most about the subject you are interested in, and you are more likely to get some specialized attention. Not much, but some.

3. Do not be intimidated by jargon. Salespeople who use excessive jargon are either from the Old School of computer selling and know everything about computers and nothing about communication, or they are from the New School and know very little about computers but are trying to conceal that fact. When in doubt about what a word or phrase means, ask. Asking may not do you any good, but don't be afraid to give it a try.

4. Get some "hands-on" experience. Don't spend a lot of time discussing the philosophy of computing and looking at full-color brochures—sit down at a computer and *play* with the thing. There's plenty of time to talk while you're pushing buttons and watching the results of that button-pushing.

See if you can spend some time alone with the computer. This usually isn't too hard to arrange. When you have enough information to attempt a solo flight, all you have to say is, "Why don't you take care of some of your other customers and come back to me later?" There are almost always other customers to be taken care of.

5. Ask a friend who knows something about computers to come along. He or she will be able to tell you (later) whether the salesperson was giving you solid information or solid, uh, disinformation. They will also be able to, once the salesperson has gone, show you some great things about the computer. (Although don't expect your friend, who runs Program A on Computer B, to know very much about running Program C on Computer B.)

6. Use the computer for what you'll be using the computer for. If you're going to use it for creative writing, write something creative. If you're going to use it for correspondence, write letters. If you'll be doing accounting, do some accounting. If you're going to use your computer as an electronic spreadsheet, bring along some numbers and project some costs. If you're going to play games, play some games.

When you're done looking at your desired application, ask the salesperson to show you what else the machine can do.

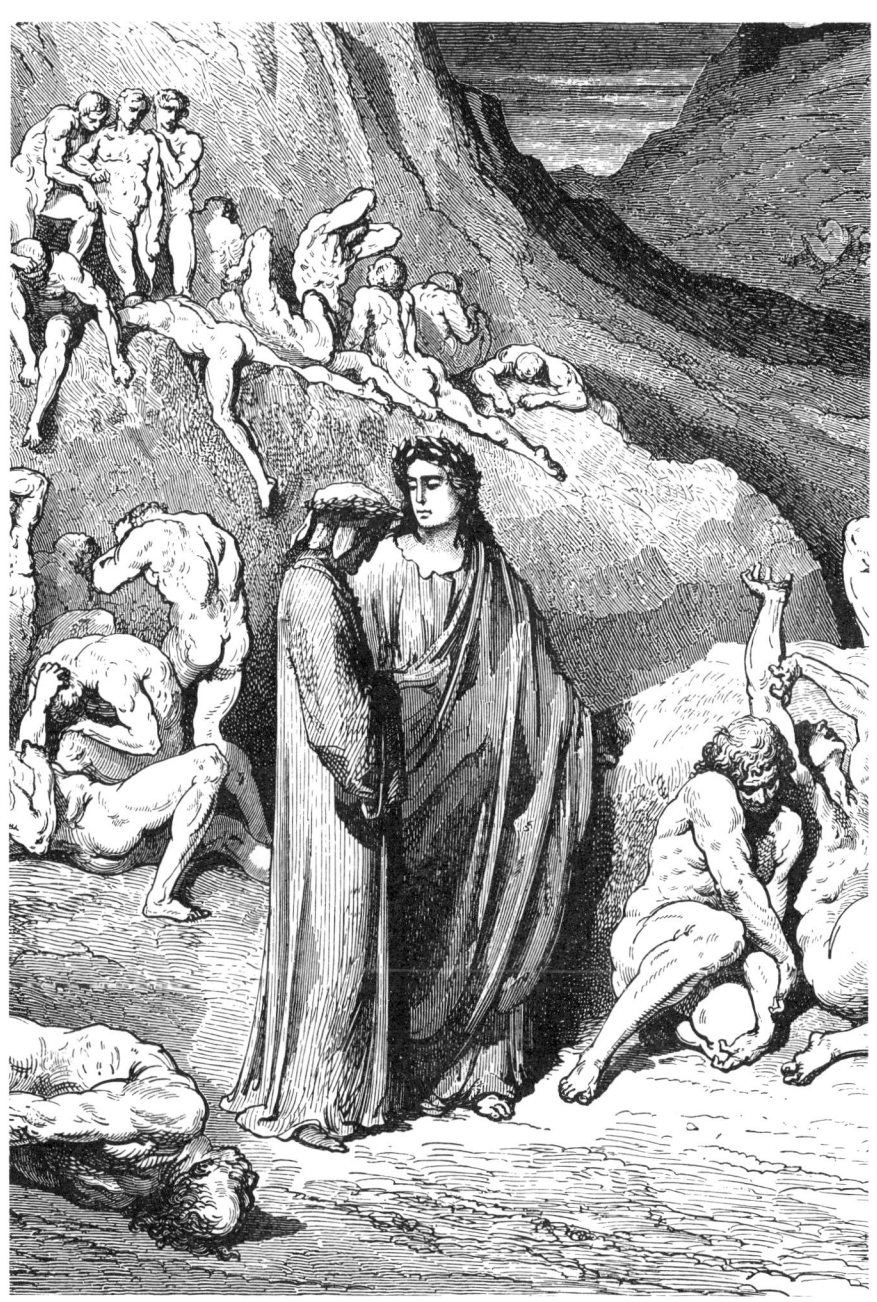

"Don't pay any attention to them. They bought the wrong computer and they're not happy about it. Serves them right, they didn't do their homework. Let's move on."

PERSONAL COMPUTERS AND THE DISABLED

7. Be on the lookout for good salespeople as well as good computers. If, while in the store, you observe a salesperson who really knows what he or she is doing, and it is clear that "your" salesperson does not, it is time for diplomacy, tact, and good old American deception. (Going from one salesperson to another is like changing dates after you're at the ball.)

First, create some emergency that needs taking care of and leave. (You have to buy your seeds for National Potato Week or something.) The longer you stay in the store, the more the not-so-hot salesperson will feel you "belong" to him or her.

Exit soon, but first find out (a) the lunch hour and (b) the day of the week your original salesperson has off. (Make it sound as though you will rearrange your schedule so as not to miss him or her.) Return to the store next at (a) that hour, or (b) that day. The better salesperson should be on duty, and you now have a new salesperson.

8. Make notes. Record model numbers, prices, salesperson's names, everything. After leaving the store, debrief yourself and note the pros and the cons of the machines and programs you've just evaluated. The things that are clear in your mind upon leaving a store will be hopelessly muddled a few weeks and a dozen computer stores later. Ask, too, for any printed literature the store can part with.

9. Trust your intuition. It's important that you feel good about the computer you purchase. Include your emotional reactions in your notes and in your decision. Just as cars are more than how many MPG they get, computers are more than how much RAM they have.

10. What happens if it breaks? Be sure to investigate what you'll have to do if the computer does not compute either in or out of warranty. Can you bring it back to the store or will you have to pack it up and ship it to California? How much time will repairs take? Are loaners available for free or at a reasonable cost? Will the store put all its promises in writing? Think about the unthinkable before you buy.

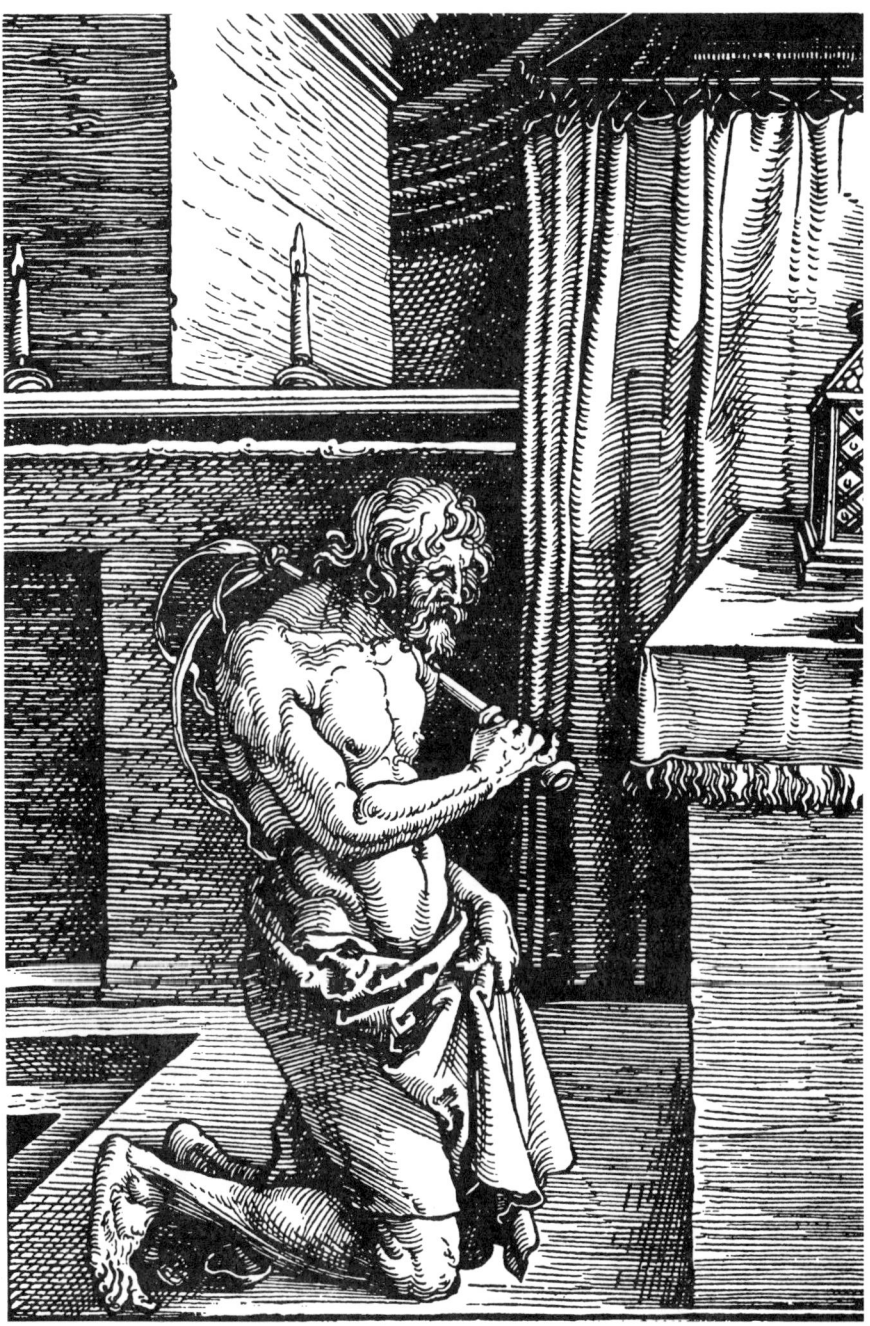
Chose your computer wisely so you won't have to regret it later.

PERSONAL COMPUTERS AND THE DISABLED

11. Take your time. Don't try to look at everything in a week. You might experience a Personal Systems Overload. Take it easy. If you must travel to The Big City to do your investigations, it's better to plan several shorter trips rather than one long one. Gather all the information you can, let it digest, and make your decision in a relaxed state of mind.

12. Enjoy yourself. Keep in mind that it's hard to lose. All personal computers have *something* worthwhile to recommend them. To paraphrase Father Flanagan, there are no bad computers. You might not buy the best computer that fills your every need for the best price, but such is life. Whatever you do buy will serve you faithfully, teach you several magnitudes more about computers and computing than you know now, and assure that your next computer purchase will be an almost perfect one. Knowing there's no way to lose, enjoy playing one of the most intricate and challenging computer games around: buying a computer.

In getting the best price on your personal computer, it pays to shop the back pages of the various computer magazines (*BYTE* in particular). There you will find mail-order companies that sell computers at rather remarkable discounts. Some computers will be there, and some computers will not. Different computer companies have different policies, and although "fair trading" (i.e., price fixing) was ruled illegal some years ago, some companies control their dealers such that you can be sure you will never find one of their products sold for less than full retail price.

If the computer store in your area offers absolutely nothing in the way of knowledge and support, or if you live a goodly distance from even the closest computer outlet, you might consider buying a computer by mail. Most mail-order computer companies have good reputations, but the unspoken agreement is, "We'll sell you a computer cheap, but you're on your own after the sale." That means that

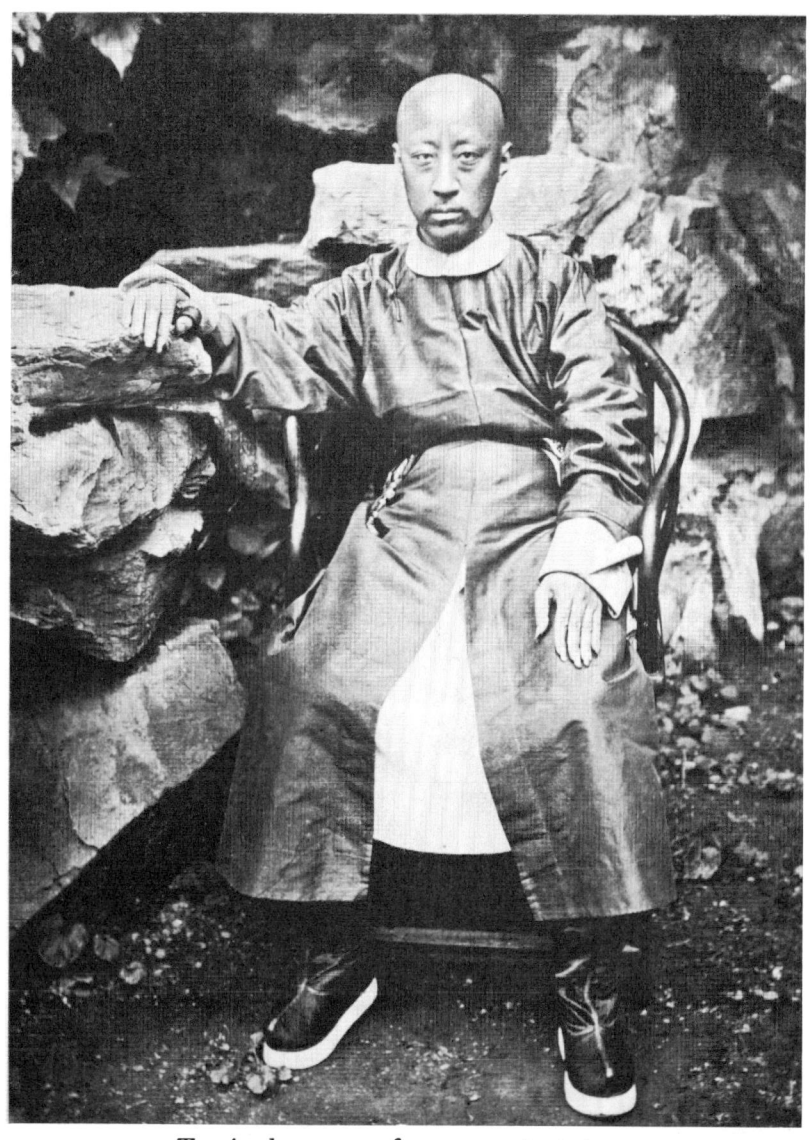
Typical owner of a computer store.

PUBLISHER'S NOTE: WE WOULD LIKE TO APOLOGIZE TO ALL COMPUTER STORE OWNERS WHO DO NOT LOOK LIKE THIS. MR. MCWILLIAMS'S CONTRACT GIVES HIM EDITORIAL CONTROL OVER THE CONTENTS OF HIS BOOKS—A MISTAKE WE DO NOT PLAN TO LET HAPPEN AGAIN.

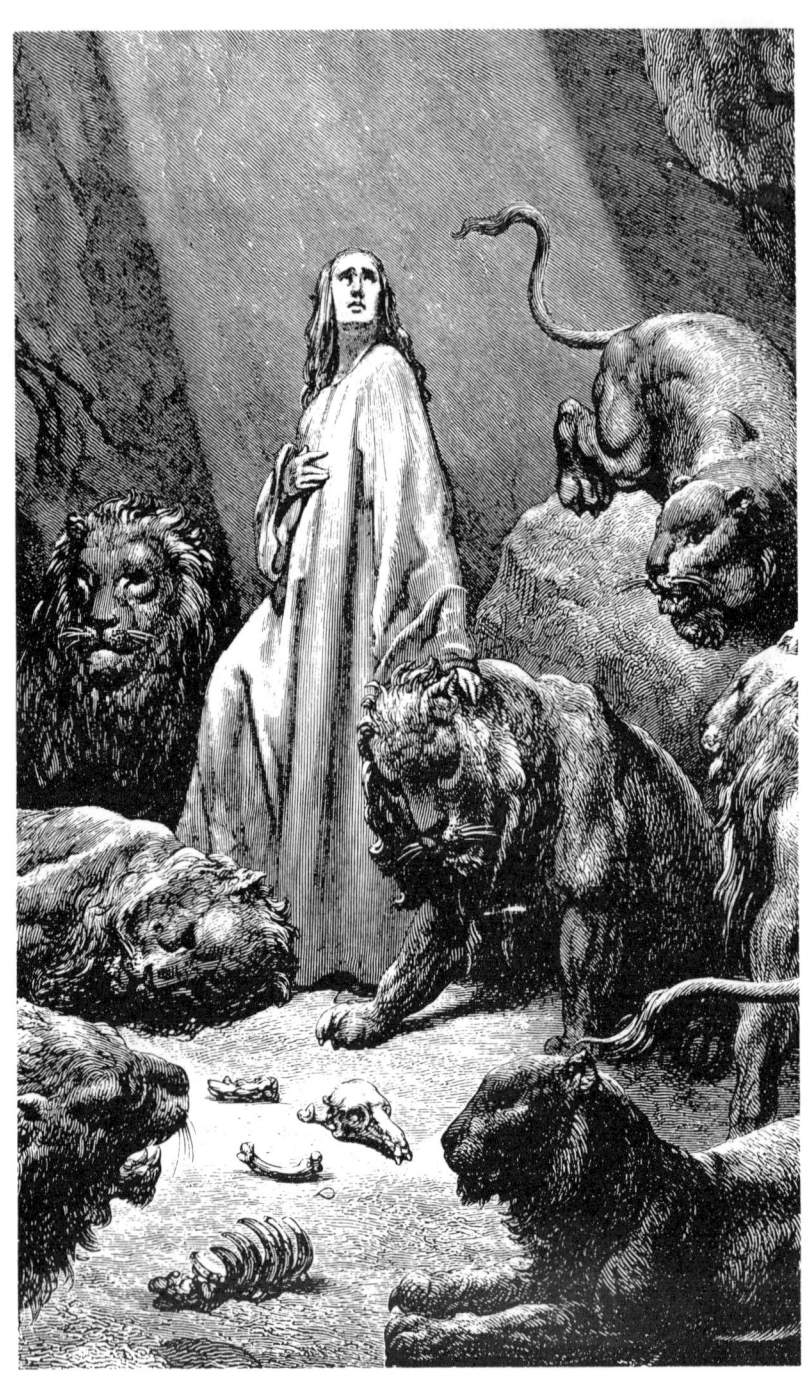
Daniel in the computer store.

fixing the computer is between you and the manufacturer (most are good at mail-in warranty repairs), and that learning the computer is between you and the Almighty.

If the computer store in your neighborhood seems to know what they're doing, can communicate that with a fair degree of intelligibility, and seems to be able to offer you after-the-sale support (a repair department, software, peripherals, maybe even classes), then buy from them.

You may or may not be able to get a lower price from the local computer store by showing them the ads in the magazines. They may give you a special "systems price," or throw in some software, or offer to come over to your house and set it up. Most stores, if they are interested in your business, will make some concession somewhere.

Don't expect them, however, to "meet or beat" the price in the mail order ad. The unspoken agreement between you and a walk-in computer store is that they will be there to serve you after the sale. This costs something, quite a lot actually, and, like a club, you pay your dues when you join.

You might, too, consider hiring your salesperson, or someone you met in your quest for RAM, as a consultant. This is especially true in a business environment. Offer them $25 per hour—or more—to review your computer purchase just before making it, set the computer up, test it out, make sure everything is working, teach you how to run different programs, and be on hand to answer any questions as they arise (and they *will* arise).

If your consultant works, say, ten hours at this task, he or she might prove to have been the most valuable $250 peripheral you could possibly have purchased.

Chapter Twelve

A Brand Name Buying Guide

To computer companies, we're all the same. Their products can be used by almost everybody, able-bodied or not. Depending on your needs, however, some computers are better than others. A great deal of software specifically for disabled individuals is written for Apple II and IIe computers, for instance, so an Apple or Apple-compatible may be the computer you need. In general, if you need a computer to run a particular program, be it word processing or environmental control, find which computers the program works on, and choose from there.

I've organized the hardware, software, and peripheral equipment information as follows. In this chapter, name brand computers are reviewed. This is the same chapter as in my other books, *The Word Processing Book, The Personal Computer Book,* and *The Personal Computer in Business Book.* Therefore, if you read the reviews in any of those books, you can simply skip to the next section. The *Hardware, Software and Computer Services* section covers specific items that may be useful to a disabled individual. Also there, you will find any additional information on computers that this first part does not cover. (There is a special model of the Radio Shack Model 100 computer, for instance, whose control and shift keys stay down, allowing for mouthstick or one finger operation. This kind of information, you will find there.) You will also find companies who will modify computers to individual needs.

Buying guides are, by their very nature, incomplete and obsolete. Even as I write, computers are being introduced, and improvements are being made on personal computers already on the market.

When all makes and models are accounted for, there are something like 200 personal computers on the market. This does not include software, printers, or other peripherals.

PERSONAL COMPUTERS AND THE DISABLED

To spend just one day with each of these computers would take me the better part of a year, and to devote but one page to each of them would take the better part of this book.

I am reminded of a *Ripley's Believe It or Not* item from my childhood. It said that if the population of China were to line up and march four abreast past a point, the line would never end. The rate of reproduction was faster than the number of people moving past the point. (I wondered, precocious youngster that I was, how they could reproduce that fast while standing in line.)

Reviewing computers, I fear, would have the same effect. By the time the 200 days were done, there would be another hundred computers to look at, and by the time I got through those, it would be time to start all over with revisions and improvements.

During all the days spent with these machines, of course, this book would not be in your hands. I postponed the publication of *The Word Processing Book* twelve times. Every week I heard about something new, and every week I thought, "I'd better investigate this—it's worth waiting a week if I can include it."

Three months later I had to draw the line. "What I know about word processing **today** will encompass the first edition of the book, and that's that."

And so it is with this Buying Guide. What I know about personal computers now is what's in this guide.

One warning: these "reviews" are subjective and heavily biased. This chapter is nothing but my opinions and, just because they happen to be bound in a book, gives them no more credibility than anyone else's.

I have divided this section into several groups, arranged by types and needs. First, there are the home computers—computers that are under $1,000 and are suited particularly for games, introductory programming, and home accounting needs. Next come lap-sized personal computers. These are machines that weigh under 10 pounds and are meant for business or word processing use on the road.

Then come the larger, slightly more expensive computers. Most of these are geared for people who have a more active need for computing—in business or word processing. I have divided these computers into three sections: IBM and IBM-compatible computers; Apple and Apple-compatible computers; and CP/M and other computers.

All the computers listed have two disk drives, 80-column screens with at least 24 lines on the screen, a numeric keypad on the keyboard, and separate cursor keys, unless otherwise noted.

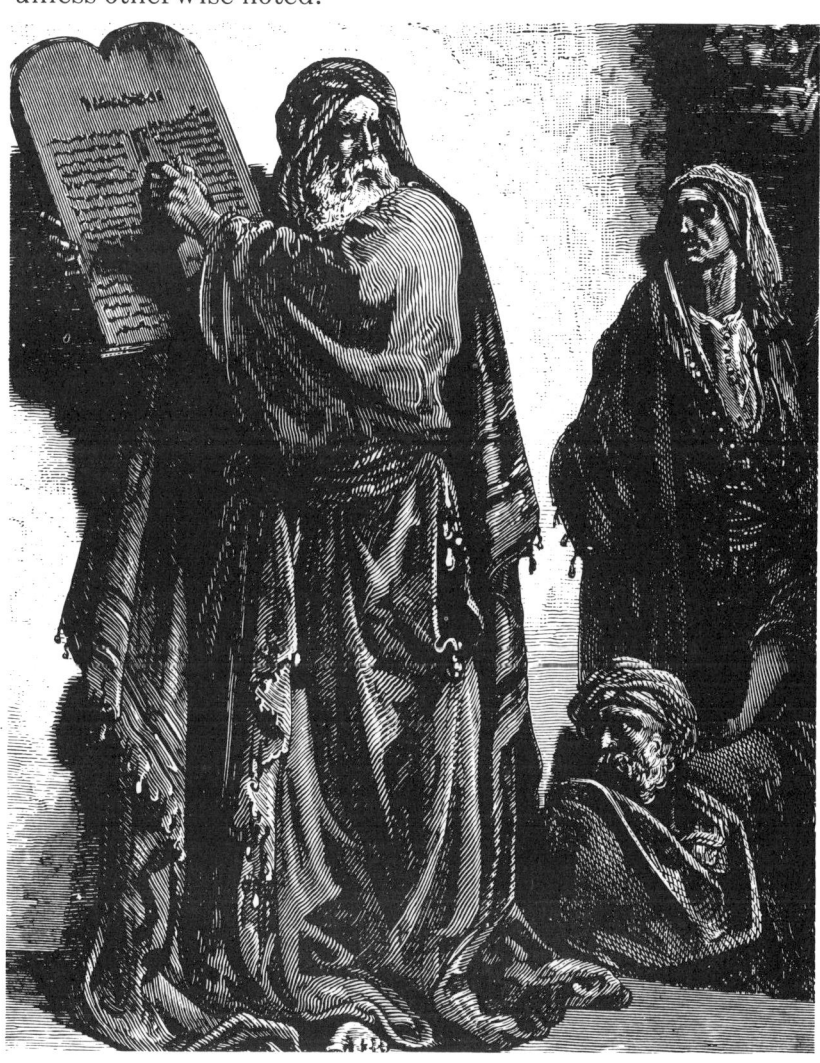

PERSONAL COMPUTERS AND THE DISABLED

Home Computers

Atari 800XL

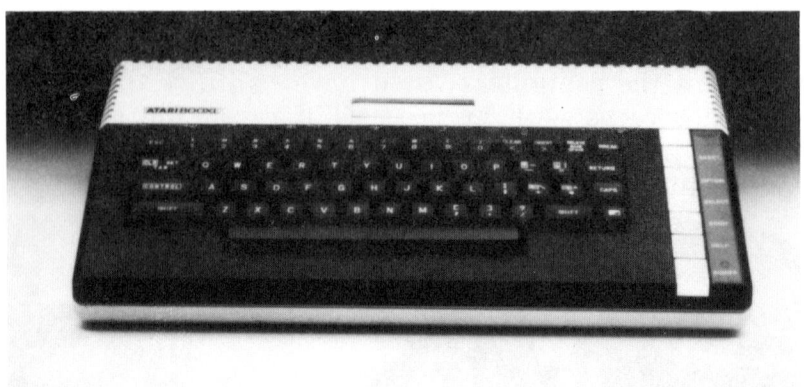

Price: $399 (no drives, no monitor)
Screen size: 40 characters x 24 lines
Screen color: color
Main operating system: Atari OS
Processor: 8-bit 6502C
Standard memory: 64K
Disk drive type: 5¼" (available for $450 each)
Capacity of formatted disks: 127K
Software included: BASIC, operating system
Keyboard:
- detachable? yes
- number of keys: 62
- number of function keys: 4

Weight: n/a

Comments: Atari dropped half its line of computers and now only sells the 600XL and the 800XL (until the 1450XLD is released). Neither are good for word processing or for business. They are home computers, geared as an introduction to computing. Atari's game cartridges are ever popular, and if games are your main interest in computing, the Ataris may fill your needs.

> And a smooth-faced Atari executive, in charge of the Home Consumer Division, tears his gaze away from his in-office video screen and game master control to grin, "I play about 20 to 30 hours a day. If I had my druthers, I'd probably play all day long."—*San Francisco Examiner & Chronicle.*

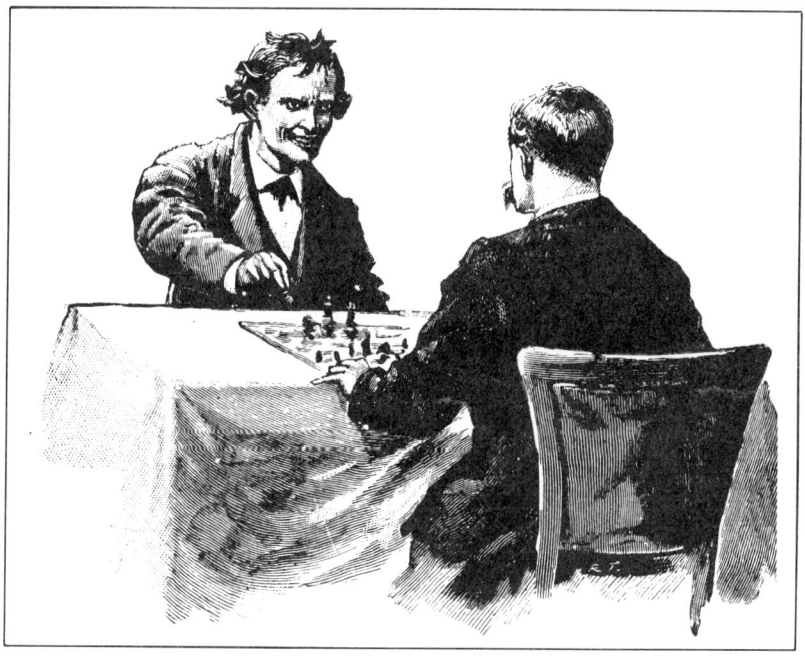

"*Atari!*"

PERSONAL COMPUTERS AND THE DISABLED

Coleco Adam

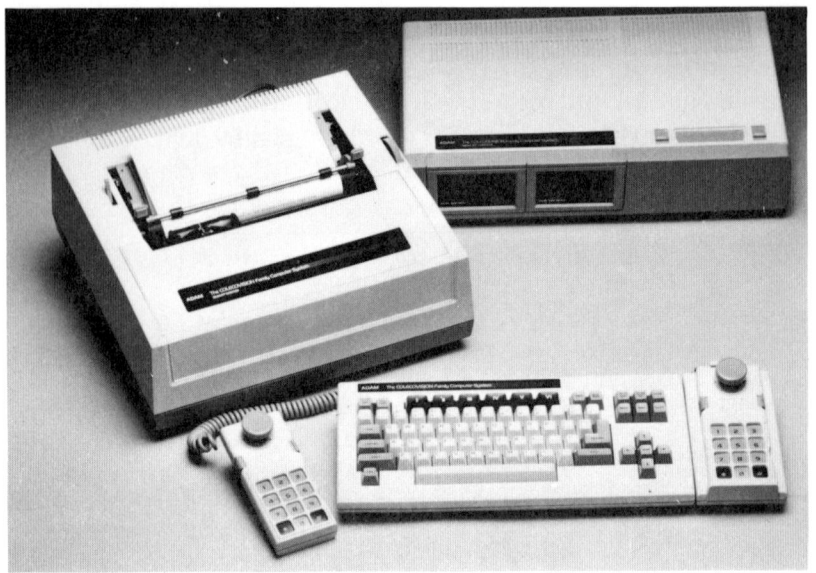

Price: $749
Screen size: (connects to TV) 68 chars x 36 lines
Screen color: color
Main operating system: CP/M
Processor: 8-bit Z80A
Standard memory: 80K
Disk drive type: cassette
Capacity of formatted disks: 256K
Software included: SmartWriter, SmartBASIC, Buck Rodgers' Planet of Zoom
Keyboard:
- detachable? yes
- number of keys: 75
- number of function keys: 15

Weight: 39 lbs.
Other: A 2 cps letter-quality printer is included.

Brand Name Buying Guide

Comments: *In the beginning, Coleco made video games, with superior graphics, and an adapter to run Atari games, and Coleco saw what it had done, and it was good.*

And then Coleco said, "Let us make a home computer system in our own image, and let it run Coleco games as well as contain all the features that will compete with Commodore and Atari." And then Coleco saw what it had done, and called it Adam.

The Adam will easily fill the needs of a "family computer." It is very easy to get acquainted with, and your kids will be using it in no time at all—if they can pry it away from you.

It comes with a full-size keyboard with six function keys, ten command keys, and two ways of moving the cursor: using the cursor arrow keys, or using one of two Coleco game controllers (included). The controllers have joysticks for games and a built-in numeric keypad.

The inclusion of a letter quality daisy wheel printer is unprecedented in the package price of a home computer system. The printer is *very* noisy and *very* slow, but adequate for those five-page school reports on George Washington. The printer can also be used directly with the keyboard as an electric typewriter (bypassing the word processing program), allowing you to type labels and envelopes.

Word processing is built right into the system. For home word processing, it can do a lot: store files, highlight text, set variable margins, number pages automatically, search and replace—even do superscript and subscript. It's modeled after dedicated word processors. Recently at a university, I overheard graduate students in a writing class considering an Adam for their dissertations. The Adam is not geared for heavy duty or professional use where long files are common. You will be disappointed if you try it. For home use, though, the Adam will do very well.

The Adam plugs into your color television set. It provides only 68 columns. As with all computers using TVs as screens, the characters are never sharp (especially when they're rainbow colored). As a consolation, Adam lets you adjust the background to colors that might please you.

PERSONAL COMPUTERS AND THE DISABLED

Like other "family" home computers, the audience for the Adam may eventually outgrow it; as youngsters become more sophisticated in their acquaintance with computers, the Adam may not be able to expand enough to meet their needs. But that's tomorrow. Today, this is a good buy.

These comments are based on the unit I used. It worked fine. The *Consumer Report* people, however, had problems with the ones they bought and according to *Time* magazine, quality defects have chilled sales and caused customers to return up to 30% of the computers. If this continues, I can't see the Adam being around much longer.

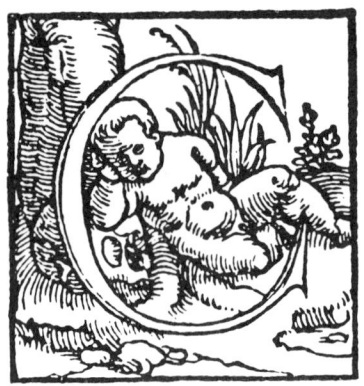 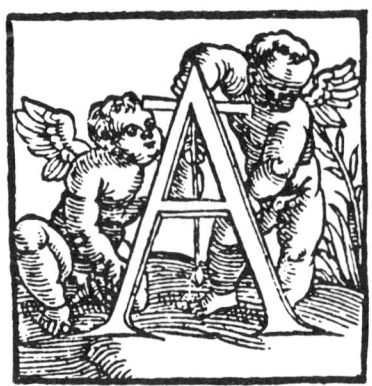

Brand Name Buying Guide

Commodore VIC 20

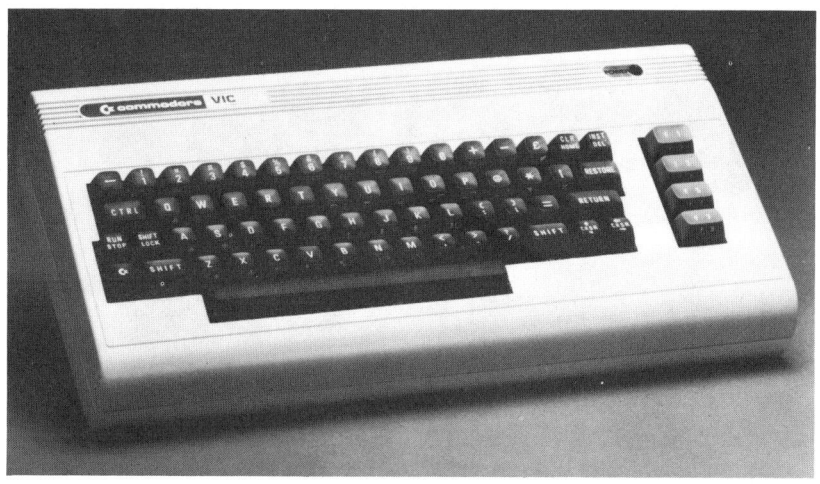

Price: $99 (no drives, no monitor)
Screen size: (connects to TV set) 23 chars x 22 lines
Screen color: color
Main operating system: Commodore OS
Processor: 8-bit 6502
Standard memory: 5K
Disk drive type: 5¼" can be added
Capacity of formatted disks: 170K
Software included: operating system
Keyboard:
- detachable? yes
- number of keys: 66
- number of function keys: 4

Weight: 10 lbs.

Comments: Commodore markets two good small personal computers, the VIC 20 and the Commodore 64. The VIC 20 is my choice in the under $200 range.

PERSONAL COMPUTERS AND THE DISABLED

Commodore 64

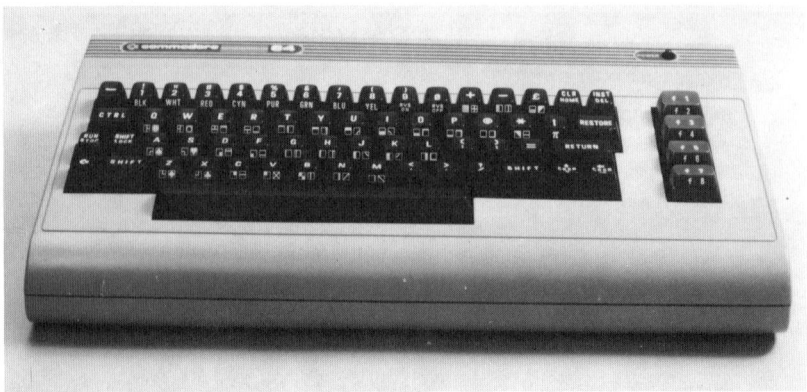

Price: $199 (no drives, no monitor)
Screen size: (connects to TV set) 40 chars x 25 lines
Screen color: color
Main operating system: Commodore OS
Processor: 8-bit 6510
Standard memory: 64K
Disk drive type: 5¼" (available at extra charge)
Capacity of formatted disks: 170K
Software included: operating system
Keyboard:
- detachable? yes
- number of keys: 66
- number of function keys: 4

Weight: 10 lbs.
Other: An all-in-one unit, called the Executive 64, has similar specifications, but comes with a 5" color monitor and one 170K disk drive, and weighs 28 lbs. Cost: $950.

Brand Name Buying Guide

Comments: The Commodore 64 is a very good hardware value (it seems to have almost every hardware feature of the Apple IIe at less than half the price). The Commodore 64 problem is one of software, a problem which extends, to a lesser extent, to the VIC 20. Neither computer should be considered for word processing or serious business computing. Time will tell how well-supported these Commodores will become. They are popular.

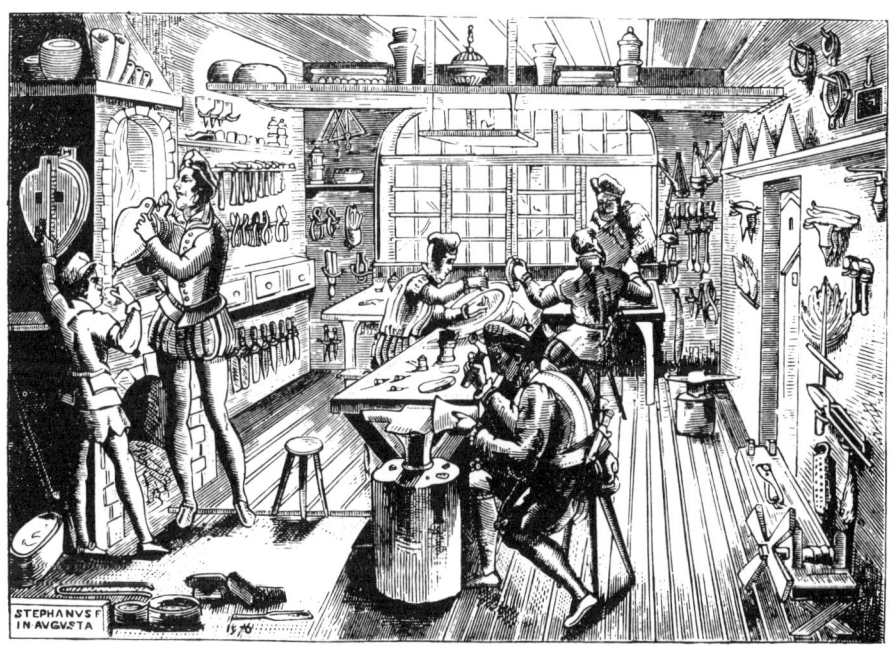

Main assembly room for the Commodore 64.

PERSONAL COMPUTERS AND THE DISABLED

IBM PCjr

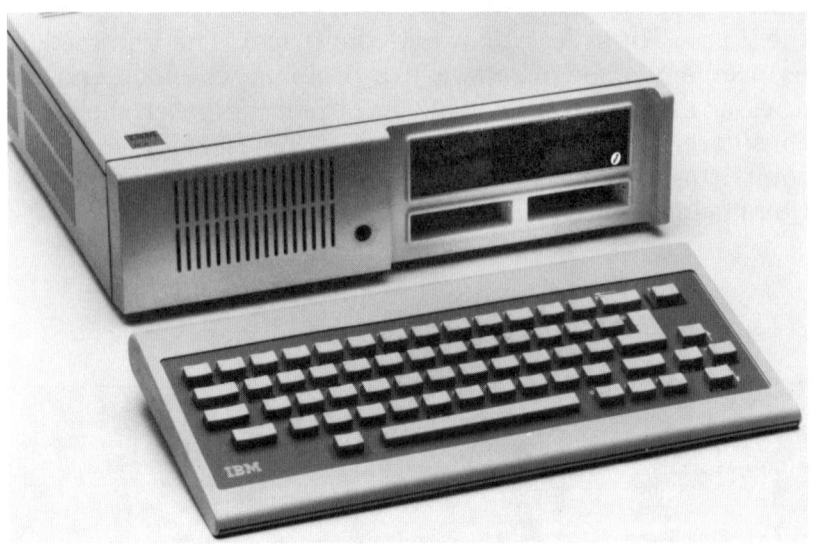

Price: $999 (one drive, no monitor)
Screen size: —
Screen color: —
Main operating system: MS-DOS
Processor: 16-bit 8088
Standard memory: 128K
Disk drive type: 5¼"
Capacity of formatted disks: 360K
Software included: none
Keyboard:
- detachable? yes
- number of keys: 61
- number of function keys: 0

Weight: 10 lbs.

Comments: Because IBM is IBM, all the software and peripheral manufacturers are figuring this is THE home computer, and they are going off and writing programs and making plug-in boards and, lo, with all that support, the PCjr *will* become THE home computer. It's a form of self-fulfilling prophecy. It will work. And no one other than IBM could pull it off.

Brand Name Buying Guide

The "Entry Model" comes with 64K of memory, two cartridge slots (for games programs, and whatever else the world dreams up), and a detachable keyboard.

The "Expanded Model," which the chart shows, has 128K of memory and a 360K disk drive. The idea behind the expanded memory and only one drive is this: The program is loaded into the memory and acts like an "A" drive. This disk drive stores the data people usually put in the "B" drive of a two-drive system. A bit more memory is cheaper than a second drive. For the home, it makes sense.

Offered accessories for the PCjr include a built-in modem ($199); a wonderful joystick ($40); a carrying case ($60—watch out Kaypro?); a cheap but terrible printer ($175); and an OK but expensive color printer ($1,999).

Both the Entry and Expanded Juniors are designed to use ordinary televisions for screen display (connector for TV: $30), although any number of houses will invest in the Ultimate PC Junior option: an IBM Color Monitor ("If you have to ask...")

The keyboard is something new. It looks like five rows of chicklets. No self-respecting middle-manager would want one on her desk. No secretary would want one on his desk. It has no numeric keypad. Obviously it's not made for business.

That aside, it's not bad to work with. I wouldn't want to write a novel on it, but a review or two would be no problem. In other words, for the kid's homework and the parent's letter to Abby, it'll do just fine. Also: unlike the PC Senior, the shift key is in the right place.

And the keyboard is THE most detachable around. There's not even a wire connecting it to the computer. It's all done by infra-red rays, just like science fiction movies (and remote control units for television). Like the ads for cordless phones, mom can take her computing by the pool without any wires getting in the way.

For a home computer—not a full-time business or word processing computer—the PCjr is definitely one to look at.

PERSONAL COMPUTERS AND THE DISABLED

Sinclair QL

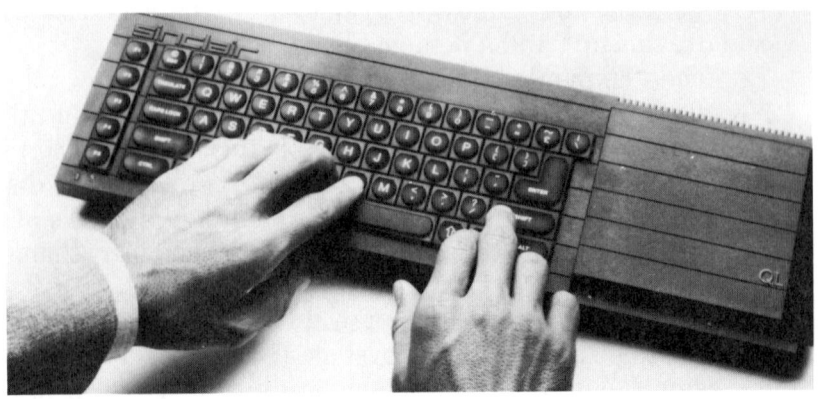

Price: $499 (announced price, without monitor)
Screen size: —
Screen color: —
Main operating system: Sinclair OS
Processor: 16/32-bit MC68000
Standard memory: 128K
Disk drive type: Sinclair wafer tapes
Capacity of formatted disks: 100K
Software included: word processing, spreadsheet, data base manager, and graphics
Keyboard:
- detachable? yes
- number of keys: 65
- number of function keys: 5

Weight: 3 lbs. (without monitor)

Brand Name Buying Guide

Comments: A short while ago, you may have heard of the Timex/Sinclair computers. You could get them just about everywhere: drug stores, department stores, hardware stores—almost every popular place where people congregated except computer stores. The price was right: $49. They became as popular as watches, and over 3 million were sold. And yet Timex/Sinclair exists no longer. The Timex people found Clive Sinclair's computers had an insufficient profit margin, so they dropped the line. Sinclair, an entrepreneur and Englander from the same cloth as Sir Freddie Laker, still ticks. He is offering his new computer by direct mail.

My mail box has not brought me one yet—at publication time, the Sinclair QLs had not yet reached these shores.

I like the idea of a powerful, portable computer using the same processor as the Apple Macintosh for under $700 (including a monitor). Today, however, success requires top-notch marketing, and with Timex out, that leaves a large dent in Sinclair's schemes. Even if the Sinclair QL becomes a wholloping success in Europe, without a distributor here, it means nothing. I seriously doubt many people would consider buying a computer by mail. Most folks fear computers as is, and buying one by mail would never be considered. To be popular, the computer must be in stores. Perhaps Sears or J.C. Penney will put their imprint on it. (I can see the ads now: A woman with a bouffant hairdo lovingly holds "The new Lady Kenmore Computer....")

PERSONAL COMPUTERS AND THE DISABLED

Lap-Sized Computers

Epson Geneva/PX-8

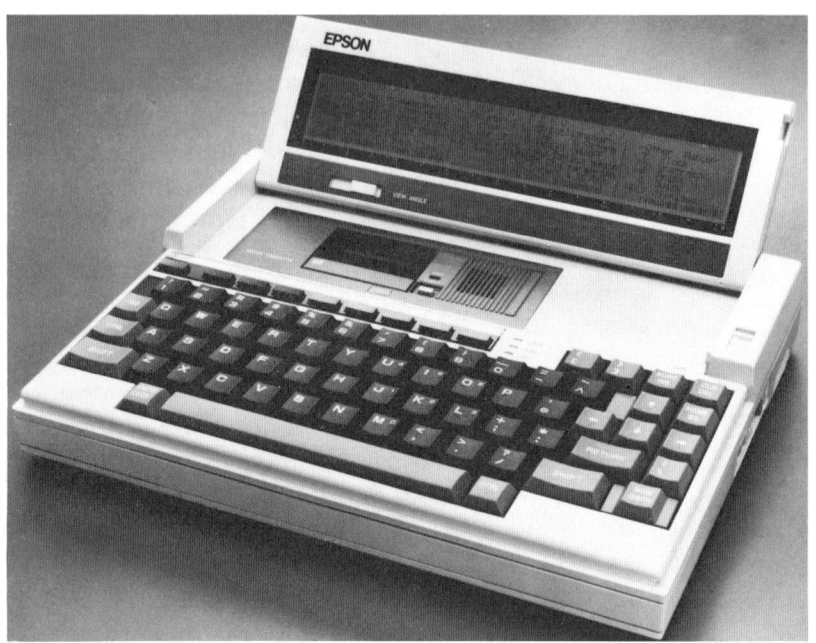

Price: $995
Screen size: 80 characters x 8 lines
Screen color: LCD
Main operating system: CP/M
Processor: 8-bit
Standard memory: 64K
Disk drive type: microcassette
Capacity of formatted disks: 128K per microcassette
Software included: WordStar, spreadsheet program, electronic appointment book
Keyboard:
- detachable? —
- number of keys: 68
- number of function keys: 5

Weight: 4 lbs.

Brand Name Buying Guide

Comments: The name of this little wonder is, technically, the PX-8 and, generically, the Geneva. (There are any number of Japanese-Swiss jokes that come to mind, all of which I will spare you.)

The point that needs to be stressed in portable computers, I feel, is the weight. I once lugged a nine-pound portable around with me on a 20-city tour and sent it packing after the first five cities. Nine pounds is a lot of pounds. Four pounds is five pounds less than nine pounds, and four pounds is not bad. Maybe the Geneva will make it to city ten on the next tour.

The batteries last 50 hours on a charge. The programs are contained in interchangable memory units (the machine can hold two at a time), allowing all 64K to be used for data files.

Those familiar with WordStar will love this machine. It's a writer's portable paradise, or, as Hemingway might say, a moveable feast. Some of the WordStar features are missing from this condensed version—most notably the display of available documents in the no-file menu—but most of WordStar survives. The spreadsheet is more than adequate, and the scheduling program beeps to remind you of impending appointments.

There is no built-in modem. I'll take the microcassettes over a built-in modem, but that's my preference. An external modem is available, as is an external 3½ inch disk drive, and a light-weight dot matrix printer.

The Geneva is a CP/M-based computer. Data files can be transferred to an MS-DOS computer, but the Geneva will not run MS-DOS programs. Epson seems to be the last of the CP/M innovators.

The price/weight/performance combination of the Epson Geneva PX-8 make it my current choice in the battle of the portables, but the battle rages on.

PERSONAL COMPUTERS AND THE DISABLED

Hewlett-Packard HP-110

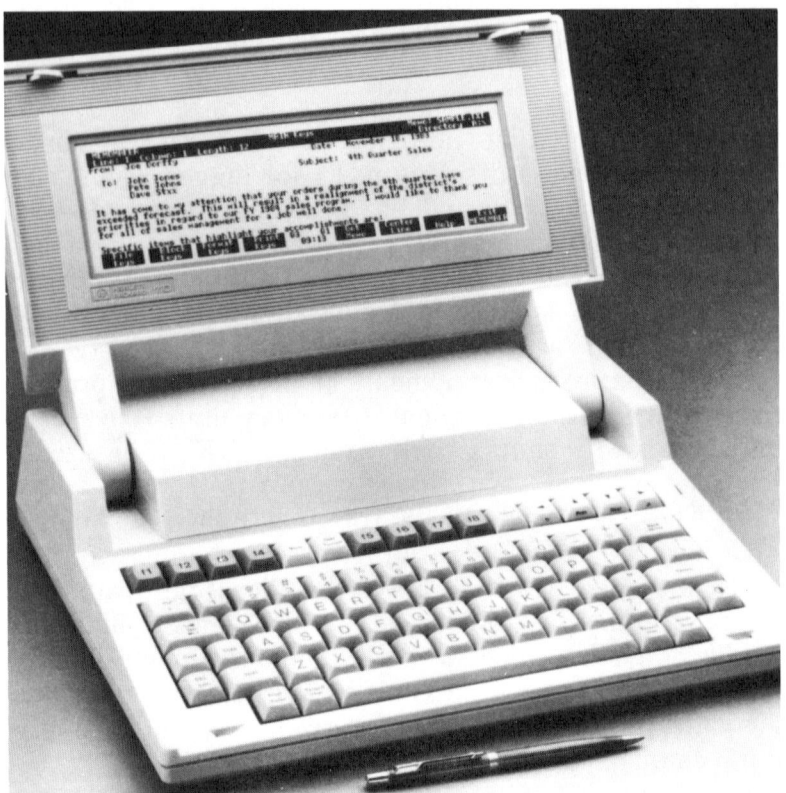

Price: $2,995
Screen size: 80 characters x 16 lines
Screen color: LCD
Main operating system: MS-DOS
Processor: 16-bit 8086
Standard memory: 272K
Disk drive type: external 5¼" drive optional ($800)
Capacity of formatted disks: 360K
Software included: MS-DOS, Lotus 123, MemoMaker
Keyboard:
- detachable? —
- number of keys: 76
- number of function keys: 8

Weight: 8.5 lbs.

Comments: The HP-110 is designed to be an exceptionally portable full-function computer, and in that regard, it does remarkably well. You type your work into the memory, and when the machine is off, the memory remains on (using very little battery power), retaining the software and your material. When you return to the office, you can connect the HP-110 to an HP-150, an IBM computer or IBM-compatible, and download or swap information. You can even use the other machine's disk drives.

Because the HP-110 uses standard MS-DOS programs, you can run anything you could on a desk-top computer. I used WordStar, and WordStar had all the same capabilities it does in a large machine.

The HP-110 has a 80 character by 16 line liquid crystal display screen. While this is still eight lines short of the standard 24 lines, it is large enough for word processing or spreadsheets.

The computer uses CMOS RAM memory, a new type of memory which takes only a small amount of electricity to keep everything in RAM. The unit has 272K of RAM for ones work. The HP-110 comes with Lotus 123 and a simple word processor called MemoMaker. These programs are in ROM, so they take none of the RAM memory storage space.

The HP-110 comes with a built-in modem, allowing you to dump its memory into the office computer while you're on the road. The price is a bit high for a portable, but so is the technology.

PERSONAL COMPUTERS AND THE DISABLED

Radio Shack Model 100

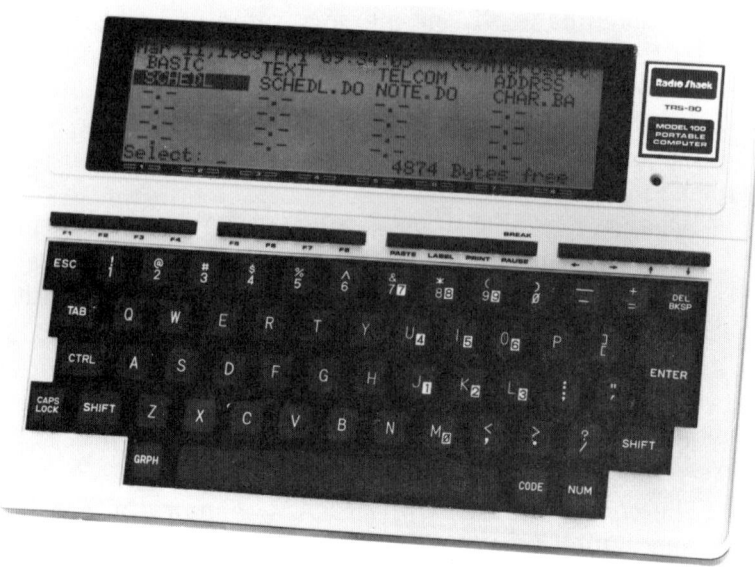

Price: $799
Screen size: 40 characters x 8 lines
Screen color: LCD
Main operating system: MS-BASIC
Processor: 8-bit 80C85 CMOS
Standard memory: 8K
Disk drive type: microcassette
Capacity of formatted disks: n/a
Software included: Text, Schedule, Addressbook, Telecommunications, and BASIC
Keyboard:
- detachable? —
- number of keys: 56
- number of function keys: 0

Weight: 4 lbs.
Other: Built-in auto-dial modem. A version with 24K of memory costs $999; 32K, $1,119. Also available is a disk-video interface for $799. It comes with one disk drive and a connection for a monitor or TV.

Brand Name Buying Guide

Comments: You wouldn't want to run your office with a Model 100, but you might want to throw one in your briefcase.

The 100 is light, compact, and highly portable. It's smaller than a three-ring binder. The full-sized keyboard has a great feel. The screen is liquid crystal (like a pocket calculator) and displays eight 40-character lines.

It's not what you'd call a word processor—more a word recorder. Whatever you store in the 100 can be transferred to another computer for later editing and revision. Documents are stored in a kind of RAM that never forgets. After files are transferred to another medium, or printed, the memory can be erased for future computing.

One of the most interesting features is a built-in modem. By plugging in a modular telephone cord, one can contact data banks or the computer in the office.

It operates on batteries that can be plugged in. The hardware design (Japanese) is first-rate, and the software (from Microsoft) is as easy to learn and use as one can ask.

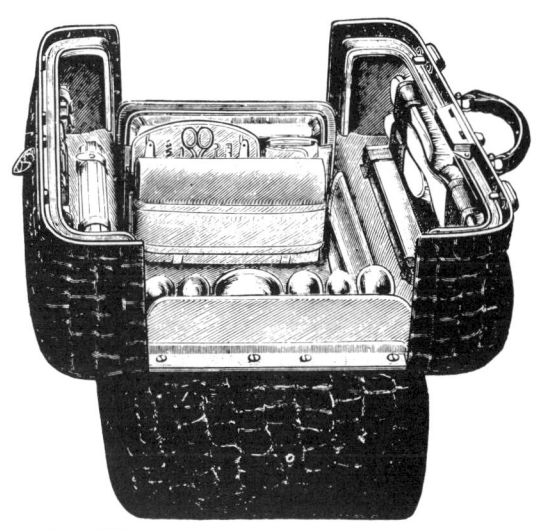

And there's still room for the Radio Shack Model 100.

PERSONAL COMPUTERS AND THE DISABLED

Teleram T-3000

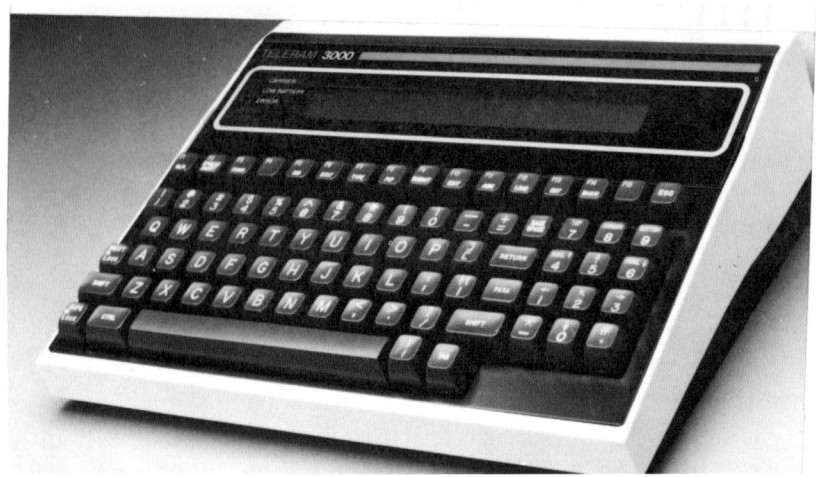

Price: $1,795
Screen size: 80 characters x 4 lines
Screen color: LCD
Main operating system: CP/M
Processor: 8-bit Z80L
Standard memory: 64K
Disk drive type: Bubble memory
Capacity of formatted disks: 128K (256K version for $2,095)
Software included: CP/M, utilities, TeleText, TeleTalk
Keyboard:
- detachable? —
- number of keys: 83
- number of function keys: 28

Weight: 9 lbs.
Other: There's a T-4000, with an 8 line screen and 128K for $1,995; and a T-5000, 16 lines and 128K, for $2,495.

Comments: The Teleram portables are the most portable full-function computers available. They come with 128K of bubble memory, and another 128K can be added. Bubble memory is user-changeable, like RAM, but it keeps the information indefinitely, even when the power is turned off, like ROM. It's a great combination of the two.

The Teleram is rugged, and full 80-character lines are displayed. Many reporters for newspapers use this computer in the field.

While one would not want to write a magnum opus on a four (or sixteen) line screen, it's possible.

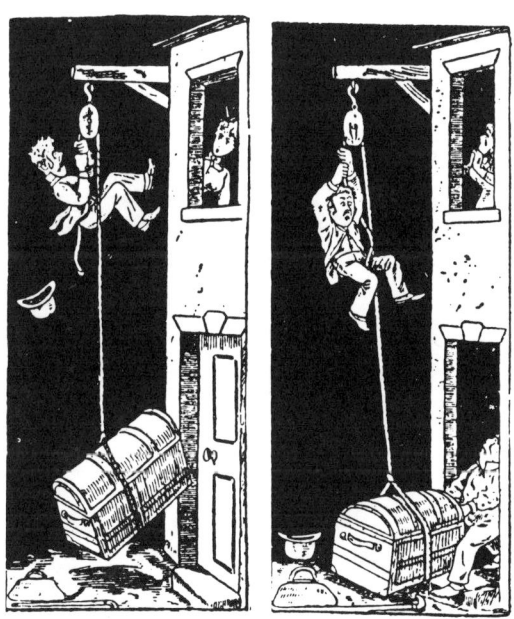

Giving her a Teleram wouldn't be this difficult.

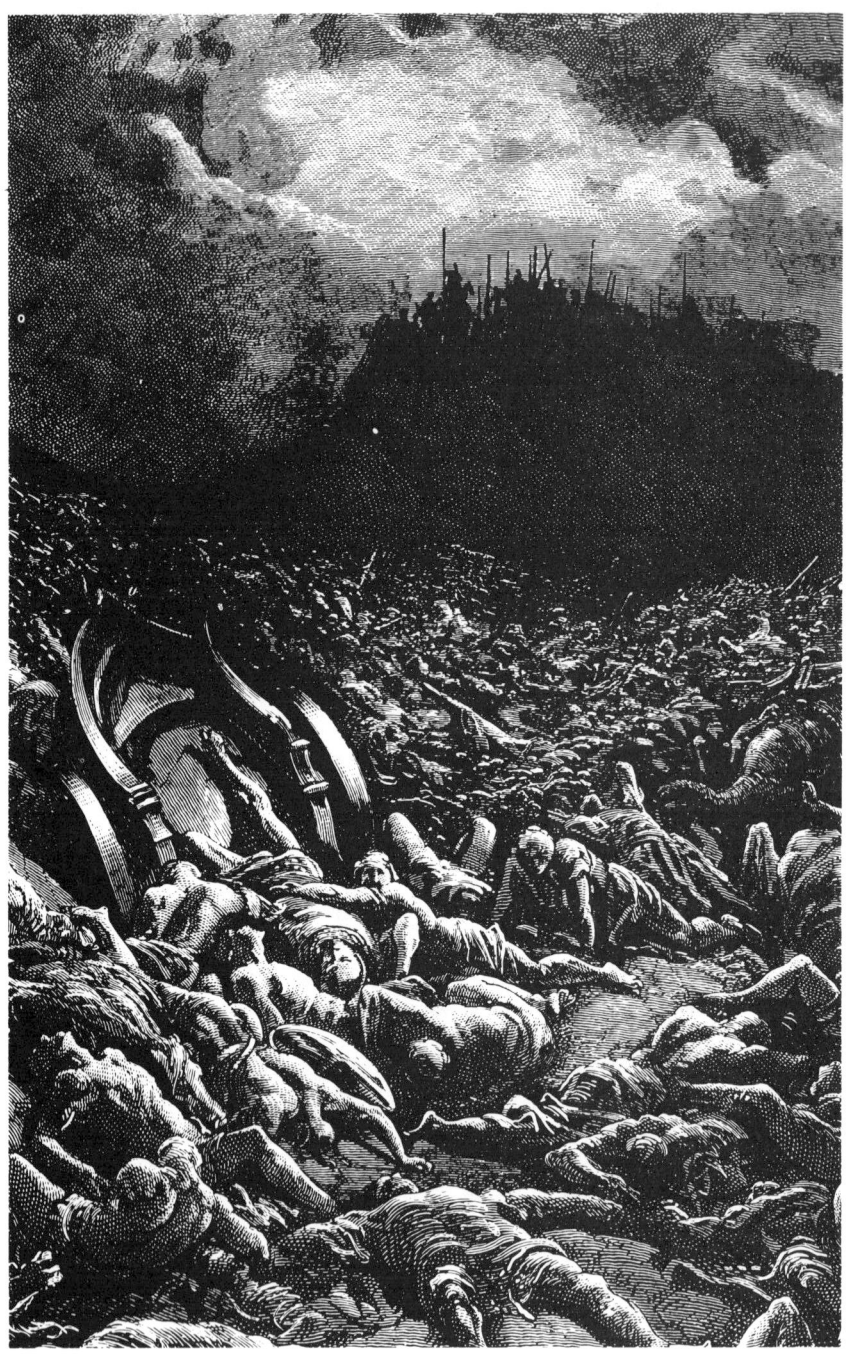

IBM and IBM-Compatible Computers

The Battle Is Over

The battle is won. It's all over but the fighting. IBM is the new standard for personal computers, and is likely to remain so for years to come.

The great Punic Wars over a standard have been raging for some time. Early battles pitted the Commodore PET against Radio Shack against Apple. Radio Shack and Apple won. Then CP/M came along and slugged it out in a tag-team match with the two winners. No clear winners in that battle. It smoldered on for years.

Someone put CP/M on the Apple, which formed an unlikely alliance, and indicated that both had won. But Radio Shack said, "We have 6,000 stores. We already won. Why don't you both go away?" The battle continued.

Noting that the real losers of this battle were really consumers, the UN (computer writers) joined in, and declared a sort-of truce: CP/M was the winner for business and word processing; Apple was the winner for games and overall expandability; Radio Shack won for being everywhere at once (there was hardly a small town anywhere that didn't have a Radio Shack store).

The treaty was never ratified by The Big Three, but at least consumers knew where to shop for what.

Then came IBM. It offered *a whole new standard*. Just what the computer world needed (he said, with no small degree of irony). But, in little more than a year, IBM won, and imposed this fourth standard as THE standard for personal computers.

The signs of an IBM victory are everywhere. Not only is almost every significant new piece of software being introduced first on the IBM, but almost every piece of software that's ever been written is being rewritten for the IBM.

Plug-in board, peripheral, and printer manufacturers are outdoing themselves in not only quantity, but also quality of product.

And, most telling of all, other computer manufacturers are turning out computers that are advertised proudly as "IBM Compatible."

PERSONAL COMPUTERS AND THE DISABLED

In the meantime, it's not certain what IBM will do about all this. Will they follow the Apple route and sue everyone in sight? Or will IBM take a smarter tack, and license its ROM to interested parties? This would lead to true compatibility, choice in the marketplace, and the final seal on the fact that the IBM Standard is the new standard for personal computers.

Does this mean you should only buy an IBM if you want to do word processing? No, not at all.

If the *only* thing you want to do with your computer is word processing, then get the screen and keyboard you like best. The fact that thousands of educational, business, and recreational programs are available for the IBM will not matter. You'll be busily writing, oblivious to the hubbub, in love with whatever computer you've bought.

I do not use an IBM. I do not plan to use an IBM in the near future. I hate the clicky sound of the keyboard. The replacement keyboard from Keytronics is quieter, but not much better. I'm more than happy writing on the first computer I bought almost three years ago. Sitting unused a few feet away is a PC IBM sent me for evaluation (along with a half-dozen other expensive "state of the art" computers from other manufacturers). I like what I've got. I'm used to it. We're comfortable together.

If, however, you plan to do things *other* than word processing on your computer, then the IBM deserves a serious look. A *very* serious look.

Also, a new generation of word processing programs is being written for the IBM. We found *scores* of them while researching *Word Processing on the IBM*. (A special edition of *The Word Processing Book* for potential IBMers.) If you think you'll want to upgrade programs, and will want to have each state-of-the-art word processing program as it comes along, then the IBM would be the best bet.

If money is an issue (and when is money not an issue?), a Morrow or a Kaypro make excellent word processing computers for about half the cost of an IBM. Don't feel you have to mortgage the ranch just to get an IBM. There's lots of word processing power to be had for lots less.

Brand Name Buying Guide

I don't want you to feel locked into an IBM. This essay is not my endorsement of IBM as *the* personal computer, it is simply my best guess as to what the future standards of personal computing will be.

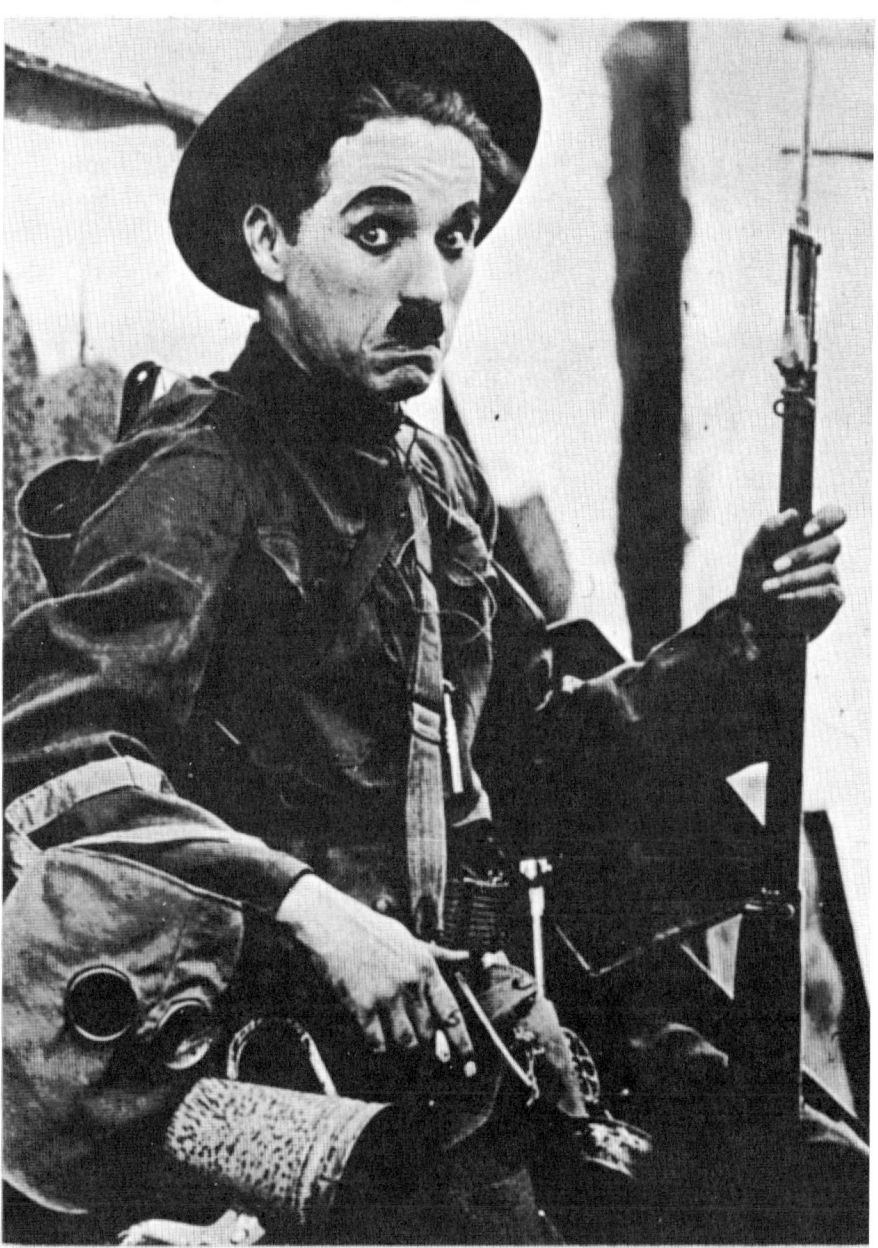

PERSONAL COMPUTERS AND THE DISABLED

The Myth of IBM Compatibility

Now that IBM has become the standard in personal computers, a lot of manufacturers are claiming their machines are "IBM Compatible."

Last year, the key selling phrase around computerdom was "User Friendly." One software manufacturer confessed, "Creating User Friendly software generally meant pulling out last year's brochures and stamping 'User Friendly' on them."

This year's selling phrase is "IBM Compatible." Whatever the minimum a manufacturer can do to call its computer IBM Compatible, it'll do.

Generally, the minimum is getting the computer to "read IBM disks." This means that if you put an IBM disk into the drive of Computer X, Computer X will be able to read information from the disk. This does not mean Computer X will be able to write information onto that disk, or that it will run a program on that disk, or that it will even be able to display the information on its video screen.

In other words, if all a computer will do is "read IBM disks," what the manufacturer is really saying is, "Please buy our computer. We're desperate."

The next level of IBM Compatibility is adding MS-DOS, which is the same disk operating system as IBM-DOS. This makes the two machines "DOS Compatible," or, as Brand Y likes to say, "IBM and us share the same operating system." This means, theoretically, that Brand Y can read IBM files and write IBM files, but not necessarily run a program written for the IBM.

Running programs written for the IBM requires that a computer, Brand Z, say, copy a good deal of the internal architecture of the IBM. Most of this is public domain, or available for license from other manufacturers. (IBM purchases a good deal of its internal workings from other manufacturers, and so could Brand Z.) If Brand Z set out to clone the IBM, it could do a pretty good job—until it got to ROM.

Brand Name Buying Guide

IBM holds a copyright on the information inside its ROM chip, and any computer manufacturer that copies an IBM copyright does so at its own peril. So IBM cloners copy a little here and a little there, but thus far no one has been courageous or dumb enough (choose your own adjective) to copy the whole thing.

Without *all* the information in IBM's ROM, a computer cannot be considered fully IBM Compatible. This is because you never know when a programmer will use some of that information in a program. If a program, written for the IBM, says, "Go into ROM and get this information," on an IBM the information will be there. On a clone, it might or it might not. If not, the program will not run.

Therefore, there is no true IBM Compatibility. Some of the programs, written for the IBM, will not run on the clones. How many? Well, the clone manufacturers usually try the top 100 IBM programs and see how many will run. They then announce "most" will run (if it's more than 51), or they say 90%, or 95%, or whatever number ran.

These high percentages are nice, but what if the program you want to run is in that incompatible 5%? And what if the program you want to run was never tried? And what if the program you want to run hasn't been written yet, but when it's written it runs just fine on the IBM, but not on Brand Z?

I report this not because I like it, only because it's true. There are too many people who paid thousands of dollars on an "IBM Compatible" computer, only to find that it's not really. As of now, if you want 100% IBM Compatible, you'll have to buy an IBM.

This is unfortunate, because many of the Compatibles are better computers than the IBM, especially when it comes to keyboards. Some of the clones have discreet cursor movement keys, and properly placed shift keys, and a quiet keyboard. Others have better color graphics, or cost less, or are portable. For your needs, maybe 90% compatibility is enough—but make that choice with your eyes open.

PERSONAL COMPUTERS AND THE DISABLED

How did IBM do it? How did it come in with a new standard and wipe out the three competing standards (Apple, Radio Shack and CP/M)?

Well, first, there are those initials, I. B. and M. No small amount of mystical power is contained in those three letters. IBM is so closely linked to computers that some are predicting "IBM" will lose its Trade Mark status and, like escalator or aspirin, become a generic term for all computers. When IBM introduced a personal computer, people LISTENED.

But IBM didn't rely on its name alone to launch the product. They came up with a brilliant ad campaign featuring Charlie Chaplin. (IBM even got permission from the Chaplin estate.) These ads were not only well done, they were everywhere—still are, in fact. Now, every time someone sees Charlie Chaplin, they think of IBM.

Then there was the computer itself. Apple was good at processing games and graphics, but poor at processing letters and numbers. Radio Shack and CP/M machines were good at processing letters and numbers, but poor at graphics and games. The IBM could do both, and do both well. Finally, somebody could do word processing AND play flashy full-color graphic games on the same computer.

Beyond that, it used a 16-bit processor, which could access more memory than Apple, Radio Shack or CP/M. This extra memory opened the door to powerful new programs. Just as people bought Apples just to run VisiCalc back in 1978, people were buying IBMs just to run 123 or Context MBA in 1983.

And, in what was probably the most brilliant (and noncharacteristic) move of all, IBM *invited* other manufacturers to make peripherals to plug into and add onto an IBM. In the past, the quickest way to void an IBM warranty was to use non-IBM products on an IBM machine. (Years ago, an IBM repairman said I shouldn't be using any ribbons but IBM ribbons on my Selectric. "Is it OK if I use non-IBM paper?" I asked.)

But with the PC, IBM made usually-secret schematics available to all, and announced to the world, "We've got five expansion slots, boys. Come on and plug on in!" And they did.

And they still are. There hasn't been this much action since the Chicken Ranch closed.

Meanwhile, Apple is talking about letting the Lisa run programs written for the IBM, and Radio Shack now offers an IBM-compatible computer. Does it sound like there's a winner to you?

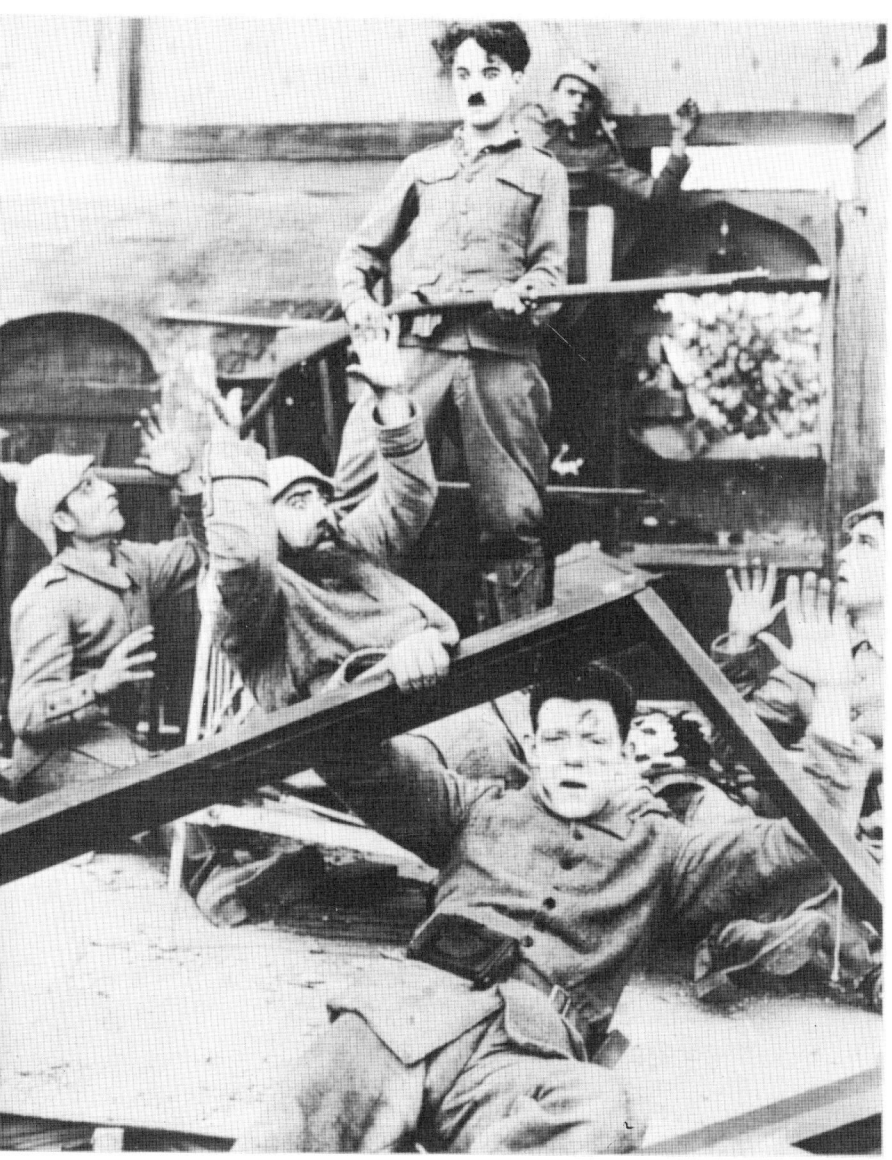

PERSONAL COMPUTERS AND THE DISABLED

IBM PC

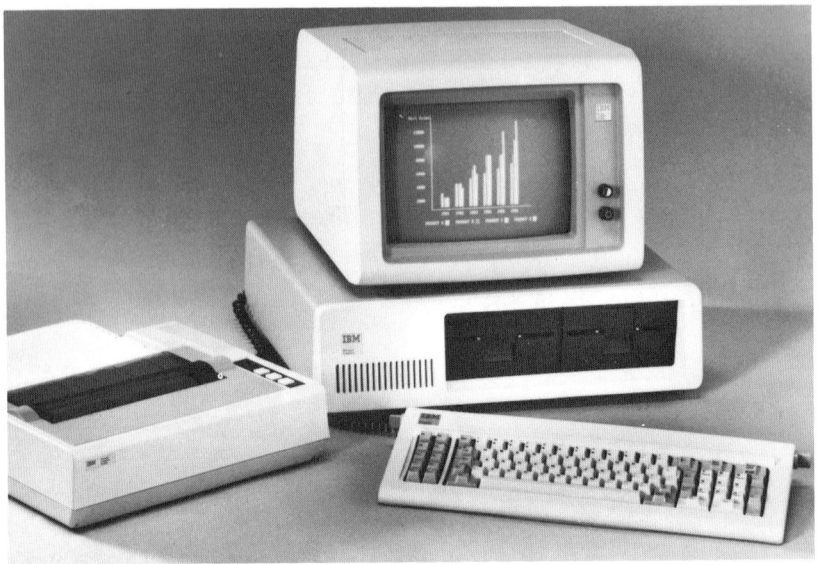

Price: $2,945
Screen size: 12"
Screen color: green (color available)
Main operating system: MS-DOS
Processor: 16-bit 8088
Standard memory: 256K
Disk drive type: 5¼"
Capacity of formatted disks: 340K
Software included: "Exploring the IBM Personal Computer"
Keyboard:
- detachable? yes
- number of keys: 83
- number of function keys: 10

Weight: 51 lbs.
Other: A hard-disk version of the PC is known as the IBM XT. The XT replaces one of the disk drives with a 10-megabyte hard disk. The price is $4,820.

Brand Name Buying Guide

Comments: IBM has built, quite simply, a great personal computer.

Rather than patch together a small computer using a little from this IBM machine and a little from that IBM machine (which they could easily have done), IBM assembled a group of engineers, designers, programmers and, yes, a few personal computer lovers, sent them all to Boca Raton, Florida, of all places, and gave them a mission: Design and build the IBM Personal Computer.

They researched everything available in the field of small computers, investigated what was new, came up with a few things of their own, massaged the information together, made a few hard decisions, and created the IBM Personal Computer.

There was fear in the land of small computers that IBM would swallow up the personal computer market. Instead, IBM has created a whole new industry. The industry is called "Supporting the IBM Computer, Inc." Everyone's getting a franchise: peripheral manufacturers, software vendors, mail-order houses, retailers—it's the IBM Personal Computer Bandwagon and everybody's welcome to climb on board.

The basic Personal Computer is rather bare. You get the CPU with two disk drives and a keyboard. The monitor and a board to run the monitor are extra (which I figured into the price on the chart to the left). Also extra is any software—including the operating system MS-DOS—and any internal memory beyond 64K.

IBM's monochrome screen is sharp, rock steady, and nice to look at. A color monitor can be added for full-color graphics, although the color screen is not as sharp as the monochrome one. If your primary interest is word processing, go with monochrome.

The keyboard has a firm and sure touch. It's detachable, although heavier than most detachable keyboards. As good as it is, the keyboard has a few drawbacks. First, the shift key is the size of a regular key, which is far smaller than shift keys usually are. This is compounded by the fact that just below the shift key is a larger key labelled ALT (for Alternate). It's very easy to

PERSONAL COMPUTERS AND THE DISABLED

hit the ALT, or any other key surrounding the shift key, because of the shift key's smaller size. Further, the shift key is not located directly next to the Z key, as is the standard, so one often hits the backslash key (which is located next to the Z) rather than the shift key. (Why the inventors of the industry standard "Selectric Keyboard" didn't follow their own standard is beyond me.)

Second, the cursor movement keys are located on the numeric keypad. This means that you can either use the cursor keys *or* you can use the numeric keypad. A special shift key must be depressed to change from one mode to the other. This could prove inconvenient in typing financial statements or documents containing many numbers.

There is an audible and tactile "click" each time a key is depressed on the keyboard. It is subtle, rather like turning a small electrical switch on and off (which is, in fact, exactly what you're doing). This is not the same as the electronic beep or boop one finds as an option on some computers. This click is built into the keys. There's no way to switch it off or get rid of it. Some people are delighted with this verification of a keystroke that can be heard and felt. Others, like myself, find it irritating. You'll have to decide if you fall into the "some" camp or "others" camp.

If there are any standards within the personal computer industry, the IBM PC comes the closest. I was sorry to see Apple develop an entirely new operating system for the Macintosh instead of working with MS-DOS. Imagine every electrical appliance you bought having a different size plug. Having standards brings down prices—and can only benefit consumers.

Brand Name Buying Guide

IBM Portable Personal Computer

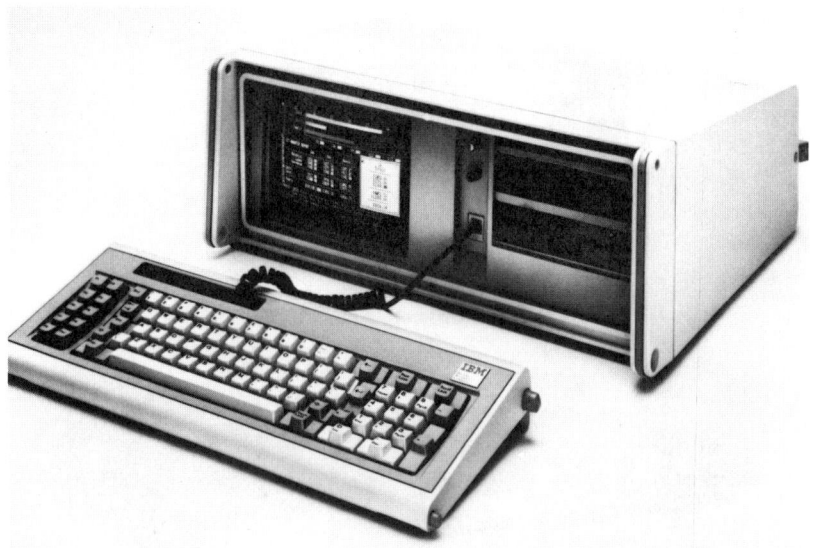

Price: $3,020 ($2,595 with one disk drive)
Screen size: 9"
Screen color: green
Main operating system: MS-DOS 2.1 (same as the PCjr)
Processor: 16-bit 8088
Standard memory: 256K
Disk drive type: 5¼"
Capacity of formatted disks: 360K
Software included: none
Keyboard:
- detachable? yes
- number of keys: 83
- number of function keys: 10

Weight: 30 lbs. (one drive)
Other: Watch out other portables!

PERSONAL COMPUTERS AND THE DISABLED

Columbia MPC

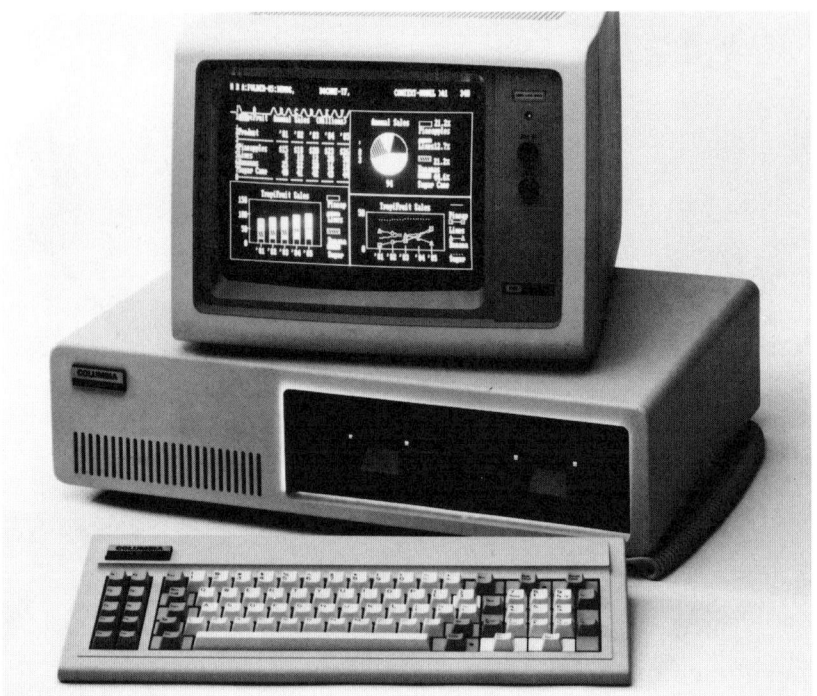

Price: $3,620
Screen size: 12"
Screen color: green
Main operating system: MS-DOS or CP/M-86
Processor: 16-bit 8088
Standard memory: 128K
Disk drive type: 5¼"
Capacity of formatted disks: 320K
Software included: Perfect Writer, Perfect Calc, Perfect Speller, Perfect Filer, Fast Graphs, Home Accountant Plus, MS-DOS, CP/M-86, communications, tutoring software, and games.
Keyboard:
- detachable? yes
- number of keys: 82
- number of function keys: 10

Weight: 46 lbs.

Brand Name Buying Guide

Comments: Columbia promotes its computers as running the 350 most popular IBM programs. The magazine *Future Computing* has similar findings and rates the machine as "quite IBM compatible," along with the Seequa Chameleon and the Compaq. I find the machine well-built, as sturdy as an IBM, employing similar expansion slots. It also has the same keyboard design flaws: the print key hangs below the vertical return key, and the alternate key lies under the shift key. At least Columbia took the clicky noises out of the keys.

Columbia's price reflects a recent increase, at the same time in which the IBM PC price went down. An IBM PC is cheaper than a Columbia, although you get a load of software with the Columbia and nothing with the IBM PC. Also, Columbia has 64K more standard memory than the IBM PC.

Columbia also has a portable computer, the VP, with similar specs as the MPC, the same software, and a nine-inch screen. Like the Seequa Chameleon, the VP runs both CP/M-80 and MS-DOS programs. Its price is $2,995.

Compaq

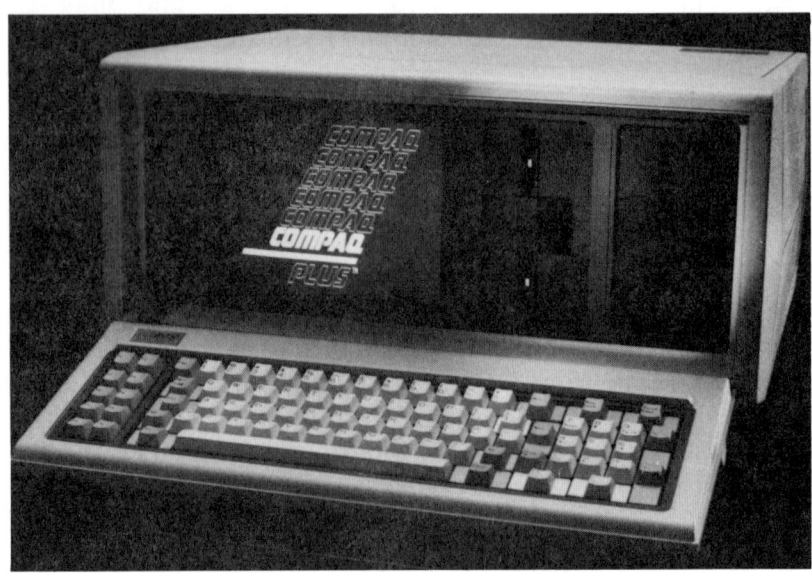

Price: $3,090
Screen size: 9"
Screen color: green
Main operating system: MS-DOS
Processor: 16-bit 8088
Standard memory: 128K
Disk drive type: 5¼"
Capacity of formatted disks: 320K
Software included: MS-DOS, M-BASIC
Keyboard:
- detachable? yes
- number of keys: 83
- number of function keys: 10

Weight: 31 lbs.
Other: A 10 MB hard-disk version, the Compaq Plus, costs $4,995.

Brand Name Buying Guide

Comments: The Compaq computer runs everything we've tried on it. A nearby computer store said they have not found an IBM program which does not work on it. Like the Columbia, Compaq has a keyboard patterned after IBM's, but has taken out the click. The keyboard has a good, solid feel. The nine-inch screen is quite sharp, though a little less so when running graphics. It is a dependable machine.

The price is just under IBM's portable, so why buy a Compaq? Well, Compaq has a few small advantages over IBM. First, Compaq's monitor is dual mode, meaning it can do both graphics and text (without needing to buy an extra graphics board). Then there's expandability—Compaq has three full-size expansion slots to IBM's one (though IBM has an additional four half-size slots.) The Compaq also comes with a parallel port for a printer. For what it's worth, Compaq has been in the portable computer market a few years more than IBM.

The Compaq Plus is a portable hard-disk model, and sells for nearly the same price as an IBM-XT (desk model).

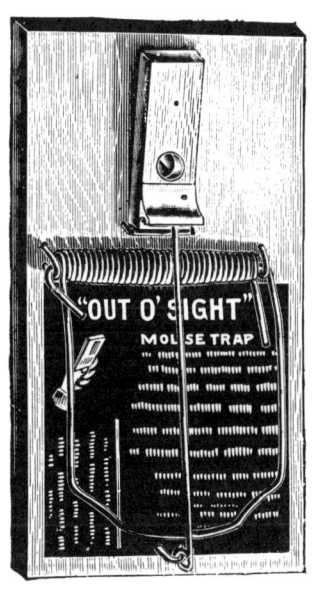

DEC Rainbow 100

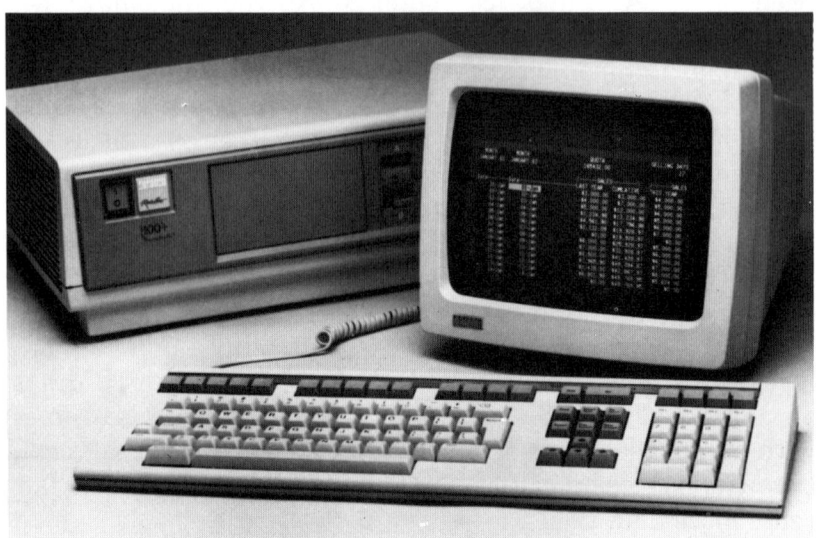

Price: $3,495
Screen size: 12"
Screen color: amber, green or white
Main Operating System: CP/M-86/80 and MS-DOS
Processor: 8-bit Z80A and 16-bit 8088
Standard memory: 128K
Disk drive type: 5¼"
Capacity of formatted disks: 400K
Software included: CP/M-86/80 and MS-DOS
Keyboard:
- detachable? yes
- number of keys: 103
- number of function keys: 36

Weight: 48 lbs.
Other: Also available is the Rainbow 100 Plus, a 10 MB hard-disk machine with two floppy drives. It costs $6,295.

Comments: In 1960, Digital Equipment Corporation (DEC) set the computing world on its ear by introducing a small computer at an outrageously low cost. Computing power had come within the reach of thousands more. The cost? A mere $120,000.

Today Digital's Rainbow computer puts computing within the reach of many thousands—perhaps millions—more.

First of all, the Rainbow keyboard is one of my favorites—the other two being the Epson and TeleVideo keyboards. (The *my* in "my favorite" is important—you'll no doubt have your favorites, too.) It has a numeric keypad with add, subtract, multiply and divide symbols, separate cursor movement keys, and more special function keys than one is ever likely to need.

The shift key, like the IBM's, is not directly next to the "Z." It is, however, larger than any other keys around it, and adjusting to the new placement is not a major hardship.

The Rainbow is an 8 *and* 16-bit machine. It will run CP/M, CP/M-86, and MS-DOS software. The memory is expandable to 896K.

A plug-in card permits high resolution graphics, and the addition of a color monitor with the card permits graphics in full color.

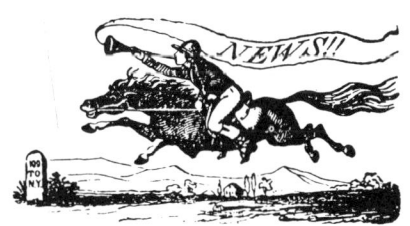

PERSONAL COMPUTERS AND THE DISABLED

Eagle PC PLUS-2

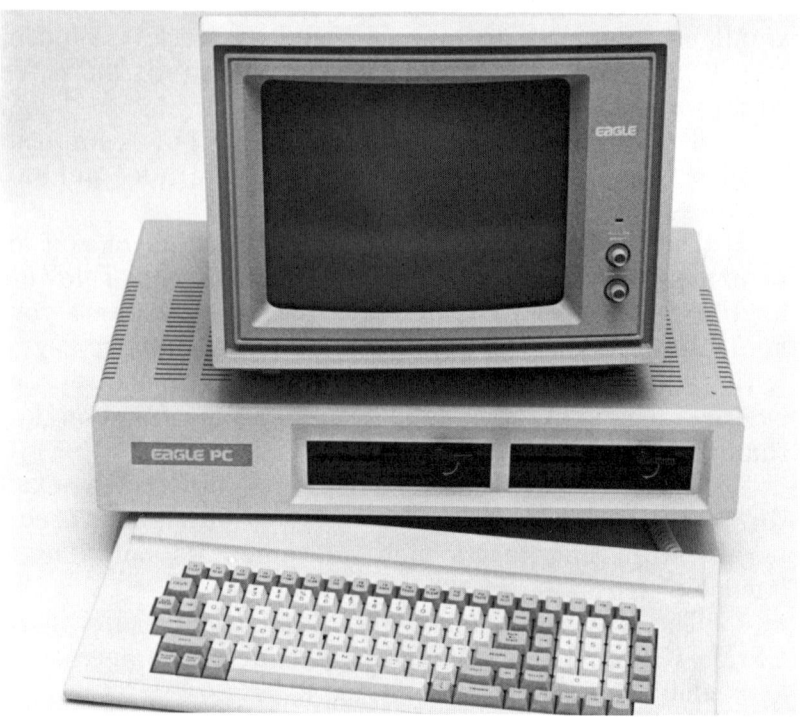

Price: $3,119
Screen size: 12"
Screen color: green (color available)
Main operating system: MS-DOS, CP/M-86
Processor: 16-bit 8088
Standard memory: 128K
Disk drive type: 5¼"
Capacity of formatted disks: 360K
Software included: MS-DOS, BASICA
Keyboard:
- detachable? yes
- number of keys: 84
- number of function keys: 10

Weight: 32 lbs.
Other: Eagle also offers the Eagle PC Turbo XL for $5,619. "Turbo" comes from its ability to operate at a speed of 8 megahertz, which would be apparent in complicated

math and business processing. 256K of memory comes standard on the Turbo, as does a 10 MB hard disk, one floppy 360K drive, a 16-bit 8086 processor, and MS-DOS and BASICA.

Comments: The Eagle PC PLUS is Eagle Computer's challenge to the IBM PC. It is virtually the same size as the IBM, and it looks a lot like the IBM. With the Eagle PC PLUS, you get a very sharp 12-inch monitor (a color monitor is also available), a 16-bit processor, and a 128K of memory. The keyboard is detachable and fits neatly inside a built-in compartment underneath the disk drives (a nice feature when desktop space is limited). And those disk drives are so *quiet!* I hate the drone of IBM's fan. Eagle took the fan out.

The Eagle PC PLUS has, in other words, all that you'd expect from a personal computer that must compete with IBM. This is one of the best IBM clones. Unfortunately, the Eagle's list price makes it as expensive as the IBM. For about the same money, a lot of people are going to choose the "real" IBM. Too bad, because the Eagle PC PLUS is in many ways a better computer.

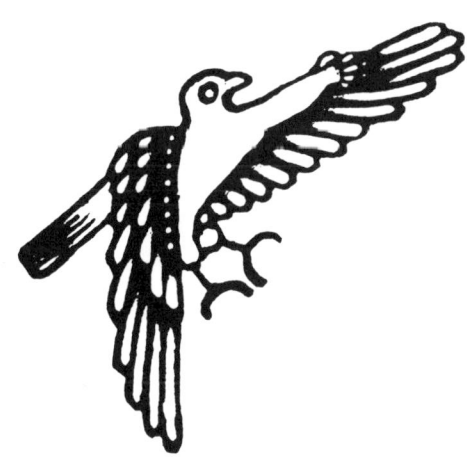

Eagle PC Spirit 2

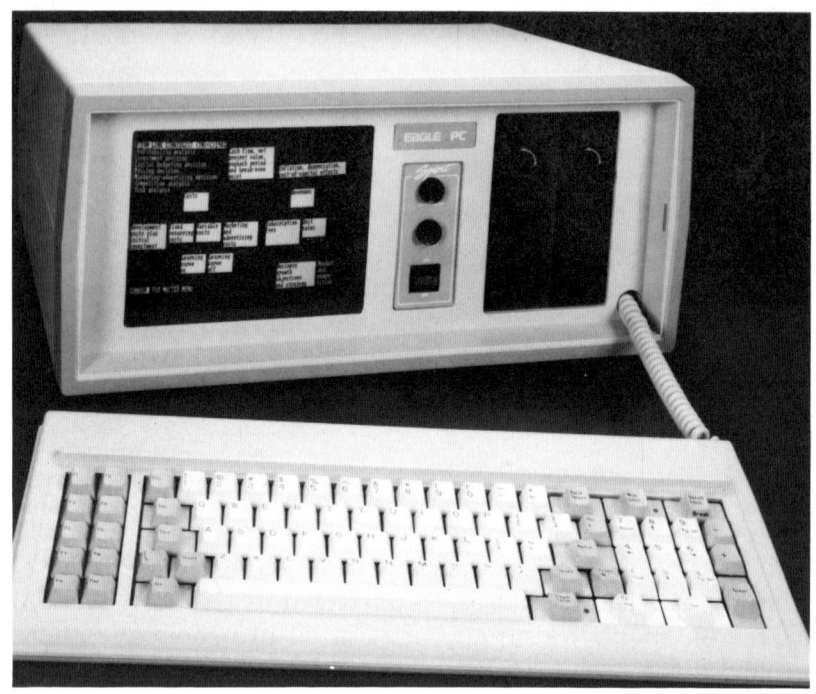

Price: $2,995
Screen size: 9"
Screen color: green
Main operating system: MS-DOS
Processor: 16-bit 8088
Standard memory: 128K
Disk drive type: 5¼"
Capacity of formatted disks: 360K
Software included: MS-DOS, BASICA
Keyboard:
- detachable? yes
- number of keys: 84
- number of function keys: 10

Weight: 28 lbs.

Comments: By discontinuing its CP/M-based IIE model, Eagle now sells only MS-DOS machines. In early 1984, Eagle had a run-in with IBM over the Basic Input Output System (BIOS). IBM charged that Eagle's BIOS infringed on IBM's copyright. Eagle had to stop shipping their computers for a short while until they could replace the BIOS chips. The new chips do not infringe on IBM's copyright, and still Eagle's computers remain highly compatible.

The Spirit is a portable computer and looks and operates quite similarly to other MS-DOS portables. One small but worthy difference becomes apparent quickly, however. Eagle placed the on/off switch on the front. No more groping at the back pushing knobs and sockets until you find the switch. This is so logical, why haven't switches been on the front before? Maybe Eagle will start a trend.

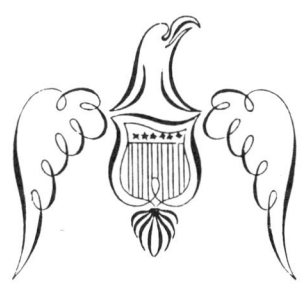

PERSONAL COMPUTERS AND THE DISABLED

Hewlett-Packard HP-150

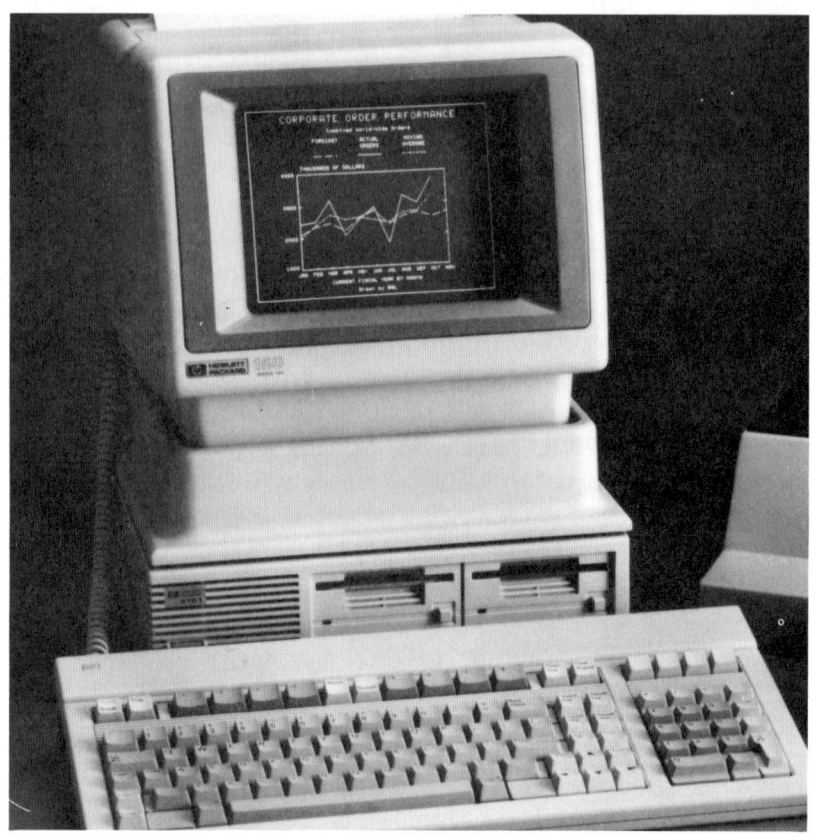

Price: $3,995
Screen size: 9"
Screen color: green
Main operating system: MS-DOS
Processor: 16-bit 8088
Standard memory: 256K
Disk drive type: 3½"
Capacity of formatted disks: 264K
Software included: MS-DOS
Keyboard:
- detachable? yes
- number of keys: 94
- number of function keys: 8

Weight: 27 lbs.

Other: It has a touch-screen, meaning you can put your finger on the screen to implement some commands. I have never found touching the keyboard difficult, but for the keyboard-phobic, this may be a good invention.

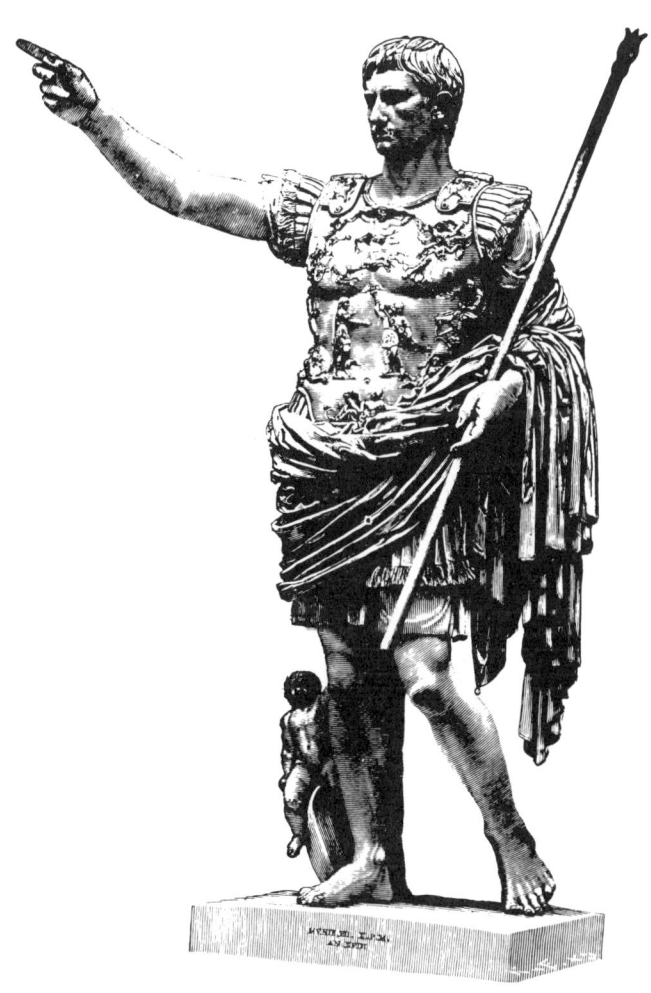

Roman Centurion waiting for the invention of the touch screen.

PERSONAL COMPUTERS AND THE DISABLED

NEC APC

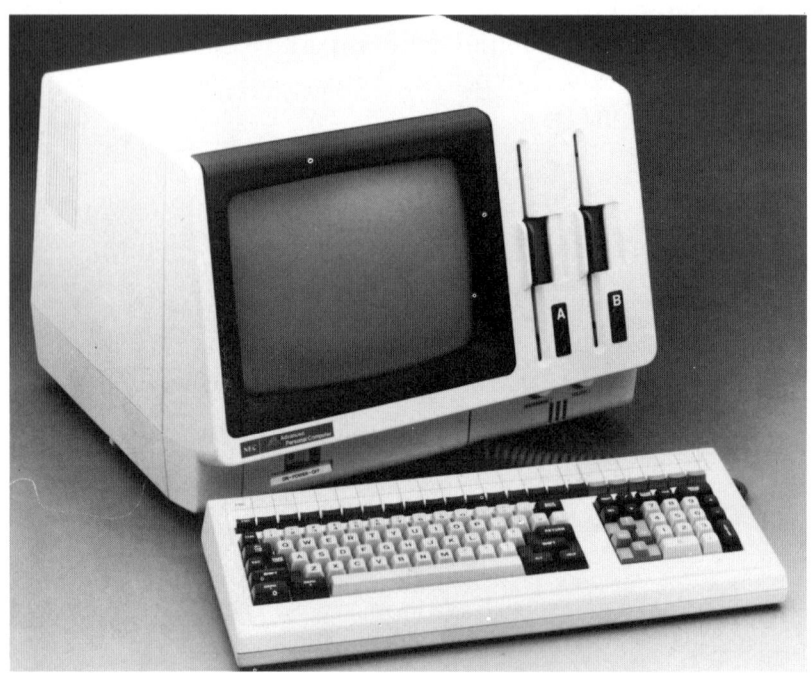

Price: $3,448
Screen size: 12"
Screen color: green
Main operating system: MS-DOS
Processor: 16-bit 8086
Standard memory: 128K
Disk drive type: 8"
Capacity of formatted disks: 1,000K
Software included: MS-DOS, WordStar, Multiplan, dBase II
  Keyboard:
  - detachable? yes
  - number of keys: 108
  - number of function keys: 22
Weight: 40 lbs.

Comments: NEC, the people who make the finest letter quality printer around, make several small computers marketed by at least two different divisions.

The one that seems to be getting the most attention is the APC, which stands for Advanced Personal Computer. As fond as I am of the NEC printers, I must admit I am not very fond of the APC.

The keyboard is solid, and the screen display is clear—but then so is the keyboard and screen display of computers costing half as much. The drives are 8-inch, and only 8-inch. They are also the noisiest drives I have heard on a small computer.

The strength of this machine seems to be when a color monitor is added. If sharp, full-color graphics are required by your business, you should certainly have a look at the APC. (And if you're someone who *must* do word processing in color, this, as well as the Texas Instruments Professional Computer, are the machines to investigate. The color monitor on the APC adds about $1,000 to the price.)

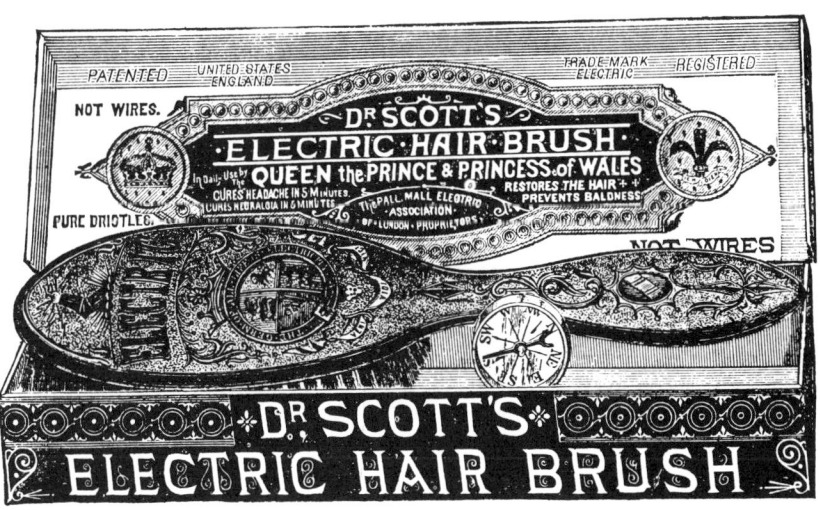

PERSONAL COMPUTERS AND THE DISABLED

NorthStar Dimension

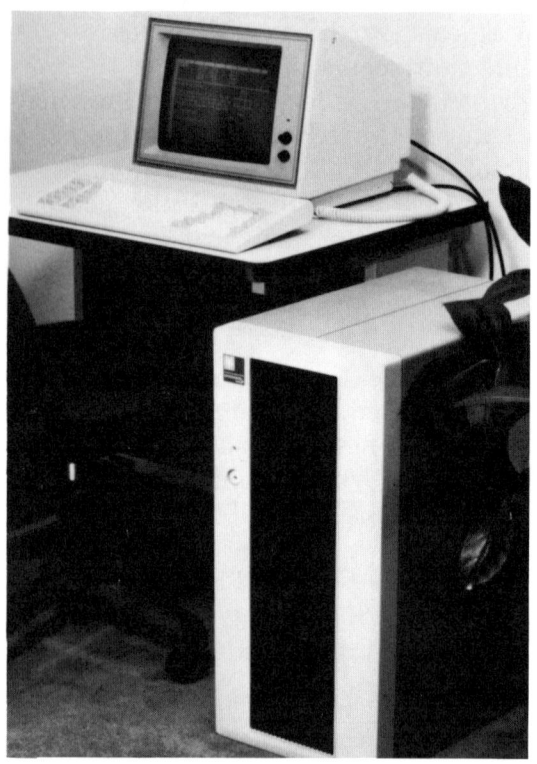

Price: $7,000 per module, $1,500 per station
Screen size: 12"
Screen color: green
Main operating system: MS-DOS
Processor: 16-bit 8088
Standard memory: 256K
Disk drive type: one 5¼" floppy drive and one 15-megabyte hard disk
Capacity of formatted disks: 360K/13 megabytes
Software included: none
Keyboard:
- detachable? yes
- number of keys: 83
- number of function keys: 10

Weight: n/a
Other: A 30 megabyte hard disk is available.

Brand Name Buying Guide

Comments: The Dimension is a multi-user-oriented system. You don't run out and buy just one Dimension as you might any other computer. You buy a module, and a module contains one CPU, two work stations, and appropriate cable and hardware to tie it all together. Additional work stations are extra for a fraction of what additional full computers might be. Up to 12 work stations can be connected to each CPU.

NorthStar felt that coming out with a basic IBM-compatible computer was asking for a great deal of competition. Competition, indeed, is brisk. NorthStar, therefore, asked itself what could it offer that no one else has offered? A multi-user network, the company decided, and so it developed the best, most economical system it could.

The system is not the same as networking individual computers together. With the Dimension system, each user has a dumb terminal—that is, a keyboard and monitor (no disk drives or CPU), just as on the Big Machines of The Corporations. This system uses easily available MS-DOS programs. Dimension, therefore, is suited for small-to-medium-sized companies.

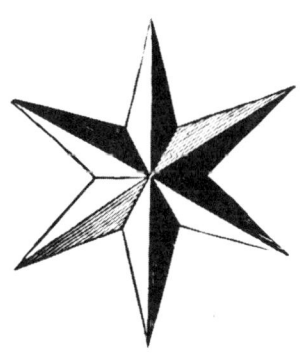

PERSONAL COMPUTERS AND THE DISABLED

Otrona 2001

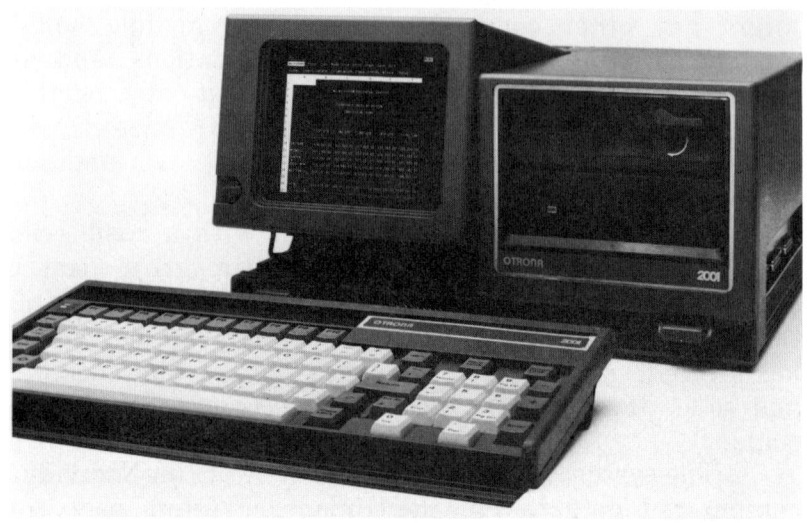

Price: $2,995
Screen size: 7"
Screen color: amber
Main operating system: MS-DOS
Processor: 16-bit 8088
Standard memory: 256K
Disk drive type: 5¼"
Capacity of formatted disks: 360K
Software included: MS-DOS
Keyboard:
- detachable? yes
- number of keys: 84
- number of function keys: 10

Weight: 19 lbs.
Other: a composite/RGB external monitor interface comes standard. Options include a 10 MB hard disk, additional memory up to 640K, Z80B processor and CP/M operating system, 8087 math coprocessor; and an internal modem.

Brand Name Buying Guide

Comments: Otrona has abandoned ship with its CP/M-based Attache computer. In Attache's place is the 2001, an advanced, well-designed MS-DOS system. While the Attache was always a bit overpriced, the 2001 enters the market with a price dead-on with its competitors. Not a carbon-copy design of many other portable computers, the 2001 has a screen which tilts up while the disk drive remains flat. I can see no practical advantage to this, but it does give it a unique appearance.

Also newly designed is the keyboard. Though it closely resembles IBM's keyboard, a few modifications make it superior: the return key is full size and moved closer to the quotation-mark key; the foreign-accent key has been moved up to a better position on the third row; and the left-hand shift key sits properly next to the Z key.

The screen-size, as you may have noted, is only seven inches. The characters produced are extremely sharp, but seven inches is too small for long-periods of use—at least for my eyes. If you truly need to carry your computer around, though, the small screen may be more than compensated by the machine's lightness. It's a full ten pounds lighter than most other full- function portable MS-DOS machines. Otrona offers a twelve-inch monitor, which attaches in seconds, to make the 2001 a desktop computer. This, naturally, adds to the price.

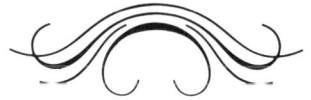

PERSONAL COMPUTERS AND THE DISABLED

Radio Shack Model 2000

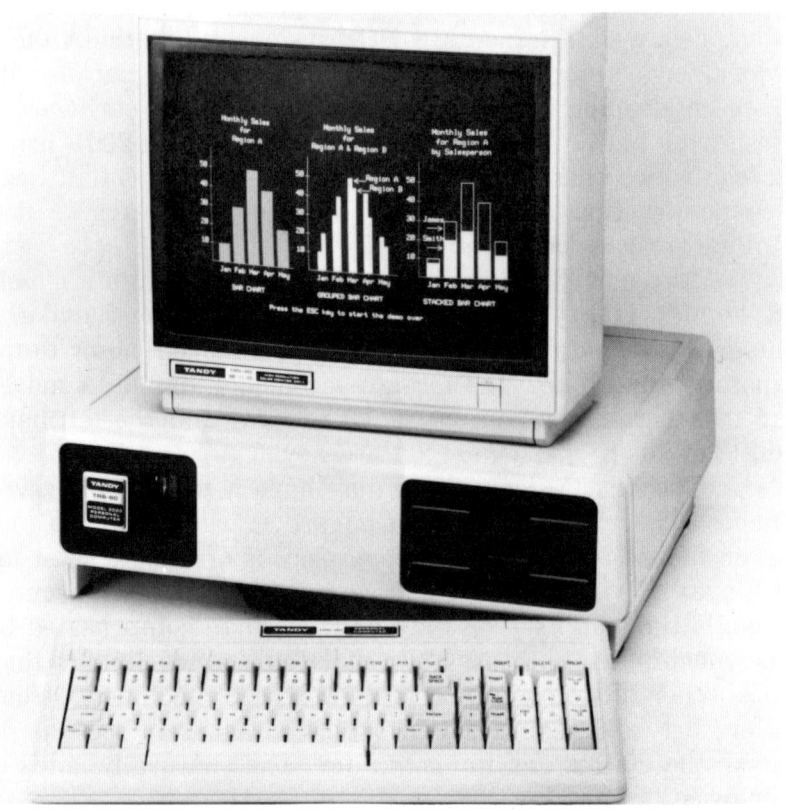

Price: $2,999
Screen size: 12"
Screen color: green (color available)
Main operating system: MS-DOS
Processor: 16-bit 80186
Standard memory: 128K
Disk drive type: 5¼"
Capacity of formatted disks: 720K
Software included: MS-DOS
Keyboard:
- detachable? yes
- number of keys: 90
- number of function keys: 12

Weight: n/a

Brand Name Buying Guide

Comments: Take note Apple: Big, behemoth Radio Shack has accepted the market trends—they came out with an MS-DOS machine. And at a reasonable price.

There are some great features here: a standard 128K of memory, a wholloping 720K of formatted disk space in each drive, and a keyboard not wedded to the IBM concept. Radio Shack's keyboard, detachable, has a full-size return key and shift keys. The cursor keys, in a diamond pattern, are separate—not part of the numeric keypad. The keys click, however, and if you're the type who doesn't like the click verification, you cannot turn it off. A mouse is optional for those who like the creatures.

The screen resolution, in both monochrome or color, is extremely sharp. The unit comes in a pleasing white styling, and inside, there are four expansion slots.

Who would have ever guessed....

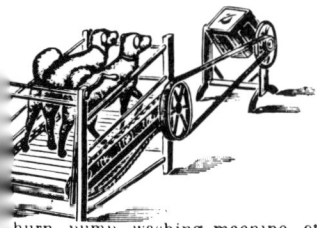

Lamb's Adjustable Animal Powers.

56830 This power is built to be operated by two dogs, sheep or goats, and will furnish sufficient power to run a "Safety" separator, corn sheller, fan mill, sawing machine, churn, pump, washing machine, etc. Balance wheel is banded for 2½ and 3 inch belt; weight, crated, 180 pounds. Price............$23.00

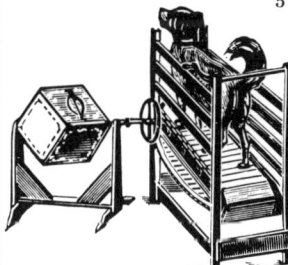

First Prize Dog Power.

53831 This power can be operated by a dog, goat or sheep; yields 25 per cent. more power from a given weight of animal than any other, and with adjustable bridge to regulate the required power and motion, a 30 pound animal will do the churning; if you keep a dog make him "work his passage." The power can be connected to any churn sold by us. Price............$15.00

PERSONAL COMPUTERS AND THE DISABLED

Seequa Chameleon Plus

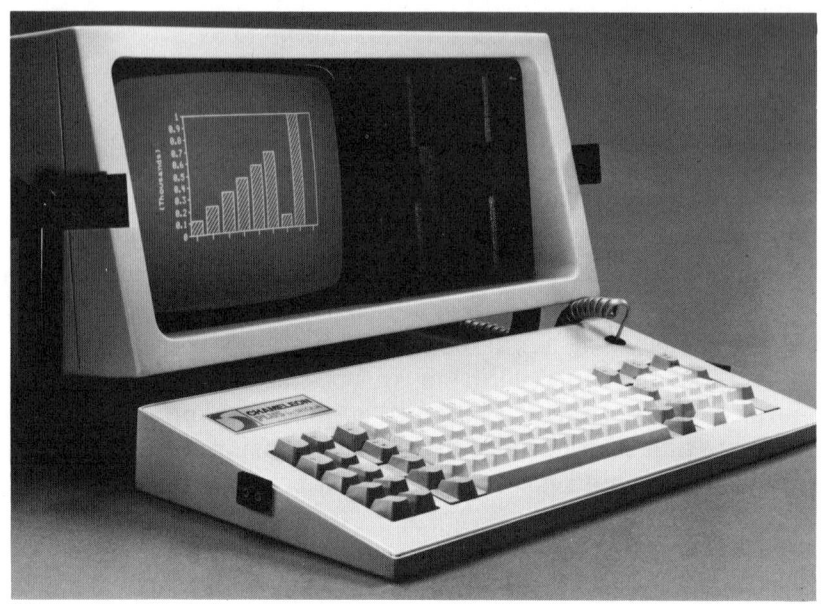

Price: $2,695
Screen size: 9"
Screen color: green
Main operating system: MS-DOS
Processor: 16-bit 8088 and 8-bit Z80A
Standard memory: 256K
Disk drive type: 5¼"
Capacity of formatted disks: 320K
Software Included: MS-DOS, Perfect Writer, Perfect Speller, Perfect Calc, M-BASIC 86, GW-BASIC, Condor-1, C-TERM, WordStar, SuperCalc 3
Keyboard:
- detachable? yes
- number of keys: 83
- number of function keys: 10

Weight: 28 lbs.
Other: CP/M software optional

Comments: The Seequa Chameleon is an MS-DOS computer touted as one of the more IBM-compatible machines on the market. With the IBM Portable Personal Computer

Brand Name Buying Guide

heading to market, all portable computers will have heavy competition. The basic Chameleon, with 128K and two 160K drives for $1,995 may fare well simply because of price. The Chameleon Plus, however, is priced only slightly less than the IBM, so people may forgo it, despite the fact that the Chameleon has two drives to IBM's one, and much software to IBM's no software.

The Chameleon's designers did a fine job on the outside. It is stylish looking with white metal casing. A standard 256K memory enables this machine to use the more powerful MS-DOS programs, such as Lotus 123 and Samna Word. Overall, it is a good value.

There are, however, a few flaws to be aware of. On the particular unit we tested, the outside was so prone to static shock that any unfortunate static contact with the Chameleon would make the screen and the program disappear and the keyboard LED's light up. I called Seequa with that information, and they said I must have an early model, one that did not have the static module. Whatever the module is, make sure the one you look at has it, and make sure the module works. I would only have to take two steps on carpeting and touch the keyboard to lose everything.

The other thing is that the 9-inch screen is not fully used. When you turn up the monitor brightness, you can see there is a healthy margin on all edges of the screen, particularly on the right-hand side. Because less area is used, the letters are smaller. This would not be so bad if the letters weren't squished and on the fuzzy side. It's like watching the credits of a Cinemascope movie on a TV set. This isn't to say letters and numbers aren't readable, but it does take more effort than on other screens.

On the positive side, the Seequa not only runs MS-DOS but 8-bit CP/M. If you want to use both types of software, this is the machine to look at. If you just need MS-DOS, its price still can't be beat.

PERSONAL COMPUTERS AND THE DISABLED

TeleVideo Tele-PC

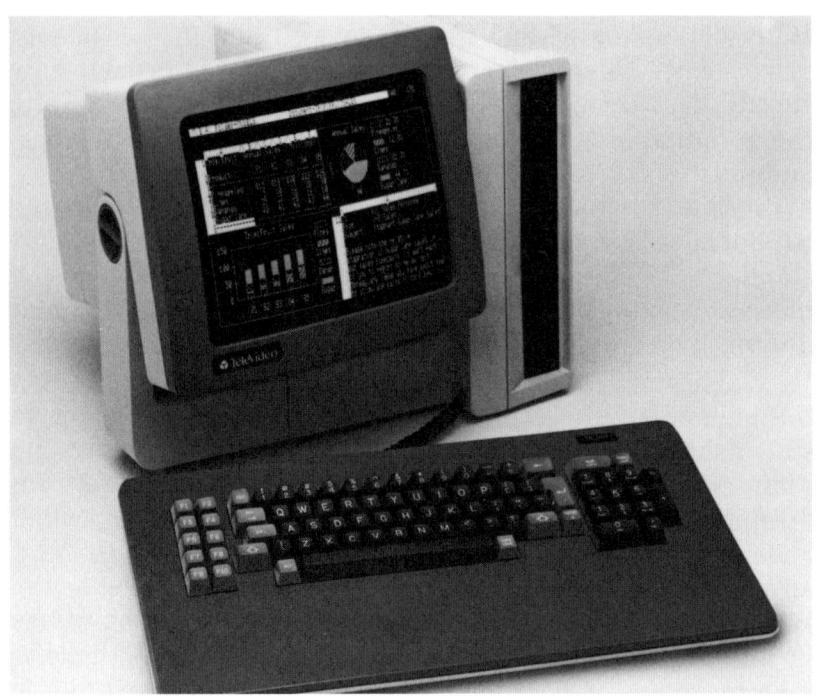

Price: $2,995
Screen size: 14"
Screen color: green
Main operating system: MS-DOS, TeleDOS
Processor: 16-bit 8088
Standard memory: 128K
Disk drive type: 5¼"
Capacity of formatted disks: 360K
Software included: TeleDOS, MS-BASIC
Keyboard:
- detachable? yes
- number of keys: 83
- number of function keys: 10

Weight: 52 lbs.
Other: A hard-disk version is called the Tele-XT, comes with 256K RAM, and sells for $4,495. A portable model with a 9" screen is named the TPC-2, comes with 256K RAM, and retails for $2,695.

Brand Name Buying Guide

Comments: The TeleVideo people have merged two good concepts into one: the splendid styling of the 803 computer with IBM compatibility. Viola! The Tele-PC.

The keyboard has the same wedge-shaped design and palm rest as the 803, but the keyboard is configured as on the IBM. That is, there are 10 function keys, and the slash key is between the shift and Z key, etc. The Tele-PC has, however, corrected a few of IBM's mistakes—the return key and shift keys are slightly larger than on the IBM.

Many items that are optional with IBM are standard here. The Tele-PC comes complete with two drives, 128K of memory, both a serial and a parallel port, and MS-DOS. As on the 803, there is no fan, just blessed silence.

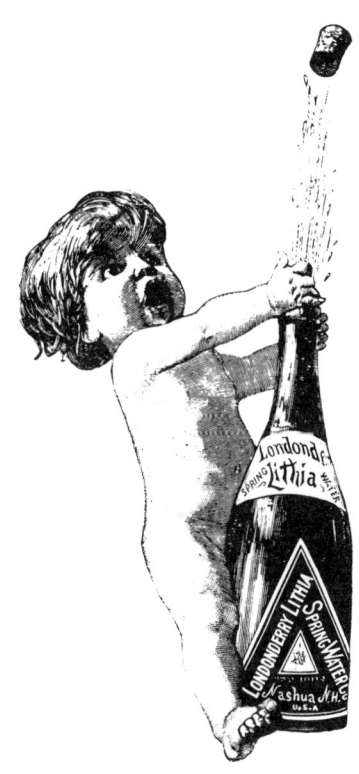

PERSONAL COMPUTERS AND THE DISABLED

Texas Instruments Portable Professional Computer

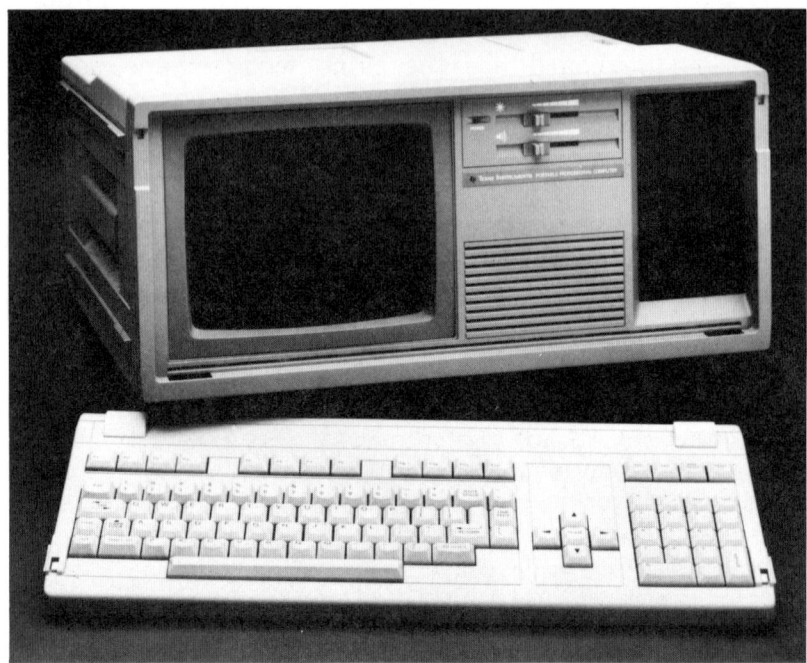

Price: $2,695
Screen size: 9"
Screen color: green (color available)
Main operating system: MS-DOS
Processor: 16-bit 8088
Standard memory: 128K
Disk drive type: 5 1/4"
Capacity of formatted disks: 360K
Software included: none
Keyboard:
- detachable? yes
- number of keys: 107
- number of function keys: 16

Weight: 37 lbs. (44 lbs. with color monitor)
Other: optional voice-recognition system

Brand Name Buying Guide

Comments: The machine I tested came with a color screen—and I was taken with its sharpness. If it were a monochrome screen, this would be very good quality. As a color screen, it's great. Texas Instruments pushes Easy Writer II as its word processing software. Easy Writer II, on this machine, turns all the letters on the screen green, as in a green phosphorous screen. I like that.

The keyboard has a good feel, the disk drives are quiet, and, in a clever design move, the machine cannot be operated without the fan door open.

Thirty-seven pounds is a bit heavy to be considered "portable."

As you may know, Texas Instruments dropped out of the *home* computer market, despite cuddly Bill Cosby as the spokesperson. I am not sure if Texas Instruments can do much better in the personal computer market, but they have a solid machine to work with.

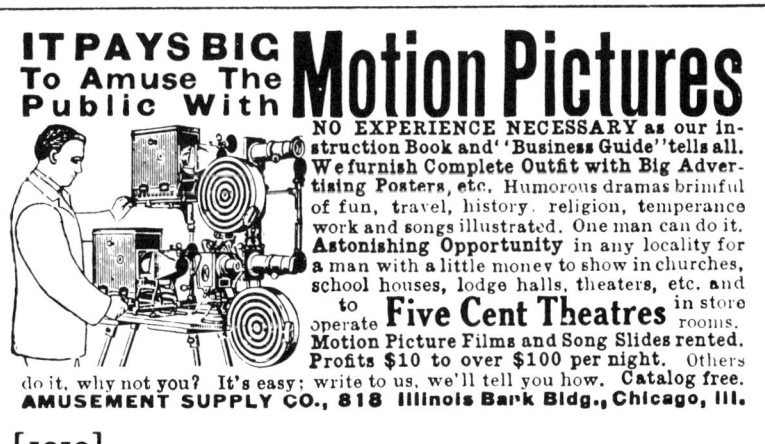

PERSONAL COMPUTERS AND THE DISABLED

Victor 9000

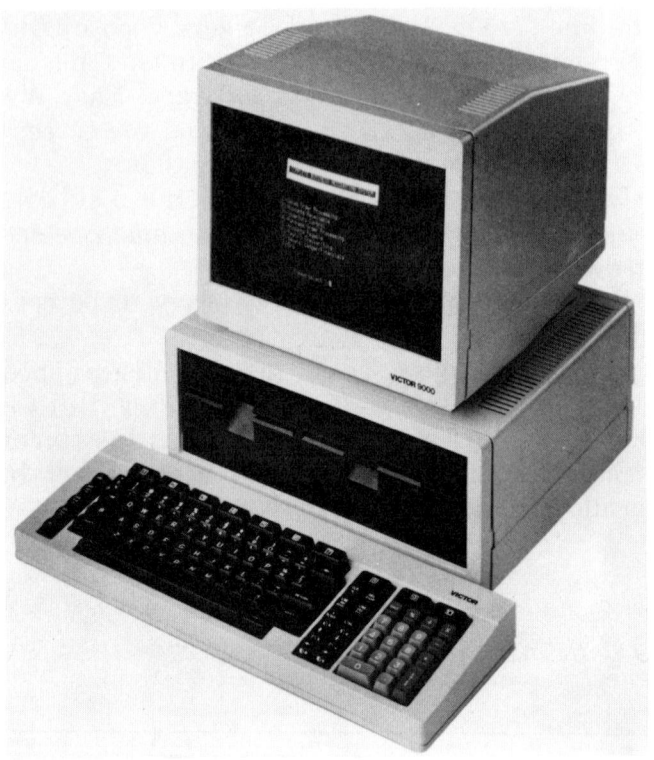

Price: $3,545
Screen size: 12"
Screen color: green
Main operating system: MS-DOS, CP/M-86
Processor: 16-bit 8088
Standard memory: 128K
Disk drive type: 5¼"
Capacity of formatted disks: 620K
Software included: MS-DOS, CP/M-86, MS-BASIC
Keyboard:
- detachable? yes
- number of keys: 100
- number of function keys: 10

Weight: 49 lbs.
Other: A double-sided disk version available. Each disk will then hold 1,240K.

Brand Name Buying Guide

Comments: The Victor 9000 is a superb computer—one of the better ones around.

The screen display is the best I've seen on a computer. Like the IBM, the characters on the Victor are made up of serifs—thicks and thins in the design of each letter. It looks more like printing than a computer display. Like the IBM, it has a green, slow-phosphor screen that's sharp and rock steady. The screen tilts up-and-down and left-to-right, and the keyboard has a palm rest, for maximum operator comfort.

The keyboard "solves" all the problems found on the IBM keyboard: The shift keys are large and the left-hand key is located next to the Z key; the return key is massive; the cursor keys are separate from the numeric keypad. Also, the keyboard is silent in operation. This will be good news or bad news, depending on your feeling about the IBM "audio tactile feedback." The keyboard is, of course, detachable.

The Victor 9000 will do color graphics with the addition of a PC PLUS board. The board will also make the machine IBM compatible. Without it, you need to get software specifically formatted for the Victor.

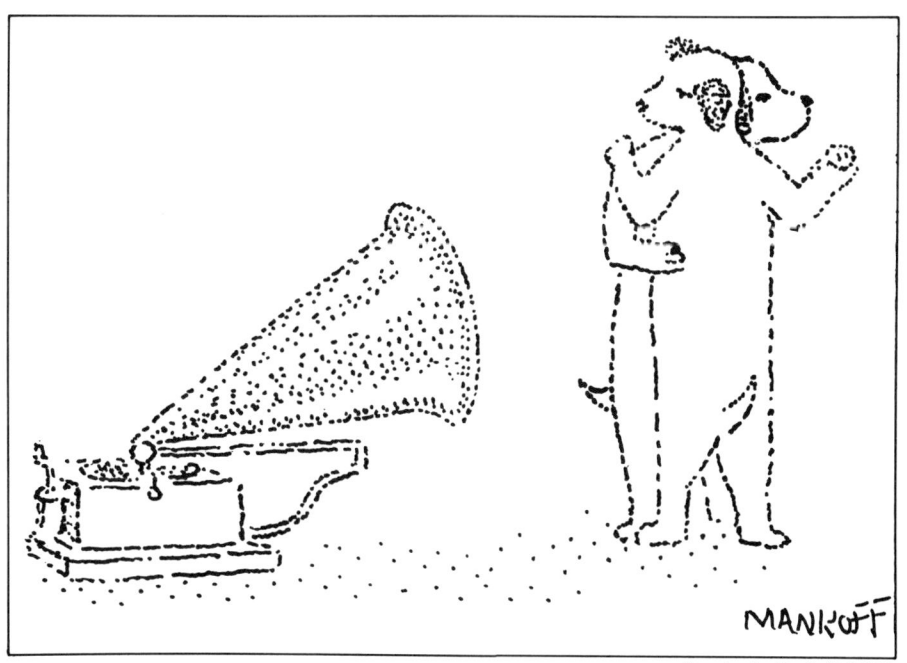

Drawing by Mankoff: © 1983
The New Yorker Magazine, Inc.

PERSONAL COMPUTERS AND THE DISABLED

Xerox 16/8

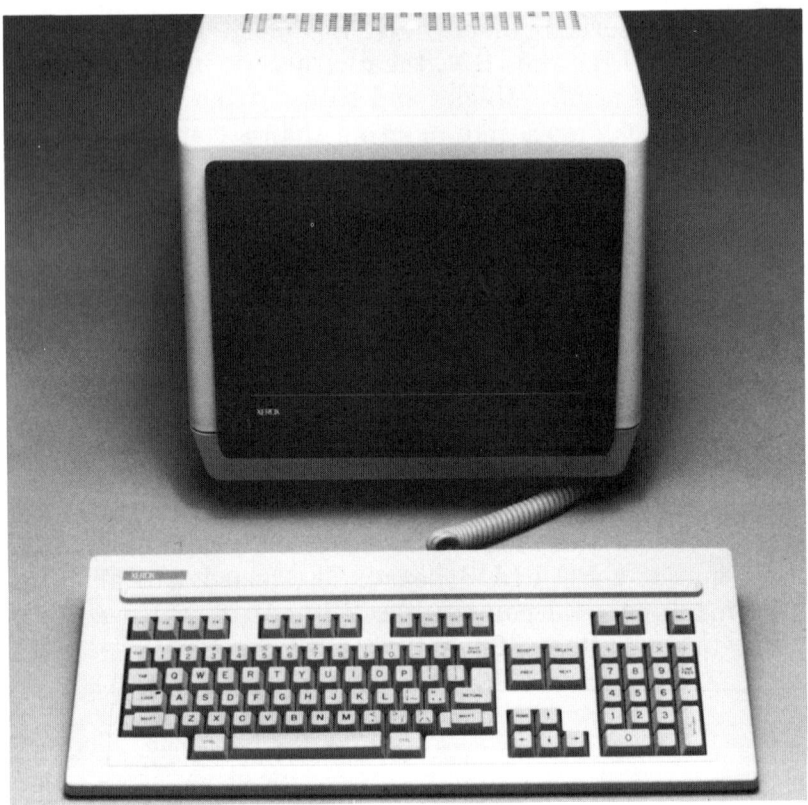

Price: $3,745
Screen size: 13"
Screen color: Black and White
Main operating system: CP/M and MS-DOS
Processor: 16-bit 8086 and 8-bit Z80A
Standard memory: 128K
Disk drive type: 8"
Capacity of formatted disks: 482K
Software included: none
Keyboard:
- detachable? yes
- number of keys: 75
- number of function keys: 18

Weight: 83 lbs.

Comments: Xerox no longer sells its 820-II computer. Instead, it is directing its marketing efforts to its other machine, the 16/8, a co-processing computer that permits use of 8-bit CP/M or 16-bit MS-DOS.

The 16/8 is a large but sturdy machine that works well. The eight-inch disks make it an odd format for an MS-DOS machine, but Xerox now offers a model with 51/4-inch drives, retailing for $3,295. A hard-disk model sells for $5,295.

If Xerox does not improve its marketing efforts, it may not be in the computer business long.

There are two X's in Xerox.

One on each end.

We're awfully tired of people spelling our name "Zerox" or "Zerocks."

It's "Xerox"—as in Xeres.

And, by the way, some of you insist upon calling photocopies made on Savin or 3m machines "Xerox" copies. Well, they're not!

Just cut it out. You think we want "Xerox" to become generic like "escalator"? So watch it. If we go under it's goodbye Masterpiece Theater and a whole lot of other good stuff on television.

XEROX

PERSONAL COMPUTERS AND THE DISABLED

Zenith Z-150

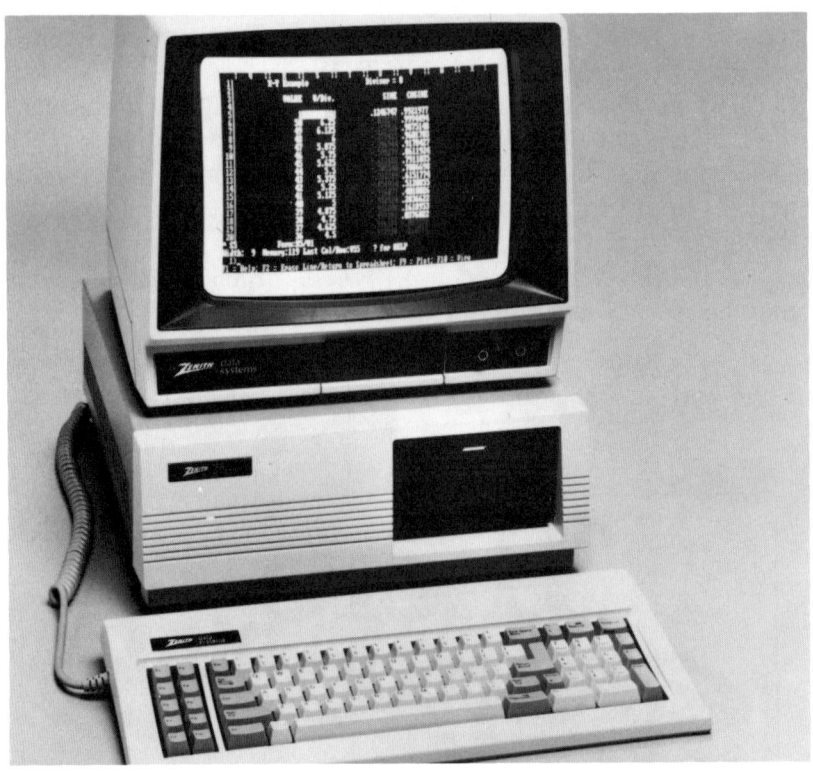

Price: $3,099
Screen size: 12"
Screen color: green
Main operating system: MS-DOS
Processor: 16-bit 8088
Standard memory: 128K
Disk drive type: 5¼"
Capacity of formatted disks: 320K
Software included: MS-DOS
Keyboard:
- detachable? yes
- number of keys: 83
- number of function keys: 10

Weight: n/a
Other: A 10.6 megabyte hard-disk version available for $4,799

Brand Name Buying Guide

Comments: Zenith is scrambling to keep up with the marketplace, and recently introduced the Z-150, and a portable model called the Z-160. The Z-89 computer has been phased out.

Though I haven't seen it yet, the Z-150 represents some better thinking on Zenith's part. The keyboard is detachable, and it does the IBM keyboard one better: Zenith has made the return key and shift keys large.

The computer is made to be IBM compatible, thus it uses MS-DOS instead of the Z-100's Z-DOS (whatever that is). Zenith tells me they have tried the 150 top-selling IBM programs, and they all run on the Z-150 and Z-160. (Hence the 150 in Z-150? Does the Z-160 run the top 160 programs? Film at eleven.)

The price for the Z-150 is slightly cheaper than the IBM, and more expensive than the Compaq or Columbia. I'm not sure what market Zenith's going for. (Why get a Zenith when you can get the real IBM?) Maybe it's for the people who bought the Zenith Space Phone, which allowed one to answer the phone through the television set.

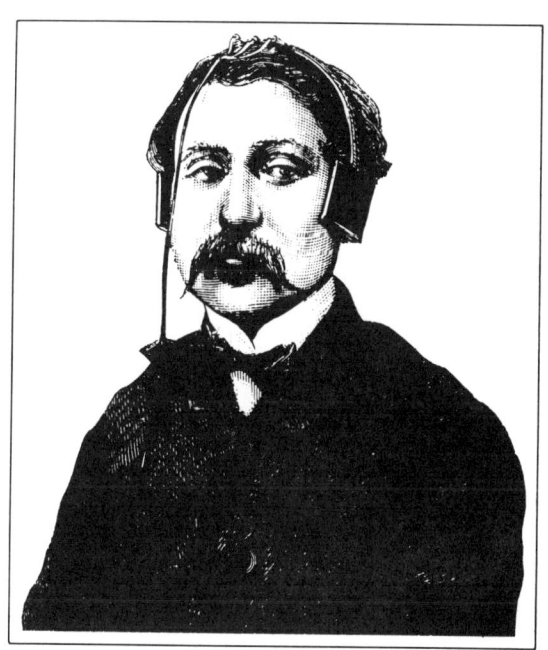

PERSONAL COMPUTERS AND THE DISABLED

Apple and Apple-Compatible Computers

Apple hasn't taken the same approach as IBM in licensing of its designs, so there are not as many compatibles. But there are a few, Franklin being the best known.

Apple IIe

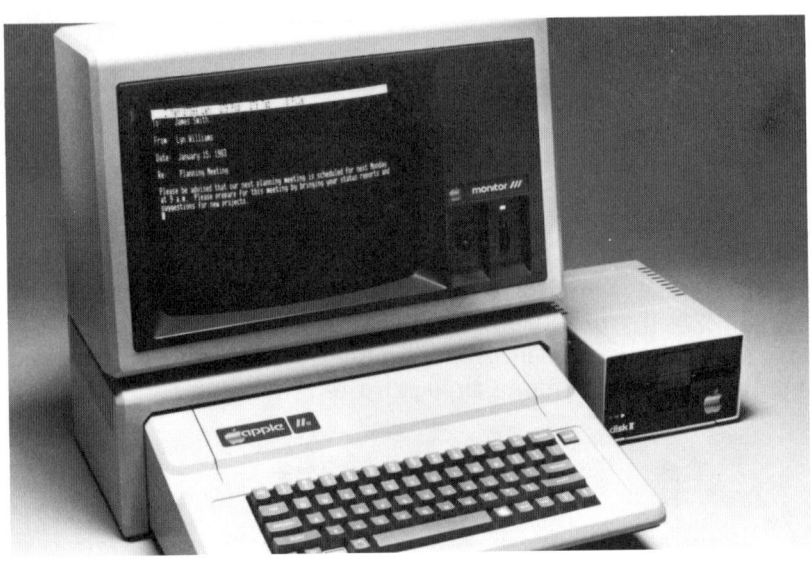

Price: $1,545
Screen size: 12"
Screen color: green (color available)
Main operating system: ProDOS
Processor: 8-bit 6502
Standard Memory: 64K
Disk drive type: 5¼"
Capacity of formatted disks: 140K
Software included: ProDOS, DOS System Master, Applesoft BASIC
Keyboard:
- detachable? no
- number of keys: 63 (no numeric keypad)
- number of function keys: 2

Weight: 31 lbs.

Comments: It's no secret that I've been dissatisfied with Apple's products in the past. Most of my criticism has been focused on their pricing. Theories of the marketplace aside, I've felt Apple tends to gouge consumers. Just a short time ago, IIes, with two disk drives and 80-column card and all, cost over $3,000. It was IBM that brought Apple to its feet.

Prices have dropped dramatically at Apple. The Lisa, which used to go for $10,000, can now be bought for $4,500, and the IIes have no list price at all—whatever the dealer wants to sell it for is fine by Apple. I've called several stores near me, and a two-drive system ranges from $1,545 to $1,699. The 80-column card is standard, as is the green monitor, and upper- and lowercase letters.

$1,545 is not a bad price. Other machines (Morrow, Kaypro, etc.) have much better prices. The machine still does not have a numeric keypad or detachable keyboard, but for a basic computer that has been around for a while and has support, the Apple IIe is, at last, a reasonable buy.

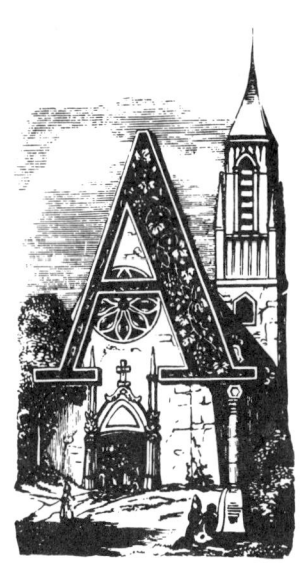

Apple IIc

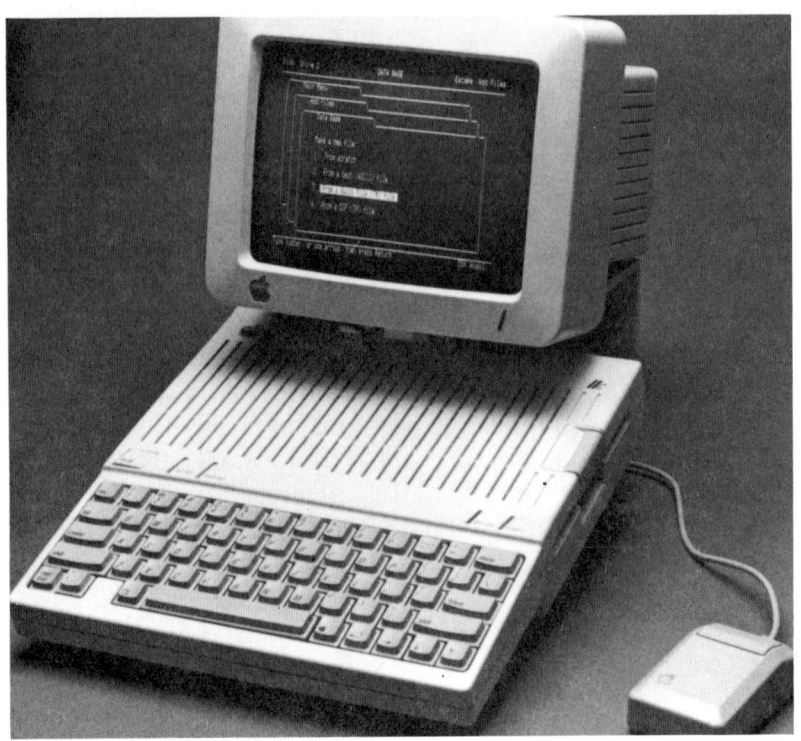

Price: $1,823
Screen size: 9"
Screen color: green
Main operating system: ProDOS
Processor: 8-bit 6502
Standard memory: 128K
Disk drive type: 5¼"
Capacity of formatted disks: 140K
Software included: ProDOS, DOS System Master, Applesoft BASIC
Keyboard:
- detachable? —
- number of keys: 63
- number of function keys: 2

Weight: 11 lbs. (with power unit, but without monitor)
Other: A mouse port and an 80/40 column switch included.

Brand Name Buying Guide

Comments: At first glance, a portable from Apple seems worth celebrating, particularly one which is advertised at $1,295. The brohaha obscures some limitations, however.

First, while 128K RAM is an ample size for memory, the IIc has no room for expansion boards, so 128K is all you can ever get. What made the desk-top Apple IIe a phenomenon originally was its expandability. Companies everywhere came up with items to plug into or onto the IIe. For this very same reason, the IBM PC blew—and continues to blow—up a storm. People are able to make their computer something more than what the factory offered them. The IIc, however, does not have this ability, so what you buy is forever what you get.

For $1,295 you get one drive and no monitor. $1,823 gives you a complete model, with two drives and the monitor. A comparably-equipped Apple IIe, at $1,545, is less expensive and offers adaptability. Other than for its semi-portability, I am not sure why anyone would want a IIc.

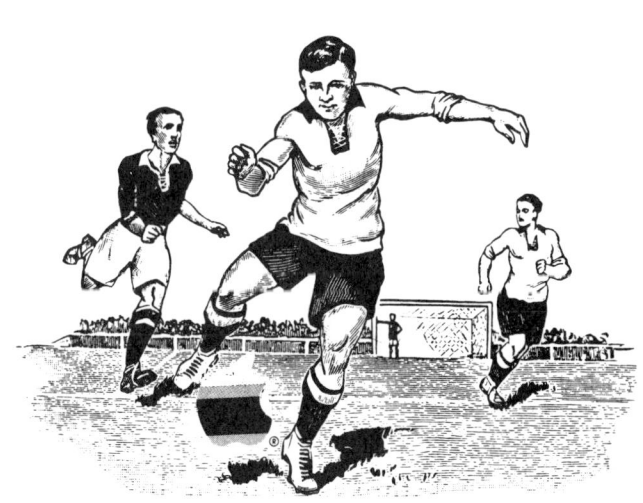

Apple Lisa 2/5

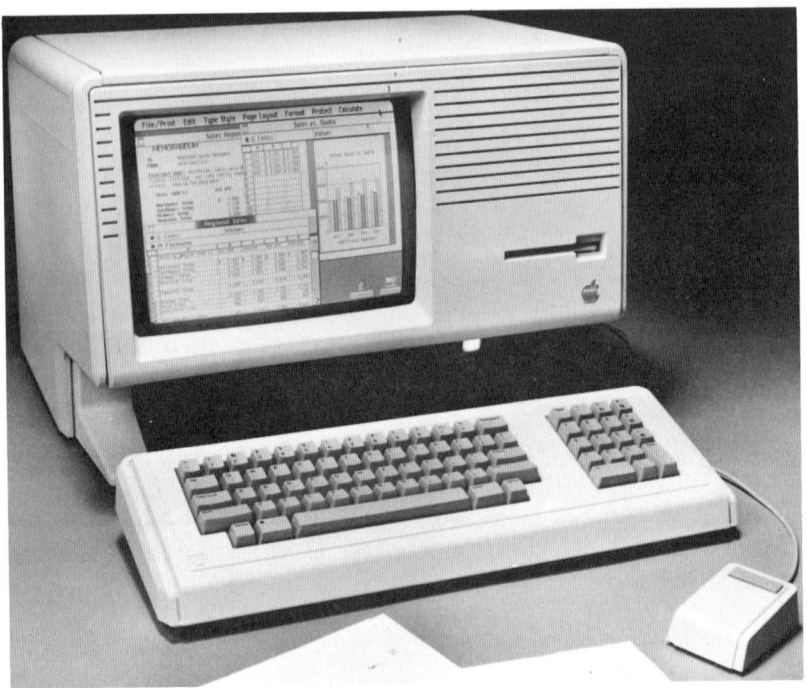

Price: $4,495
Screen size: 12"
Screen color: Black & White
Main operating system: Lisa OS, Mac OS
Processor: 32/16-bit MC68000
Standard memory: 512K
Disk drive type: One 3½" floppy and one 5 MB hard disk
Capacity of formatted disks: 400K/4.4MB
Software included: None
Keyboard:
- detachable? yes
- number of keys: 76
- number of function keys: 3

Weight: 50 lbs.

Comment: The Lisa, uh, was copied from Xerox. In December of 1979, Apple founder and chairman Steven Jobs attended a demonstration of Xerox's Smalltalk system. The demonstration was given by Xerox researcher Bruce Daniels. Six months later, Daniels (along with 20-or-so other Xerox Smalltalk researchers) was working for the Lisa team at Apple. (Apple later decided it would be best to avoid an extended legal battle and now pays Xerox a licensing fee.)

Originally, the Lisa was designed for managers and corporate gentry. Apple figured there were 30 million who could afford the $10,000 price. Perhaps their research was correct, but many of that group chose an IBM for their office. (Actually, they could buy three IBMs for the cost of one Lisa.) Besides, no one was ever fired by buying an IBM.

I think it is a fantastic machine for architectural designers and engineers—people who have use for ultra-sophisticated graphics. For others, the power will never be used, or can't be. The best business programs are written for the IBM, and the IBM is cheaper. If that weren't enough, the catalog of software available for the IBM is inches thick, while the offerings for the Lisa fit on a few pages. This means if you have an unusual need, you are more likely to find a program for an IBM than a Lisa.

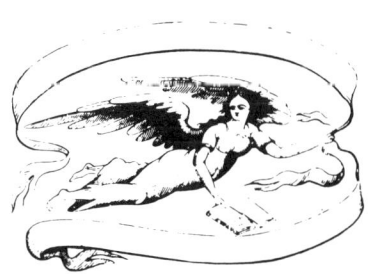

PERSONAL COMPUTERS AND THE DISABLED

Apple Macintosh

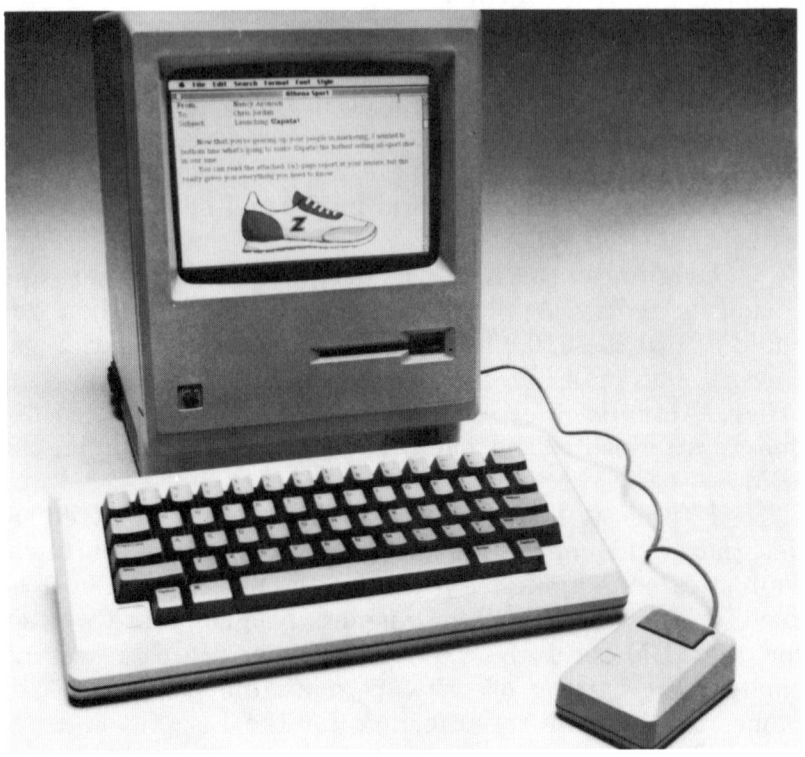

Price: $2,980 ($2,495 for one drive)
Screen size: 9"
Screen color: black and white
Main Operating System: Mac OS
Processor: 32/16-bit 68000
Standard memory: 192K
Disk drive type: Sony 3½"
Capacity of formatted disks: 400K
Software included: built-in Mac OS
Keyboard:
- detachable? yes
- number of keys: 58
  (no numeric keypad or cursor movement keys)
- number of function keys: none

Weight: 22 lbs.
Other: mouse included

Comments: Apple has blitzed the airwaves and print with how the cute, cuddly Macintosh is the computer of today. The advertising is visual and clever, and Apple promotes itself as being the concerned David in a Goliath industry. This obscures some basic facts about the Macintosh—most of which parallel my comments on the Lisa.

First, let me start with the positive. MacPaint is a terrific graphics program. This will sell lots of machines to people who will never use it, and it will also sell lots of machines to people who will. It's great fun, and is an excellent example of hardware-software integration. If the Macintosh is a success, much of the credit is due to Bill Atkinson, the author of that program. Architects, designers, and those who make black-and-white drawings regularly are encouraged to look at this program and seriously consider the Macintosh.

From there, the software goes downhill. The word processing program, MacWrite, is mediocre. Okay for memos and homework, but not powerful enough for business or professional writing. Better word processing will be available, but the Macintosh will not accept a letter-quality printer(!). One must use dot matrix, which is still not acceptable for most business correspondence.

The Macintosh is incompatible with every other computer in the known world. Even the Apple II, IIe, III and Lisa software won't run on the Macintosh. Most importantly, software written for the IBM won't run on it. IBM is now the standard, certainly for business and professional computing.

The Macintosh screen is not in color, and is not likely to ever be in color. I'm not a great fan of color myself, but if you are, know that there is more color on a Macintosh T-shirt than on a Macintosh screen.

The Macintosh keyboard has no numeric keypad (though you can buy a separate, optional keypad). For work with numbers, I recommend a computer that offers a numeric keypad.

The disk drives are non-standard. Sony is selling Apple 3½" drives AT COST, hoping that the smaller standard will catch on. After turning out some of the most

PERSONAL COMPUTERS AND THE DISABLED

resoundingly unsuccessful computers in recent memory, maybe Sony, like Apple, is desperate for market share.

Given that a comparably-equipped Macintosh is only a few hundred dollars less than an IBM, and given the reputation, support and software of the IBM PC, which would you choose?

In short, though the Macintosh does exceptionally well with a few things—namely graphics—it is severely deficient in other areas, particularly with business and word processing applications. Especially for the price.

Will there be a new standard, the Macintosh standard? Time will tell, and here's how to tell: if Apple sells 500,000 Macintoshes in 1984 and one million in 1985, then it has successfully established a new standard. There will still be a few million less Macintoshes than IBMs and IBM compatibles, but a standard will be created.

If Apple doesn't meet these sales figures, I wouldn't suggest buying one.

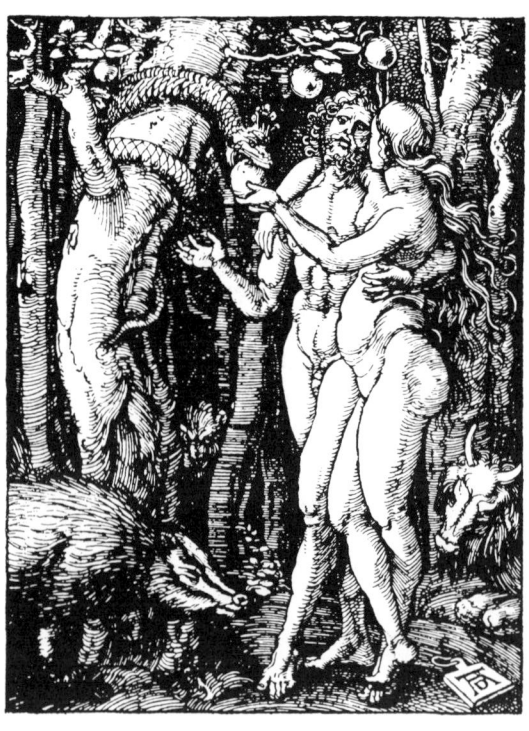

Brand Name Buying Guide

Franklin Ace 1200

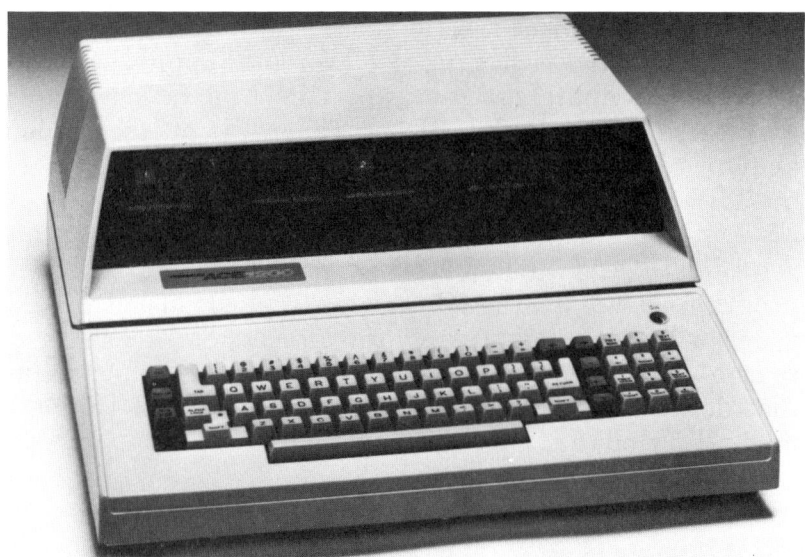

Price: $2,154
Screen size: 12"
Screen color: green
Main operating system: Apple DOS and CP/M
Processor: 8-bit 6502 and 8-bit Z80B
Standard memory: 128K
Disk drive type: 5¼"
Capacity of formatted disks: 143K
Software included: CP/M, Ace DOS, WordStar, MailMerge, Ace Calc, C-BASIC, tutorial program
Keyboard:
- detachable? no
- number of keys: 72
- number of function keys: 0

Weight: 35 lbs.

Comments: If you need to use one or more Apple programs, and still want to do some serious word processing or business applications, you might look at the Ace 1200. It has better keyboard than the Apple IIe, including a numeric keypad. A less expensive model, without CP/M, is the Franklin Ace 1000.

PERSONAL COMPUTERS AND THE DISABLED

CP/M and Other Computers

This is the last section, but certainly not the least. Apart from all the hoopla of IBMs and Apples are some fine, solid computers, those using CP/M operating systems and those from Radio Shack. There is a tremendous amount of software written in CP/M and a barrelful for the TRS-80 machines.

If your main interest in computing is business, and you don't need the powerful and complex graphing programs made for the IBM, consider a CP/M machine. If your primary interest is word processing, there is no reason you have to spend hundreds more for a machine that does the same tasks as those in this section. Some of my best friends are CP/Mish.

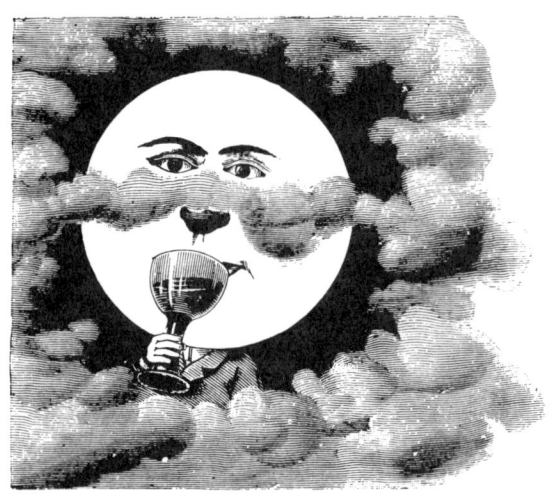

Brand Name Buying Guide

Cromemco C-10

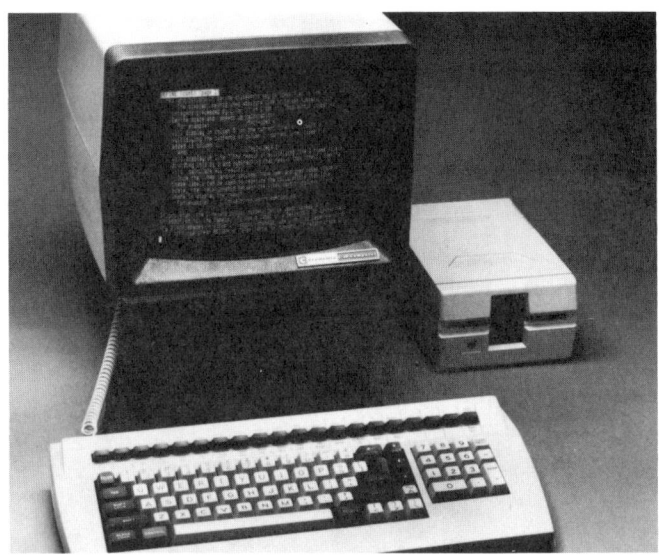

Price: $2,380
Screen size: 12"
Screen color: green
Main operating system: CP/M
Processor: 8-bit Z80A
Standard memory: 64K
Disk drive type: 5¼"
Capacity of formatted disks: 390K
Software included: WriteMaster, PlanMaster, CalcMaster MoneyMaster, Screen Editor, Chess, BASIC
Keyboard:
- detachable? yes
- number of keys: 97
- number of function keys: 20

Weight: 40 lbs.
Other: WordStar/MailMerge/InfoStar/CalcStar package available

Comments: When this computer first came out, it did not have a numeric keypad on the keyboard. Now the keyboard has one, making this a good, full-featured machine, albeit on the expensive side.

PERSONAL COMPUTERS AND THE DISABLED

DECmate II

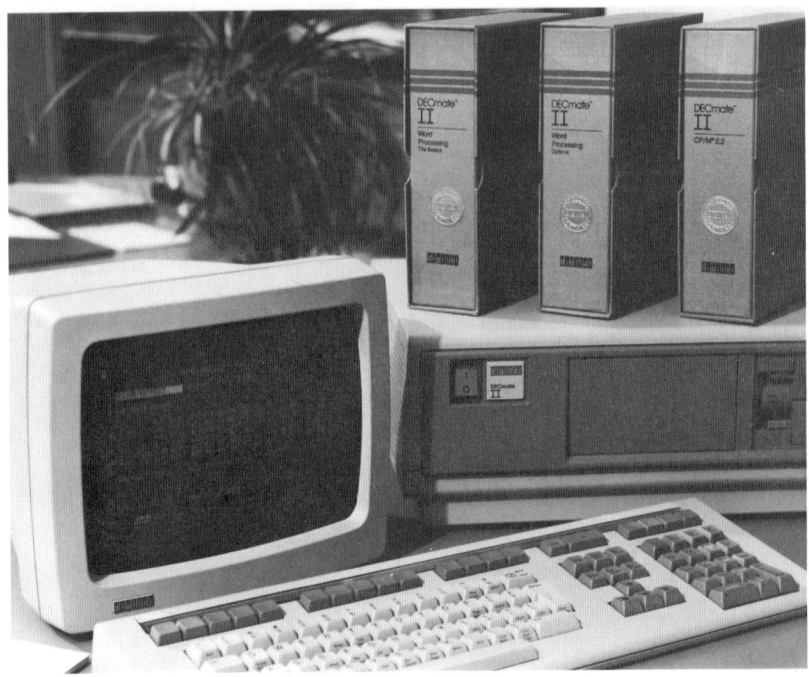

Price: $3,745
Screen size: 12"
Screen color: black and white
Software included: COS-310, WPS-8
Processor: 12-bit 6120
Standard memory: 96K
Disk drive type: 5¼"
Capacity of formatted disks: 800K
Software included: COS-310
Keyboard:
- detachable? yes
- number of keys: 105
- number of function keys: 20

Weight: n/a

Comments: This is designed solely for word processing, although it will run other programs. The DECmate II is very much like the Rainbow, except the processor is the Digital 6120, which is made to run Digital's existing word processing program. It is (get this) a *twelve*-bit processor (just when I was getting used to eight and sixteen). But don't worry. For a few hundred dollars extra you can have a CP/M auxiliary processor installed and run 8-bit CP/M. The CP/M plug-in card also adds an additional 64K of RAM.

The price of the DECmate II is a fraction of the traditional Wang-Lanier-IBM Displaywriter (etc.) stand-alone machine prices. It directly rivals the $8,000 to $15,000 stand-alone word processors sold by the Other Guys.

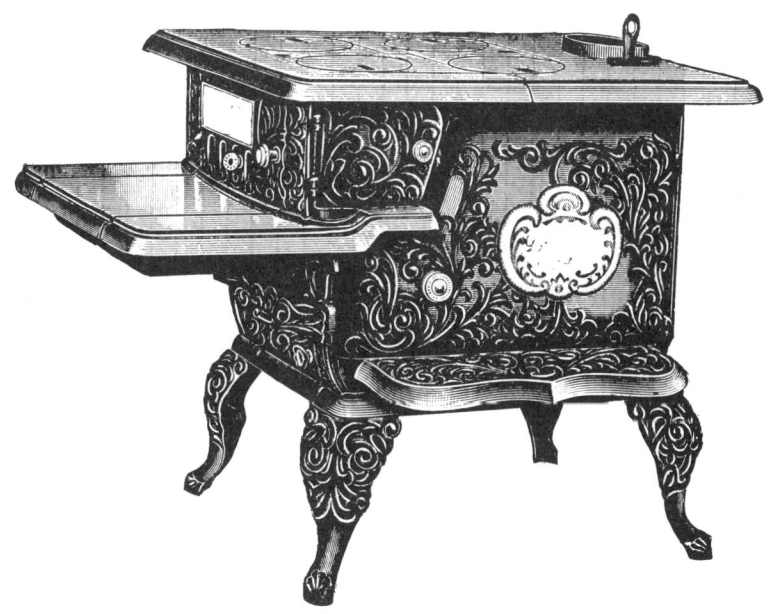

Computer stand

PERSONAL COMPUTERS AND THE DISABLED

Epson QX-10

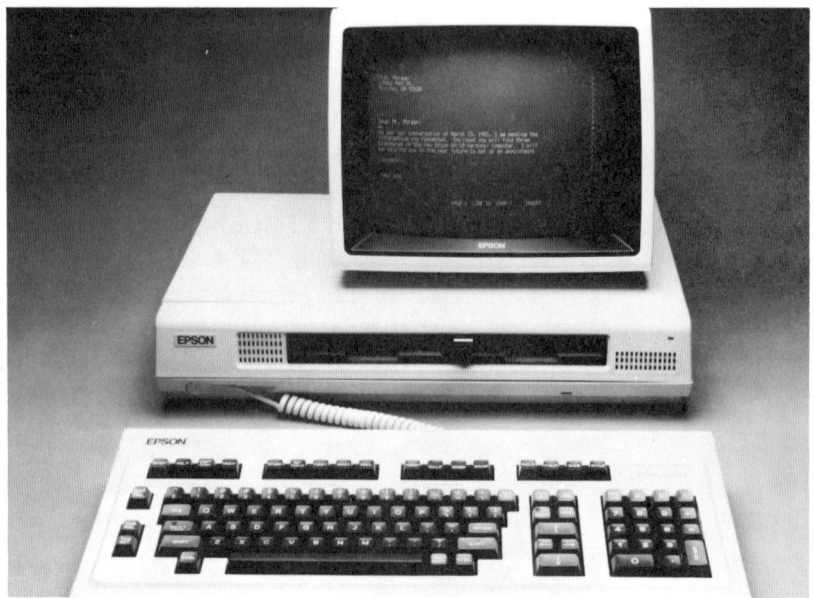

Price: $2,995
Screen size: 12"
Screen color: green
Main operating system: CP/M
Processor: 8-bit Z80A
Standard memory: 256K
Disk drive type: 5¼"
Capacity of formatted disks: 376K
Software included: Valdocs, CP/M, Time-management program, and games
Keyboard:
- detachable? yes
- number of keys: 104
- number of function keys: 20

Weight: 38 lbs.

Comments: With the Epson comes a green, exceptionally sharp 12-inch screen which is capable of high-resolution graphics. The keyboard is a pleasure to work with. It is, of course, detachable. The overall design (that is, the way the QX-10 looks) is delightful.

Brand Name Buying Guide

The Valdocs word processing software has all the features one might expect from a state-of-the-art word processing program including sub- and superscripting, and mail-merging. The one problem with Valdocs, until now, has been its speed. Because of its ease of use and user friendliness, Valdocs has tended to be slow in executing commands. Not slow enough that a novice would notice, but slow for experienced computer users. The new Series Two generation (Valdocs 2.0) promises to be much swifter. It also allows for spelling checkers to be used, including the Word Plus.

The Valdocs software does some things that few word processing programs do. In addition to its ease of learning, it will display bold words in bold on the screen. Also, italicized words in italics. It will even display words in bold italics. If that weren't enough, character pitch (that is, the size of the letters) can be altered and mixed on screen.

The computer has a clock that remembers day, date, and time—even if the machine is unplugged for shipping. The day and date is automatically added to the index. The index is made up of whatever name you wish to assign your files. No longer are you limited to one-word descriptions. You can rhapsodize about the contents of a file using, if you like, about twenty words. To find a file, for later editing or telecommunication, all you need remember is any *one* of the words. The computer will display all files with that word in the index.

The computer has some considerate features. For example, if you are working on something you don't want someone else to see, all you have to do is push the CONTROL and STOP buttons. This blanks out the screen display until the person has gone. Hitting any key on the keyboard brings back the screen display. When you depress the "Calc" button, a full spreadsheet is displayed.

Unlike when the QX-10 first came out, it now supports many, many printers, including Comrex, Diablo, NEC, and of course, Epson. It runs almost all CP/M software.

The whole package to me represents a good value.

PERSONAL COMPUTERS AND THE DISABLED

Jonos C2150

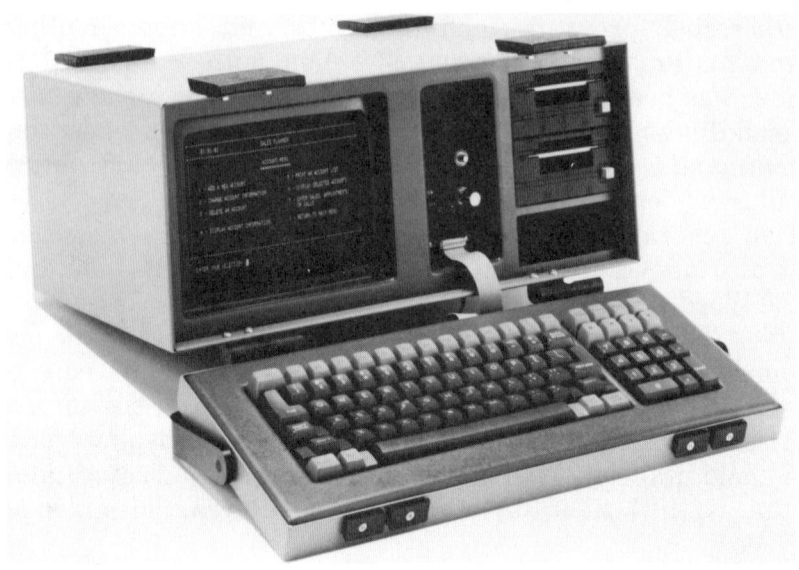

Price: $3,395
Screen size: 9"
Screen color: green
Main operating system: CP/M
Processor: 8-bit Z80B
Standard memory: 128K
Disk drive type: Sony 3½"
Capacity of formatted disks: 322K
Software included: CP/M 3.0
Keyboard:
- detachable? yes
- number of keys: 92
- number of function keys: 10

Weight: 28 lbs.
Other: STD-bus based—room for 4 extra cards

Brand Name Buying Guide

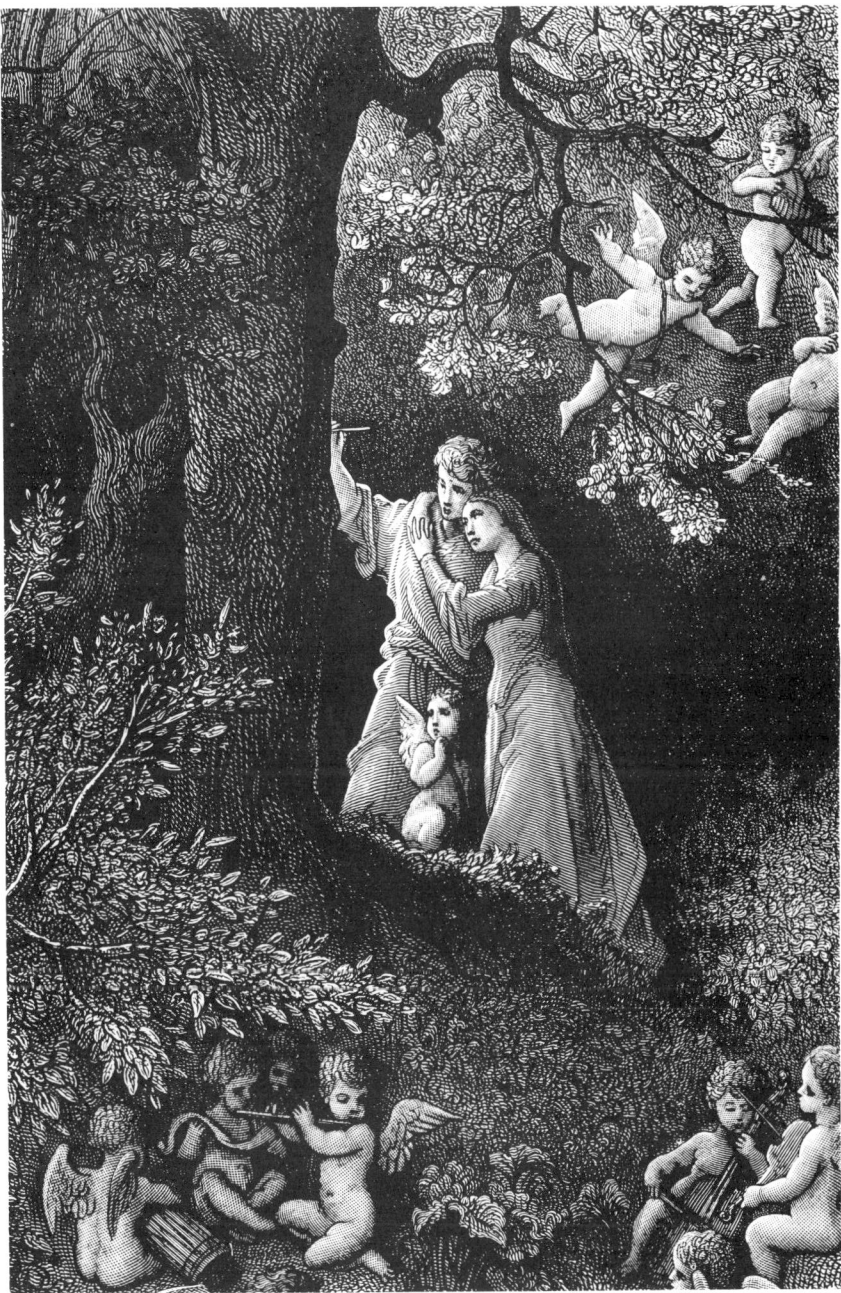

Mother Earth News *is marketing a personal computer in the shape of a tree. Here a young couple use a light pen to check the price of soybeans on the organic commodities market.*

PERSONAL COMPUTERS AND THE DISABLED

Kaypro II

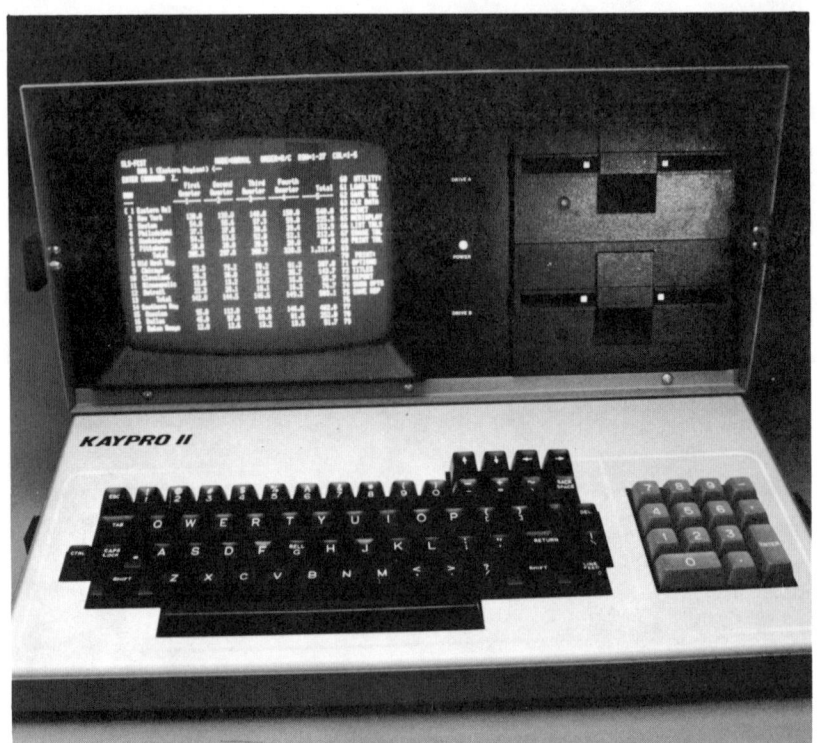

Price: $1,295
Screen size: 9"
Screen color: green
Main operating system: CP/M
Processor: 8-bit Z80A
Standard memory: 64K
Disk drive type: 5¼"
Capacity of formatted disks: 192K
Software included: CP/M, WordStar, The Word Plus, DataStar, SuperSort, MailMerge, CalcStar, Profit Plan, M-BASIC
Keyboard:
- detachable? yes
- number of keys: 76
- number of function keys: 0

Weight: 26 lbs.
Other: high-resolution screen, as on the Kaypro 10

Brand Name Buying Guide

Comments: The Kaypro computer is the Volkswagen Beetle of computers. It's not an elegant-looking machine, but it gets the job done. Though Osborne (now defunct) may have been the first to bring affordability into the world of computing, Kaypro was the first to add quality to price.

In the past, Kaypro has been quite responsive to the comments of the marketplace. They've been constantly adding and refining their list of free software. They've developed and offered machines with more power (Kaypro 4, 10, etc). They are also becoming a bigger company, and I am concerned with their quality control. In their eagerness to get new machines out, a shipment of bad disk drives found their way into Kaypro 4s. Quality control missed them. For a while, there were problems with the hard-disks in the 10. These problems have since been corrected. I just hope the Kaypro management doesn't lose sight of the quality they were built on. The Kaypro II, which has been around longer than many personal computers on the market, is a solid machine.

Kaypro's competition in affordability and dependability are the Morrow computers. Especially if your main interest in computing is word processing, please examine both Kaypro and Morrow. Also know that Kaypro offers the Kaypro II-X, which is a Kaypro II with two double-sided drives (as on the 4 or 10). It does not have the internal modem or all the software of the 4 or 10, but only costs $1,595.

PERSONAL COMPUTERS AND THE DISABLED

Kaypro 4

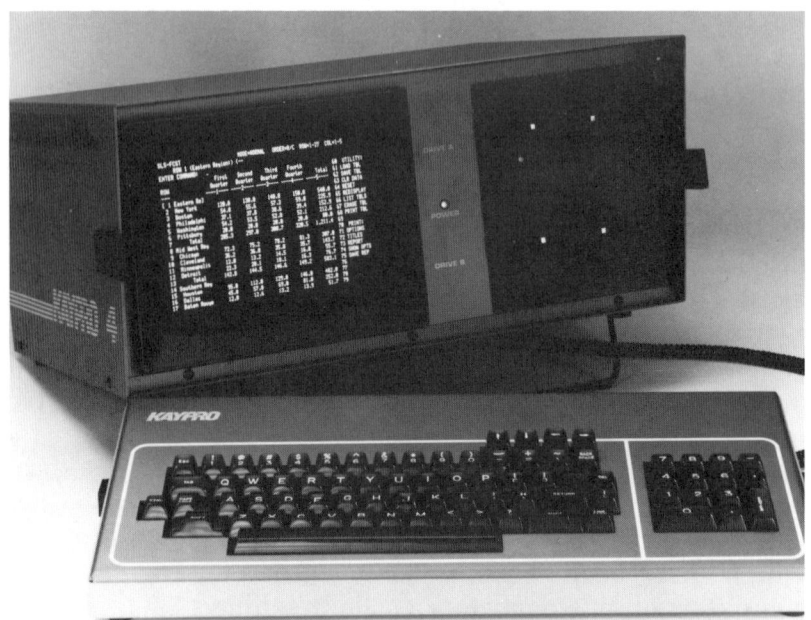

Price: $1,995
Screen size: 9"
Screen color: green
Main operating system: CP/M
Processor: 8-bit Z80A
Standard memory: 64K
Disk drive type: half-height 5¼"
Capacity of formatted disks: 384K
Software included: CP/M, WordStar, The Word Plus, dBase II (with tutorial), InfoStar (integrates DataStar and ReportStar), MailMerge, CalcStar, Microplan, M-BASIC, S-BASIC, C-BASIC, Suprterm
Keyboard:
- detachable? yes
- number of keys: 76
- number of function keys: 0

Weight: 27 lbs.
Other: Also included: a built-in auto dial/auto answer modem and a real-time clock

Comments: The Kaypro 4 is similar to the Kaypro II. Instead of single-sided disk drives, the 4's drives are double-sided, giving more disk storage space. It also has an extra serial port, a built-in 300 baud modem, and a real-time clock (which shows the time on the screen). The software package is slightly different, adding a few pieces such as dBase II and InfoStar. All the software is name brand and powerful—making for one of the most impressive free-with-purchase offerings around.

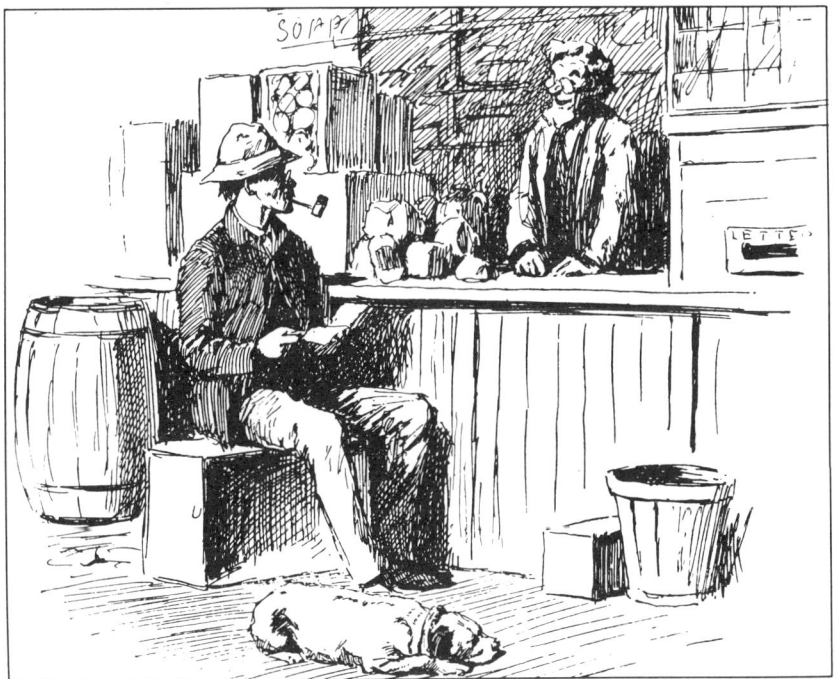

"Got a special today on a 64K, double-density, 8-bit sweetheart of a computer."

Kaypro 10

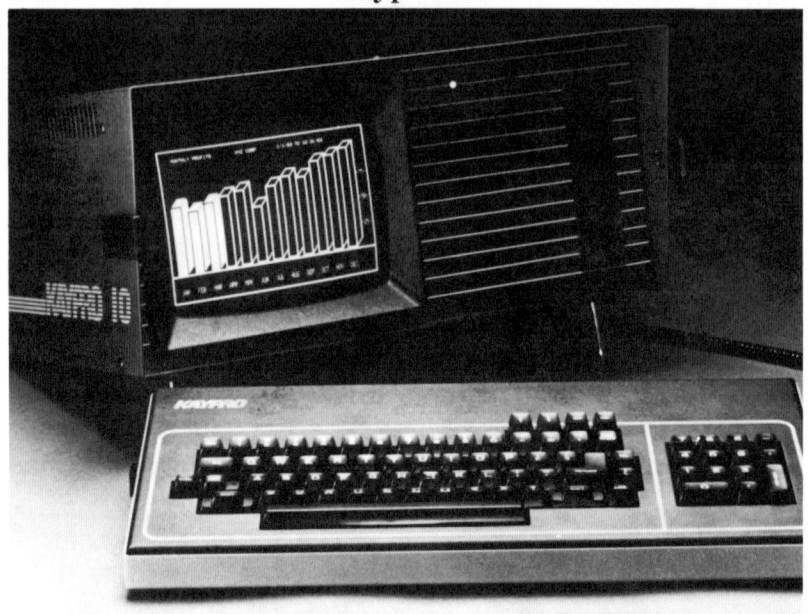

Price: $2,795
Screen size: 9"
Screen color: green
Main operating system: CP/M
Processor: 8-bit Z80A
Standard memory: 64K
Disk drive type: one half-height 5¼" and one 10MB hard disk
Capacity of formatted disks: 384K/8.3MB
Software included: CP/M, WordStar, The Word Plus, dBase II (with tutorial), InfoStar (integrates DataStar and ReportStar), MailMerge, CalcStar, Microplan, M-BASIC, S-BASIC, C-BASIC, Suprterm
Keyboard:
- detachable? yes
- number of keys: 76
- number of function keys: 0

Weight: 32 lbs.
Other: Also included: a built-in modem, and a real-time clock

Brand Name Buying Guide

Comments: The Kaypro 10 is very much like the Kaypro 4, except the Kaypro 10 has one floppy disk drive and a built-in 10 megabyte hard disk.

The machine is wonderful, a superb value, and all that, but I have one major concern: the hard disk. In the world of personal computers, hard disks are considered delicate beasties, who must be treated gently, and with the respect that's due anything that can destroy on whim 5,000 typewritten pages of information.

When a hard disk is put in a *portable* computer, considering the knocks and bangs portable anythings are subjected to, I become worried. I'm told the disk drive is of a new design and double-shock mounted and on and on. Still, in the testing stages, my Kaypro 10 went out twice. Two friends of mine have had problems with the 10. Kaypro tells me we're in a quite small minority, that problems the public has had with the machines have been quite few. I hope so.

This leads me to an important concept: as with any computer, hard-disk or otherwise, one should back up information on a regular basis. This is good advice, and like all good advice, seldom taken. A 10 megabyte hard disk holds the same amount of information as twenty-five Kaypro 4 disks, or *fifty* Kaypro II disks.

Granted, one will seldom have 10 full megabytes of information that will need frequent backing up. Much of the disk will be empty, or filled with programs that are already on master disks somewhere. But, still, the idea of making even 10 back-up disks on a regular basis is, well, not appealing.

Please understand that these are subjective, primordial, emotional reactions, like the fear of flying. (99.9999% of all airline flights are completed safely. 50,000 more people die in traffic accidents every year than in plane crashes. Then why am I afraid of going on an airplane and not afraid when I get behind the wheel of my car? It's not logical, especially the way I drive, but there it is.)

You see, as long as it works, the Kaypro 10 is a great computer. It has a sharp screen display, has an

PERSONAL COMPUTERS AND THE DISABLED

attractive blue-grey bushed metal case, has all the software of the Kaypro 4.

This computer is heaven-sent for people with tens of thousands of things to file. The titles of whole *libraries* or bookstores or auto parts companies or baseball card collections can be put on this computer.

Ten megabytes could handle the accounting, inventory, and word processing needs of a good-sized company, and still leave room for the boss's computer games.

Then why am I afraid? Why do I fear the letter that says: "I took your advice and I bought this thing and after five months of putting everything I know on it, it broke and I hate you forever"?

Ten megabytes is a lot. It's very powerful, but very dangerous. *Please*, with this or any computer, *back up your irreplaceable information regularly*. Back-up information is like wearing a seat belt: If it's only used once in ten years, it was worth the effort.

Maybe the Kaypro 10 and I should get away somewhere, take a long trip or something, and maybe we can work on my anxiety together.

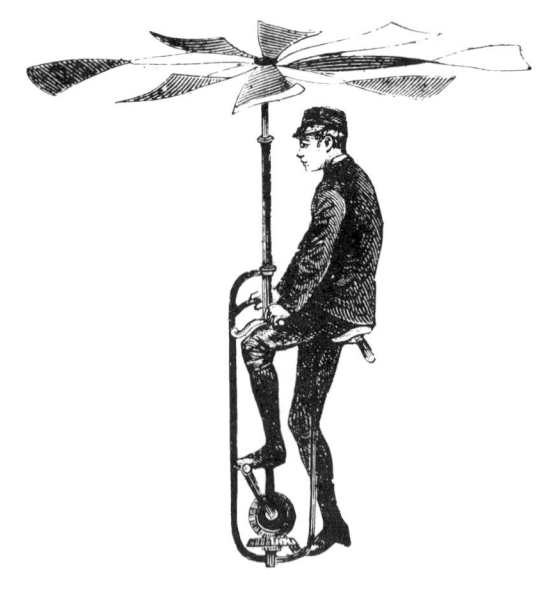

Brand Name Buying Guide

Lanier TypeMaster

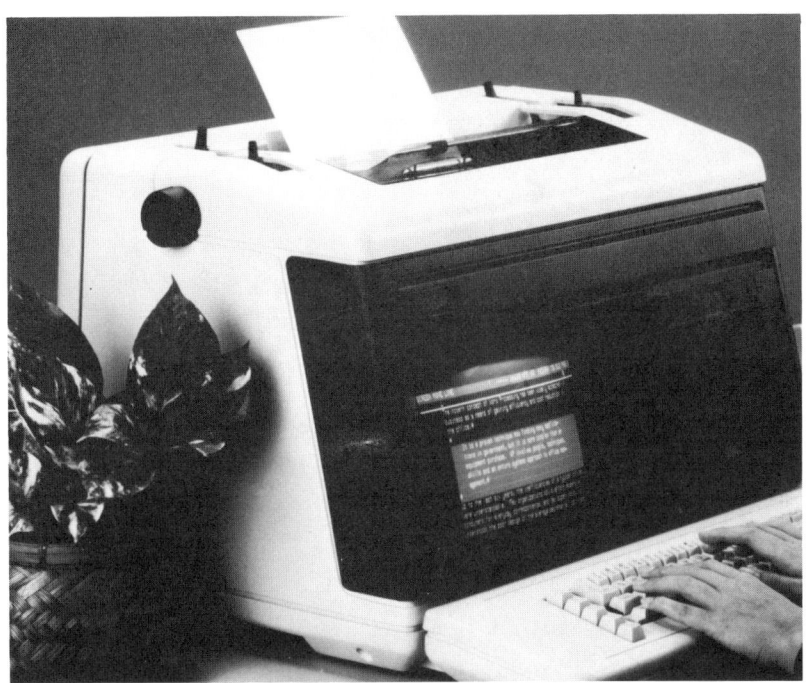

Price: $3,495
Screen size: 9"
Screen color: green
Main operating system: AES
Processor: 8-bit Z80
Standard memory: 64K
Disk drive type: 5¼"
Capacity of formatted disks: 70K
Software included: word processing
Keyboard:
- detachable? no
- number of keys: 83
- number of function keys: 30

Weight: 60 lbs.
Other: The printer's included, right in the top, and paper spurts out like toast. All-in-one has never been—and pray Heaven never again will be—taken this far. Note that the 70K disk capacity is quite small.

PERSONAL COMPUTERS AND THE DISABLED

Morrow MD-2/MD-3

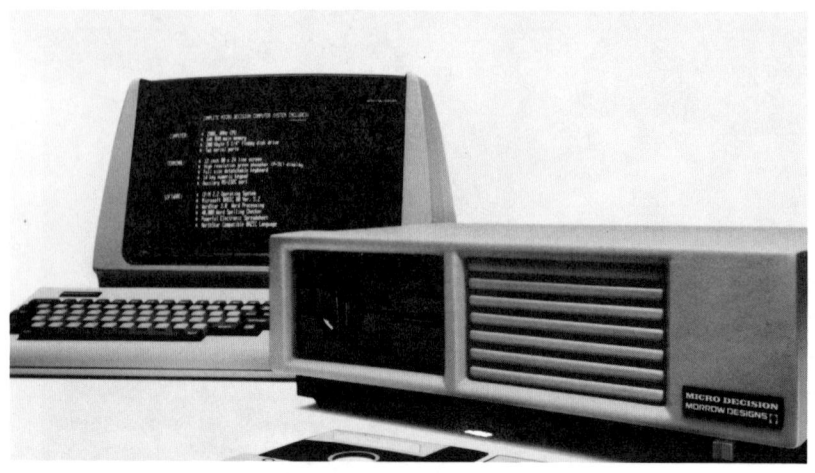

Price: $1,699/$1,999
Screen size: 12"
Screen color: green
Main operating system: CP/M
Processor: 8-bit Z80A
Standard memory: 64K
Disk drive type: 5¼"
Capacity of formatted disks: 186K/384K
Software included: CP/M, NewWord, List Manager, Correct It, SuperCalc, M-BASIC 80, Pilot, SmartKey (Also included with MD-3: Personal Pearl, Quest)
Keyboard:
- detachable? yes
- number of keys: 92
- number of function keys: 0

Weight: 48 lbs./44 lbs.
Other: A portable version of the MD-3, called the MD-3P, has the same specifications as the MD-3, except it is a single unit with a 9" green screen, weighs 26 lbs, and costs $1,899. The MD-3E has all of the MD-3 except the software only includes CP/M, NewWord and Correct It. The price for the MD-3E is $1,499.

Brand Name Buying Guide

Comments: These are fine computers and excellent values. They're in the same league as Kaypro, price and quality, yet, having larger and highly legible screens, make great desk models.

Everything about the Morrows I like: the keyboard has a good, solid feel; the software is name-brand and abundant. (NewWord, a word processing program, was developed by a group of people who split off from MicroPro; the command structure is virtually identical to WordStar, and has more help files. Beginners may find it easier to use.)

For companies considering multiple purchases or networking, look into the Morrows. The per-unit cost is far below an IBM or IBM-clone system, and with a hard-disk MD-11 in there, you will have plenty of storage space.

I first heard about Morrow a few years ago the way I heard about most things: a letter from a reader. The reader wrote:

"The company is MORROW DESIGNS out of San Leandro (California) and seems to be a well-established producer of hard disks and S-100 type board components. DUN'S Directory tells me they have thirty-five employees and the listed officers are all named Morrow. I have traced their ads back to 1979."

Now, of course, the company is much bigger than that. I don't know how many employees it has, but I do know the chairman is named George Morrow, an affable, pleasant man. The company has a good reputation and has been around the computer world longer than I have. It is a solid organization and will no doubt stand behind its products.

The Morrow computers are well worth your consideration.

PERSONAL COMPUTERS AND THE DISABLED

Morrow MD-11

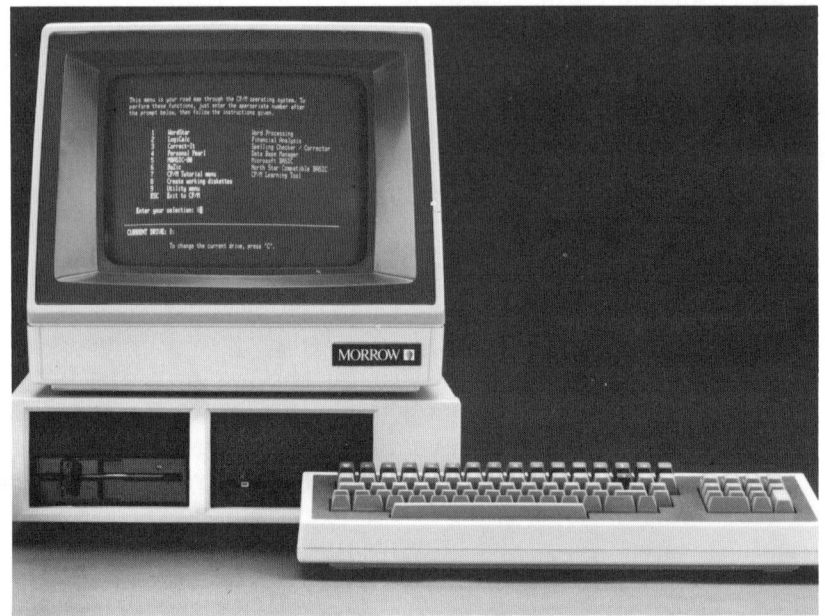

Price: $2,995
Screen size: 12"
Screen color: green
Main operating system: CP/M 3.0
Processor: 8-bit Z80A
Standard memory: 128K
Disk drive type: one 5¼" and one 11MB hard disk
Capacity of formatted disks: 384K and 10.1MB
Software included: CP/M Plus, New Word, SuperCalc, Personal Pearl, Quest, M-BASIC 80, and tutorial disk
Keyboard:
- detachable? yes
- number of keys: 91
- number of function keys: 9

Weight: 52 lbs.

Comments: The MD-11 is a tank—large, solid, reliable. It has a few features other CP/M-based machines don't have. First of all, it uses the new, more powerful CP/M 3.0. This allows for faster execution time, erase protection on individual files, and permits the machine to work with 128K of memory. After formatting is done, there is over 10 megabytes of useable storage area, which is almost 2 megabytes more than the space on the Kaypro 10.

The MD-11 comes with a utility program called Pilot. When you turn the machine on, Pilot gives a menu of all the bundled software. Next to each software program is a number. If you then want to use New Word, for instance, you press the number "1," and soon you are within the New Word program. It's handy, especially for those new to computers.

You won't see this machine on the cover of computer magazines as the Macintosh has been, but with the MD-11, you'll find power and reliability.

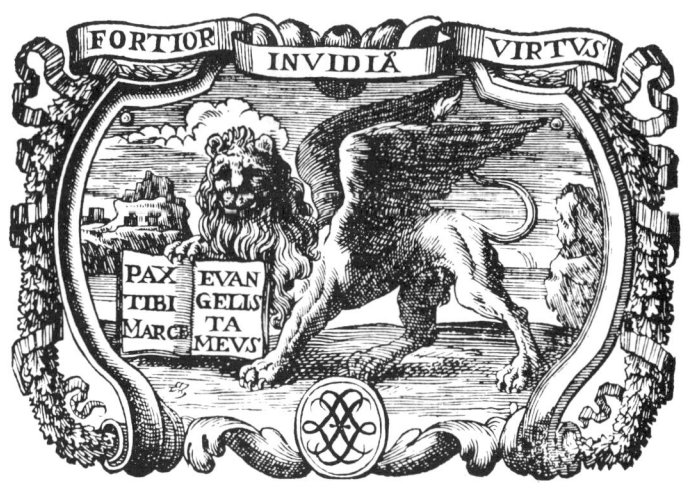

NorthStar Advantage

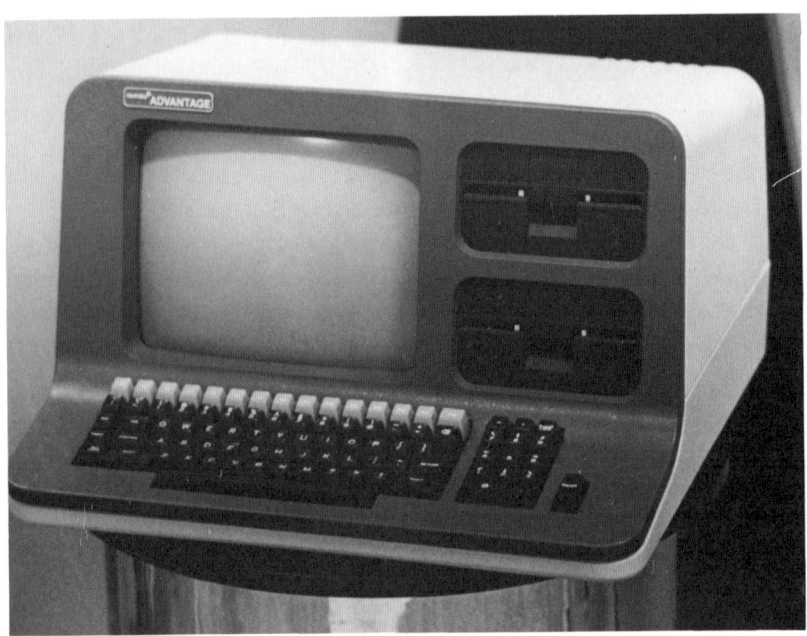

Price: $2,600
Screen size: 12"
Screen color: green
Main operating system: CP/M
Processor: 8-bit Z80A
Standard memory: 64K
Disk drive type: 5¼"
Capacity of formatted disks: 360K
Software included: CP/M, Graphics
Keyboard:
- detachable? no
- number of keys: 87
- number of function keys: 15

Weight: 43 lbs.

Brand Name Buying Guide

Comments: NorthStar has been making computers for a number of years, its Horizon being one of the most respected and dependable ever made. (I still use one.) The Advantage is NorthStar's first "all-in-one" computer—a fine machine, reasonably priced. Unfortunately, NorthStar took the concept of all-in-one too far: the keyboard is not detachable.

The Advantage has one advantage: it does high-quality computer graphics. Any business that needs graphics would do well to consider the machine. Also, take a look at NorthStar's networking system—the company's main market now is in networking.

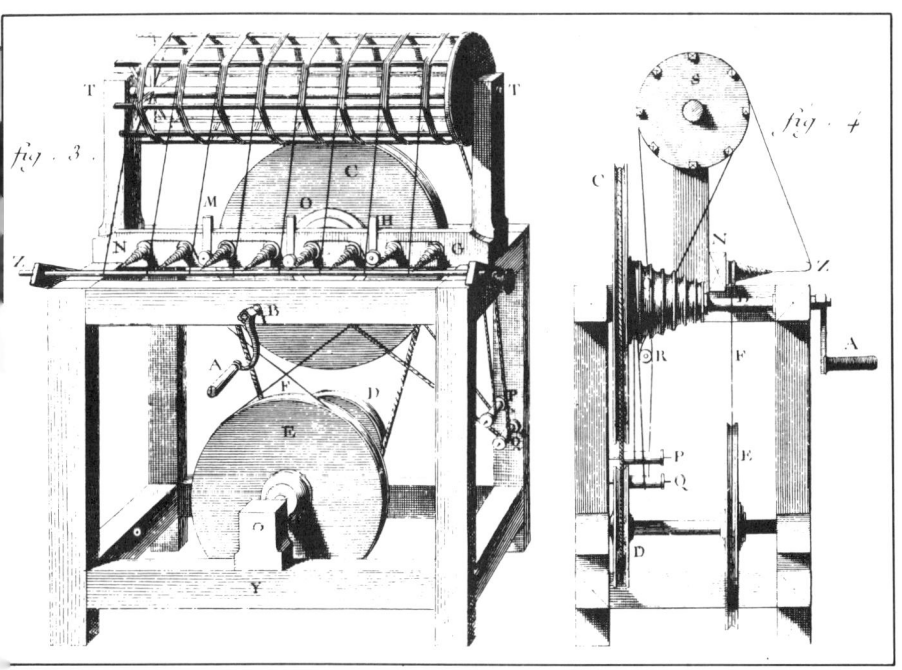

A hand-powered floppy disk.

PERSONAL COMPUTERS AND THE DISABLED

Radio Shack TRS-80 Model 4

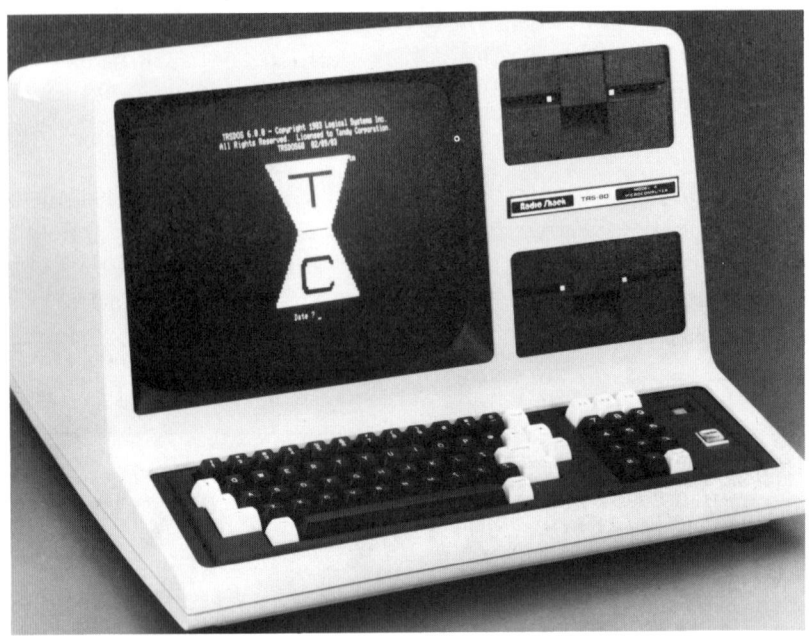

Price: $1,999
Screen size: 12"
Screen color: black and white
Main operating system: TRS-DOS
Processor: 8-bit Z80A
Standard memory: 64K
Disk drive type: 5¼"
Capacity of formatted disks: 184K
Software included: BASIC, TRS-DOS 6.
Keyboard:
- detachable? no
- number of keys: 70
- number of function keys: 3

Weight: n/a
Other: A portable version, the Model 4P, has a 9" black-and-white screen, two 184K disk drives, a detachable keyboard, and weighs 26 pounds. It retails for $1,799 and is a better computer.

Comments: The one great thing about Radio Shack is that, like Earl Scheib Auto Paint, they are just about everywhere. I even saw a Radio Shack off the beaten path in Lake Tahoe. For small towns without a variety of computer stores, Radio Shack isn't so bad. And if you move a lot, you'll always know where to get your machine repaired.

The Model 4 is the least expensive of Radio Shack's full-line computers. Two disk drives, attached keyboard. Nothing great, but it's OK.

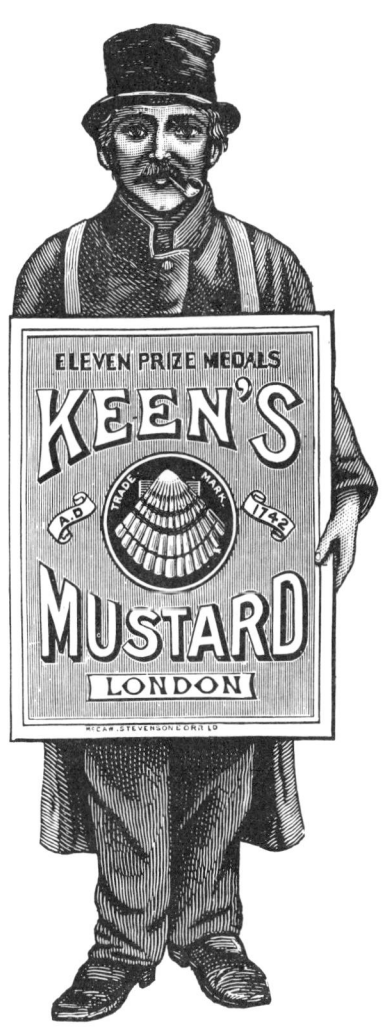

PERSONAL COMPUTERS AND THE DISABLED

Radio Shack TRS-80 Model 12

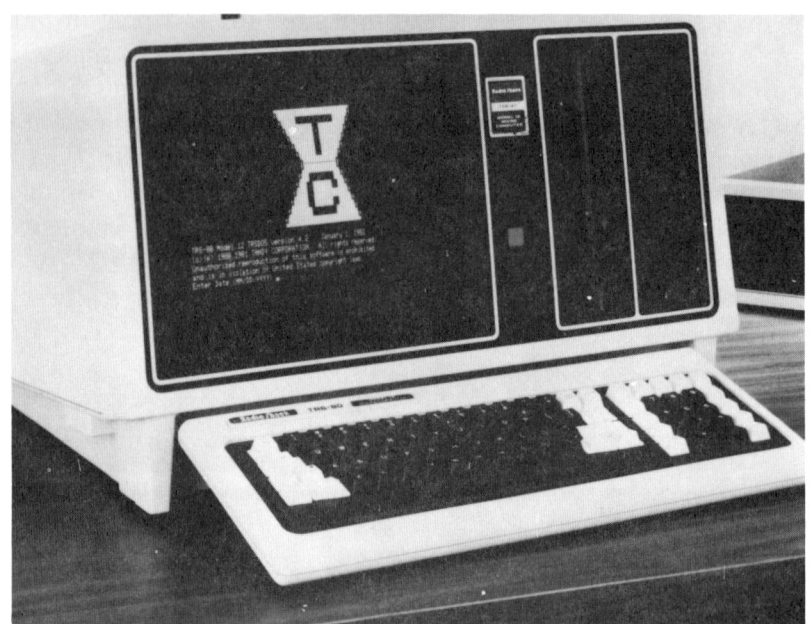

Price: $3,499
Screen size: 12"
Screen color: green
Main operating system: TRS-DOS
Processor: 8-bit Z80A
Standard memory: 80K
Disk drive type: 8"
Capacity of formatted disks: 1,250K
Software included: TRS-DOS and BASIC
Keyboard:
- detachable? yes
- number of keys: 82
- number of function keys: 8

Weight: n/a

Comments: This is one model I'd recommend for word processing. The whole unit seems a bit bland, a bit big, and a bit overpriced (Radio Shack is the Chevrolet of computers), but if Radio Shack is the only computer store in town, you could do worse for word processing or general office computing than the Model 12. (You could do worse without leaving Radio Shack.) The Model 12 does represent an overall improvement for the store, and they deserve a qualified pat on the back. (Pat, pat.)

Now that the Model 2000 is out (see review in IBM compatible section), the Model 12 seems outdated and that much more overpriced.

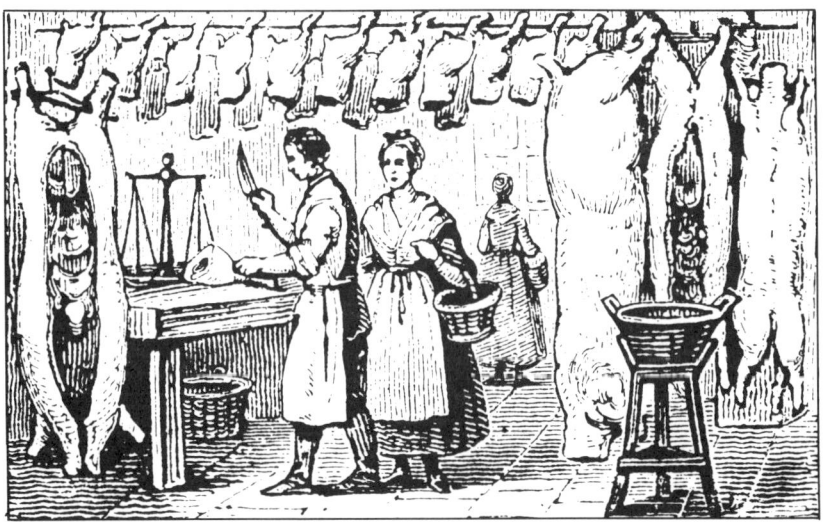

"Excuse me, please. I seem to be lost. Which way are the printers?"

PERSONAL COMPUTERS AND THE DISABLED

Radio Shack TRS-80 Model 16B

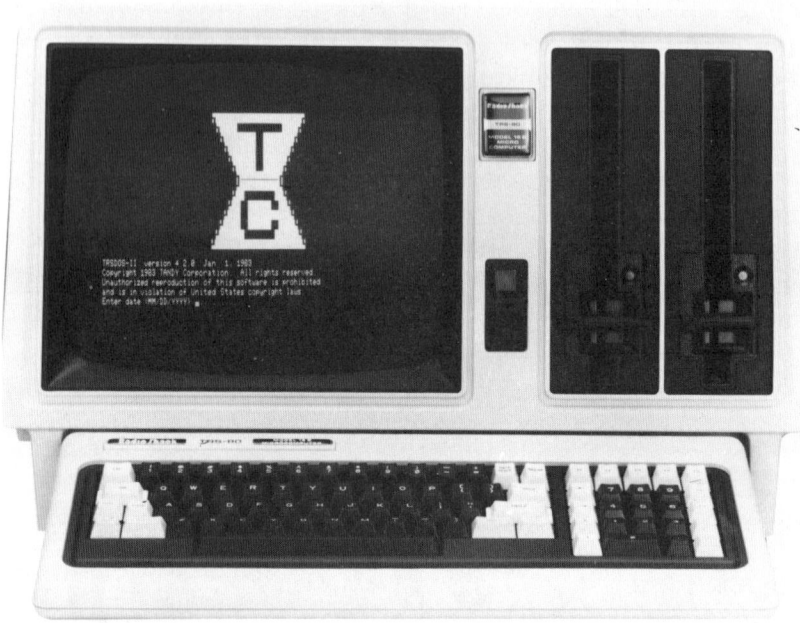

Price: $4,699
Screen size: 12"
Screen color: green
Main operating system: TRS-DOS, TRS-Xenix multi-user
Processor: 16-bit MC6800 and 8-bit Z80A
Standard memory: 256K
Disk drive type: 8"
Capacity of formatted disks: 1,250K
Software included: TRS-DOS, BASIC, TRS-XENIX
Keyboard:
- detachable? yes
- number of keys: 82
- number of function keys: 8

Weight: n/a
Other: A powerful machine, but overpriced.

Brand Name Buying Guide

Sanyo MBC-1150/1250

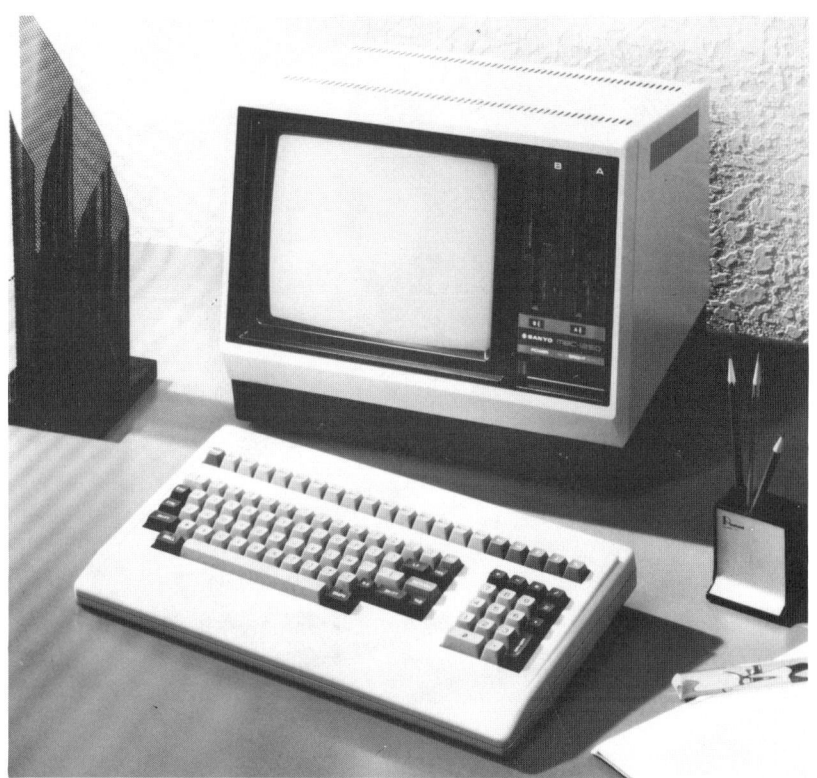

Price: $2,099/$2,599
Screen size: 12"
Screen color: green
Main operating system: CP/M
Processor: 8-bit Z80A
Standard memory: 64K
Disk drive type: 5¼"
Capacity of formatted disks: 326K/640K
Software included: CP/M, S-BASIC II, WordStar, CalcStar, MailMerge, SpellStar, InfoStar
Keyboard:
- detachable? yes
- number of keys: 100
- number of function keys: 15

Weight: 35 lbs./38 lbs.

PERSONAL COMPUTERS AND THE DISABLED

TeleVideo 802

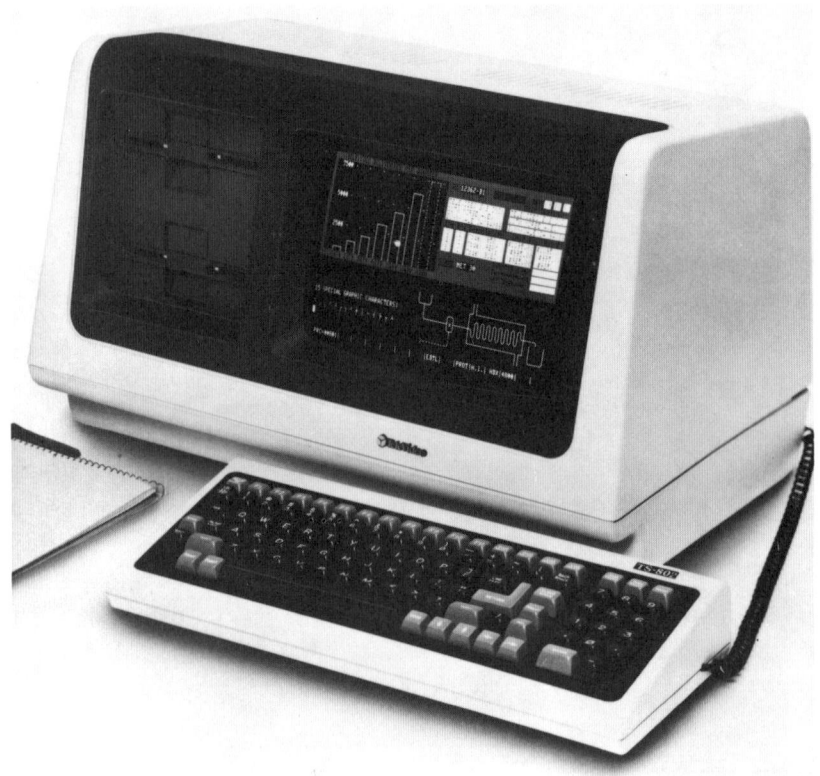

Price: $3,495
Screen size: 12"
Screen color: green
Main operating system: CP/M
Processor: 8-bit Z80A
Standard memory: 64K
Disk drive type: 5¼"
Capacity of formatted disks: 340K
Software included: CP/M
Keyboard:
- detachable? yes
- number of keys: 101
- number of function keys: 22

Weight: 44 lbs.
Other: Hard-disk version available for $5,995.

Brand Name Buying Guide

Comments: TeleVideo built high-quality, low-cost terminals for years before they manufactured full computers. To build a personal computer, TeleVideo began with the best: their own 950 terminal. The 950 is the top of the line of a dozen-or-so models.

I used to recommend the TeleVideo 802 as a good value, until an even better value came along: the 803. The 802's price now is high.

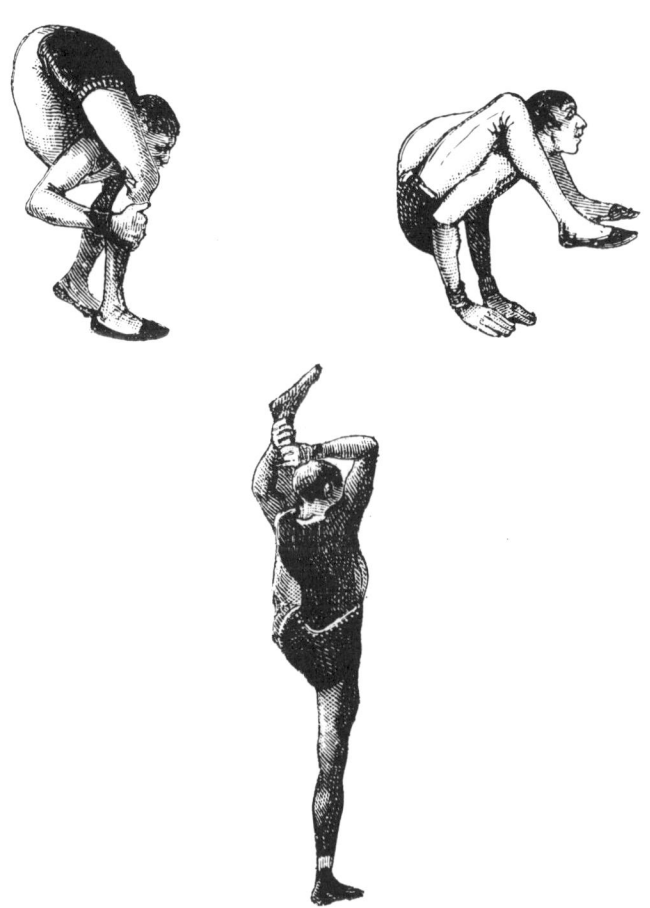

Exercises to combat keyboard fatigue.

PERSONAL COMPUTERS AND THE DISABLED

TeleVideo TS-803

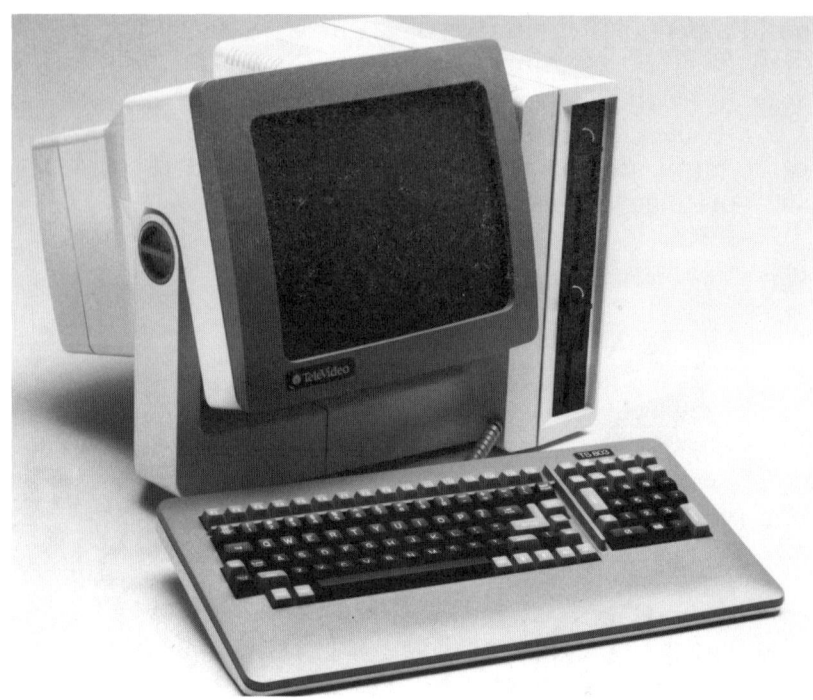

Price: $2,495
Screen size: 14"
Screen color: green
Main operating system: CP/M
Processor: 8-bit Z80A
Standard memory: 64K
Disk drive type: 5¼"
Capacity of formatted disks: 368.6K
Software included: CP/M and TeleSolutions (word processing, spreadsheet and graphics)
Keyboard:
- detachable? yes
- number of keys: 111
- number of function keys: 16

Weight: 52 lbs.
Other: A portable version of this, called the TPC-1, has the same specifications as the 803, but comes in a 32 pound all-in-one unit. It costs $1,999.

Brand Name Buying Guide

Comments: The "TS" in "TS-803" stands for, I think, Tres Sexy. This latest computer for TeleVideo is the sexiest thing this side of Euphoria.

The design is, how you say, ohh-lah-lah. If this computer does not win some design award somewhere, there is no justice. Aesthetics aside, the 803 is a powerful full-featured computer at a great price.

TeleVideo, more than any other company I know, has no fear of making the computer they introduced only a few months before nearly obsolete by the introduction of a totally new computer.

The company began with the 801, which basically added a processor, memory and two disk drives to their already popular 950 terminal. In its day, it was a good value. Then came the 802, which housed all the personal computer elements in one sleek package. Suddenly the 801 seemed a bit clunky.

Now, with the 803, which looks as though it was designed by Maserati, with more features, and far less expensive than the 802, well, is there any doubt which consumers will choose?

The screen is green phosphor and measures not 12, but 14 inches. (Does this mark the beginning of a size war among manufacturers?) The screen tilts up and down.

The screen has every key imaginable, plus sixteen special function keys, labeled word processing keys, and a numeric keypad. TeleVideo has made some of my favorite keyboards, and this one is no exception. Rather than end suddenly below the spacebar, as most keyboards do, this one slants gradually down, providing a place for a typist to rest the heels of the hands. As with most design innovations, some people will like this, others won't, and most people won't notice.

There is no fan, so the unit is quiet, silent in fact. For those deep thinkers who prefer creation without the whir of white noise, this machine is certainly worth listening to.

Although on the whole I am enthusiastic about the TeleVideo 803, I have a few reservations. Although the silence of no fan is nice, the disk drives, when they

PERSONAL COMPUTERS AND THE DISABLED

operate, sound a bit like muffled coffee grinders, and not the sort that Bessie Smith sang about. This is a minor distraction, as the disks seldom turn when any "serious" computer input is going on.

Also, the 803 has a slight electronic click each time a key is hit. Some people, especially touch typists, like this. The 802 has a switch in the back to turn the keyclick off, but I could find no such switch on the back of the 803. I'm sure that some technical type somewhere knows how to turn it off.

While I find the larger letters on the 14-inch screen easier to work with, they aren't as sharp as on the 802. A check of the specifications shows why. The 802 has a character resolution of 10x14 with a 7x10 dot matrix, while the 803 has a 8x10 resolution with a 7x9 dot matrix.

The decreases are not significant, but, when combined with the larger character size on the screen, the degeneration of character quality is noticeable. I should point out that the screen display is perfectly readable, and anyone who did not have the 802 display to compare it with would probably never know a dot here and a dot there were missing.

These few cavils should be considered minor complaints, especially when the price of the unit is taken into account.

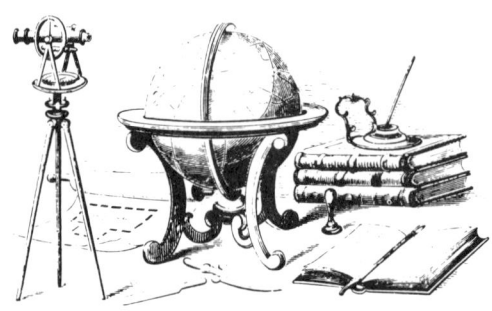

Brand Name Buying Guide

Toshiba T-300

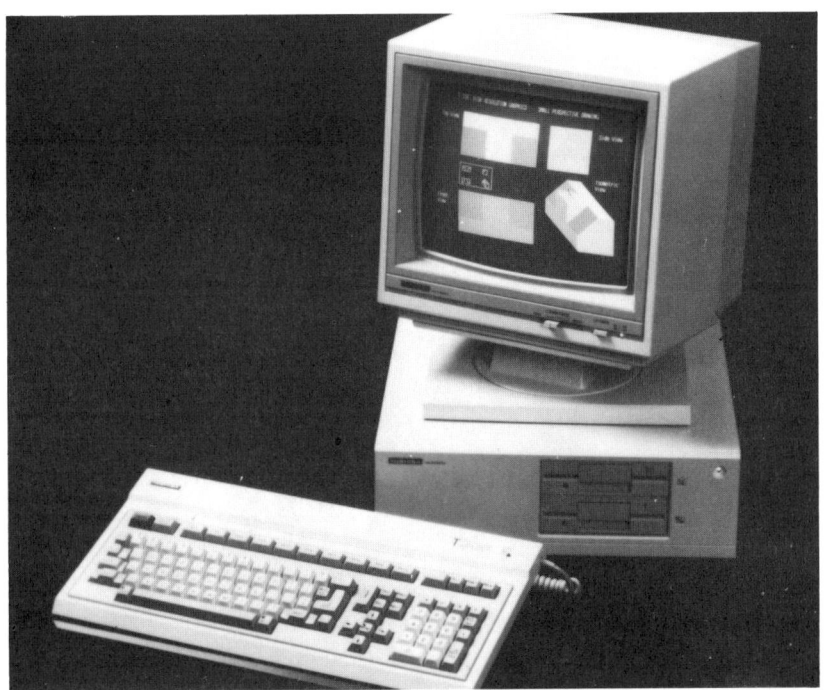

Price: $3,090
Screen size: 12"
Screen color: green (color available)
Main operating system: MS-DOS
Processor: 16-bit 8088
Standard memory: 192K
Disk drive type: 5¼"
Capacity of formatted disks: 640K
Software included: T-BASIC 16
Keyboard:
- detachable? yes
- number of keys: 103
- number of function keys: 10

Weight: n/a
Other: Toshiba has phased out its T-100 computer, an 8-bit model, and this replaces it.

PERSONAL COMPUTERS AND THE DISABLED

Zenith Z-100 (Heath HZ-100)

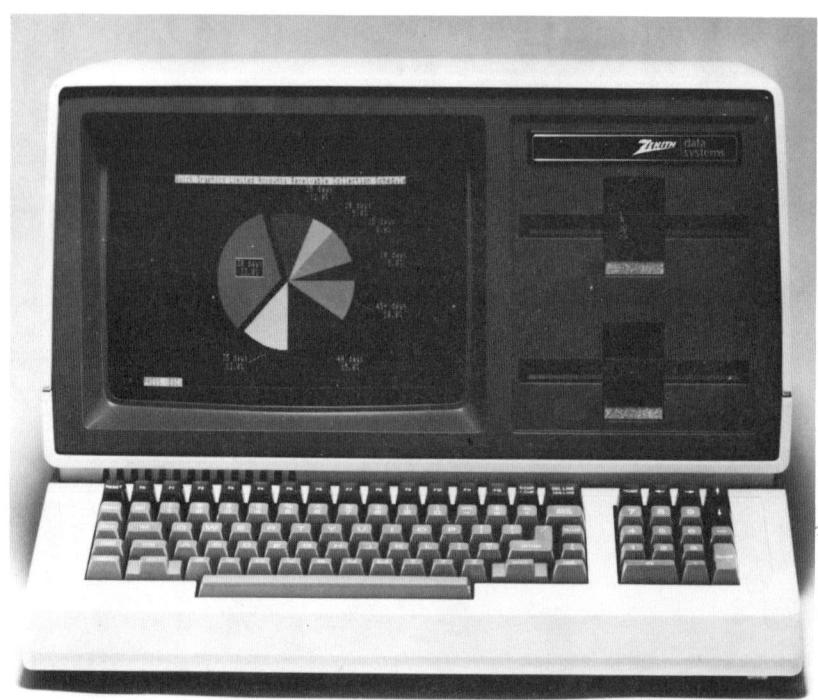

Price: $3,729
Screen size: 13"
Screen color: green
Main operating system: Z-DOS
Processor: 8-bit 8085, 16-bit 8088
Standard memory: 192K
Disk drive type: 5¼"
Capacity of formatted disks: 320K
Software included: Z-DOS
Keyboard:
- detachable? no
- number of keys: 108
- number of function keys: 13

Weight: n/a
Other: The Heath HZ-100 is in kit form

Brand Name Buying Guide

Comments: For a "state-of-the-art machine," and one with which Zenith and Heath hope to conquer the vistas of computerdom, the Z-100 is surprisingly primitive. The screen display is not very good. The keyboard is non-detachable. It is an 8- and 16-bit machine, but the amount of software that will run on it seems limited.

It has some good points. It uses an S-100 bus, for example. The S-100 bus is a standard for which hundreds of plug-in expansion boards are available. This provides great flexibility, but I'm afraid it requires a tinkerer's mentality. This machine, then, is right up a Heathkit lover's avenue. I'm not sure how well it will fare in business or word processing, where non-tinkerers abound. It's not exactly inexpensive, either.

If you own a Z-100, or are considering one, Hugh Kenner has written a great users' guide for the machine. It is published by the R. J. Brady Company.

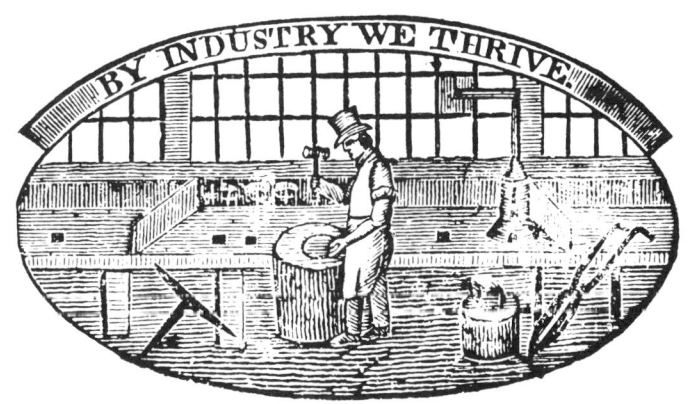

PERSONAL COMPUTERS AND THE DISABLED

PRINTERS

The next consideration is that of a printer. There are two kinds to consider, dot matrix and letter quality. Dot matrix printers cost less to buy and print faster, yet the quality of their finished pages leaves much to be desired. Letter quality printers cost more to buy and print more slowly, but the quality of their finished pages rivals that of the best electric typewriters.

Which is best for word processing? Clearly, letter quality. Correspondence, manuscripts, term papers—almost anything but in-house financial statements and invoices—look unbearably chintzy when printed on most dot matrix printers.

One of the bigger trends is that dot matrix printer manufacturers are advertising "correspondence quality." I must say, the print is getting better, but it's not as sharp as true letter quality printers. At best, the characters on dot matrix machines look like a typewriter with a thick nylon ribbon—which is saying a great deal. This quality may be enough for many people, and just below par for those sending important letters or manuscripts. Therefore, I still recommend letter quality printers.

But which letter quality printer? There are basically three kinds: daisy wheel, thimble, and converted typewriters.

Daisy wheel printers are so named because the printing element is a metal or plastic circle with "petals" Salvador Dali might mistake for a flower. Similarly, thimble printers use a print element that resembles a thimble, providing that the tip of one's finger is two inches wide. (Who names these things anyway?)

Metal daisy wheels give better print quality than do plastic daisy wheels, but plastic daisy wheels print faster than metal ones. Thimble printers combine maximum speed (55 characters per second, or about 450 words per minute) with maximum print quality. Thimble printers tend to be slightly more expensive than their daisy wheel cousins.

If money is a major factor in your decision, you can save quite a bit of it by buying a daisy wheel or thimble printer that prints at 35 cps or less rather than at 55 cps. Everything will take longer to print, but you'll initially save $1,000 or more.

Epson FX-80

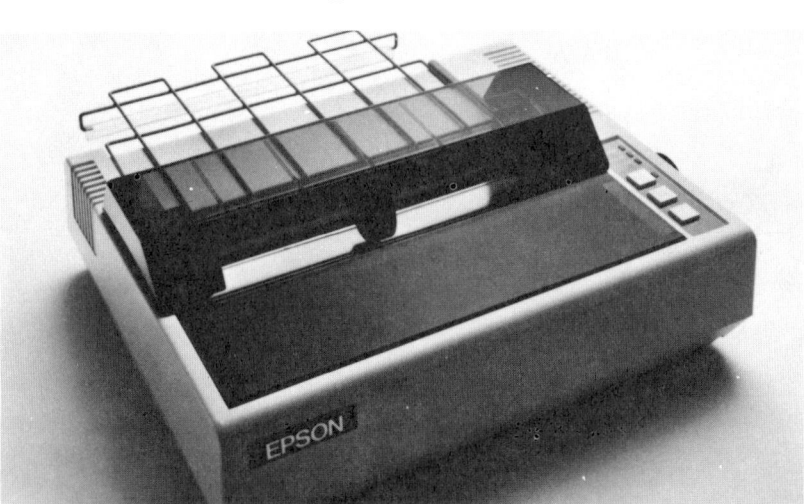

The Epson FX-80 is generally considered the leader in dot matrix printing for its price range ($500 — $1,000). Of all the inexpensive dot matrix printers available, IBM chose the Epson as the printer for the IBM Personal Computer.

A dot matrix printer, for reasons I gave above, should be considered for word processing only if the final appearance of printed copy need not look impressive. (The FX-80 does not do the "near letter quality" that newer printers are doing. Epson's LQ-1500 does this nicer printing, but it also costs $1,395.)

The Epson FX-80 is extremely rugged. I've carried it all over as a travelling printer (with my portable computer) and it withstands all the bumps I give it. It weighs only 15 pounds.

The printing speed of the FX-80 is 160 cps. The list price is $599.

PERSONAL COMPUTERS AND THE DISABLED

Mannesmann Tally 160L

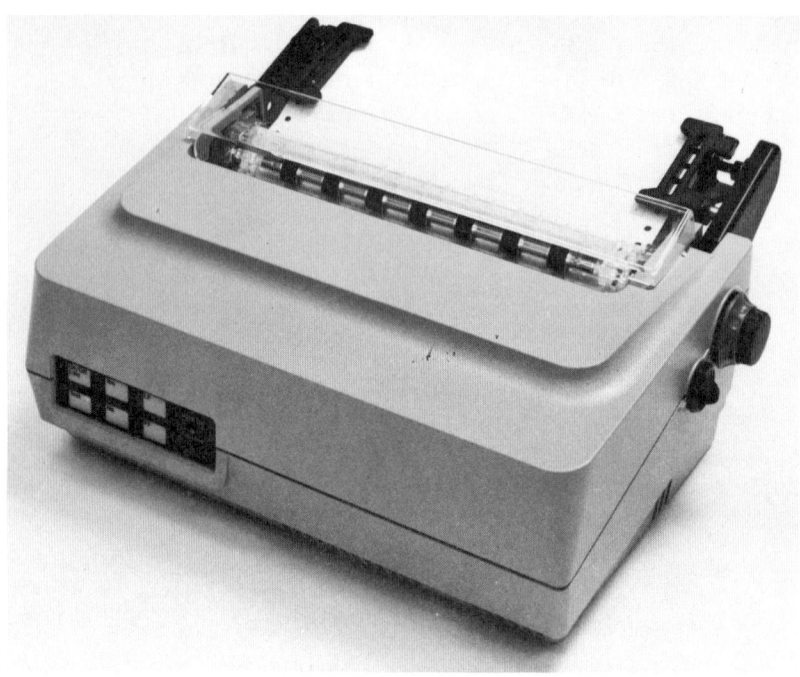

One of the new generation of dot matrix printers entering the market, the Mannesmann Tally 160L gives you a choice of 160 characters per second in the regular dot matrix "draft" mode, or near letter quality at 40 characters per second.

The letter quality is accomplished by two passes of the print head. The quality of the print is excellent, and only someone scrutinizing the type would notice how it was done.

```
     This is a sample of the Letter
  Quality mode of the Mannesmann Tally
      This is a sample of the Draft
   Quality mode of the  Mannesmann Tally
```

The Mannesmann has another new feature which should become standard on other printers. With most printers you have to face a myriad of little switches and search through a manual to set up the printer for your computer. The Mannesmann simply asks you questions in plain English on plain paper. You answer "yes" or "no." It's that simple.

Another advantage is the size of the printer. It measures just 14 inches wide and 9 inches deep. That even fits on *my* desk.

The printer comes with parallel and serial interfaces, and form feed tractor. All seems complete. There are a few drawbacks to consider, however. Single sheet paper can be next to impossible to load. Don't consider printing on your own letterhead unless it's tipped for form feed. If you use textured paper, the type can become smeared. Ribbons are expensive, around $15, don't last long and are hard to find. (They can be ordered from the manufacturer.)

The price is around $800. When you can spend more than $2,000 for both a dot matrix and letter quality printer combined, this could be one alternative.

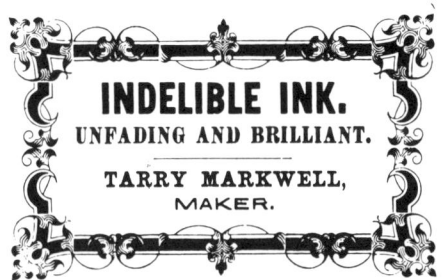

PERSONAL COMPUTERS AND THE DISABLED

Okidata

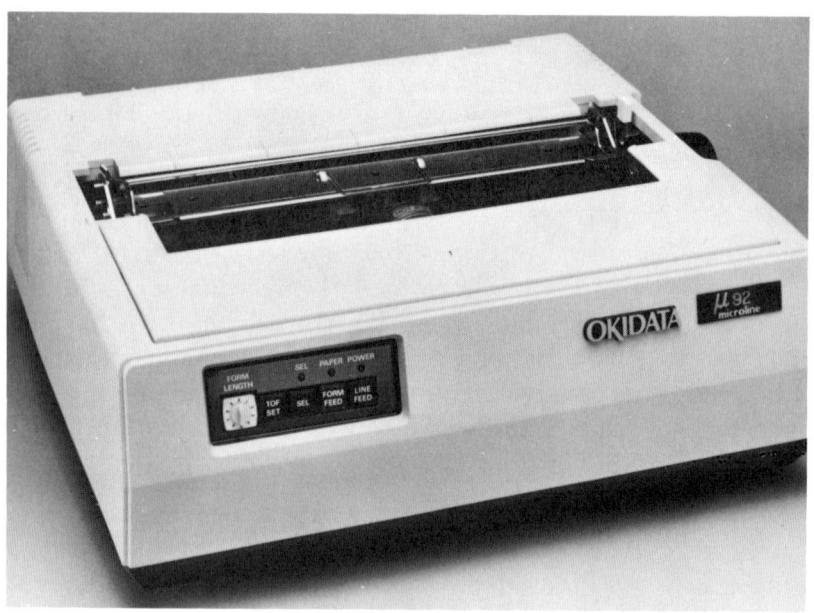

The Okidata Microline 92 is a rose among the new printers on the market. Small and offering the speed and print quality of an Epson FX, the Okidata also includes a "correspondence" grade print capability.

How does this correspondence grade look? Though it is still dot matrix, it's quite good. I think the type quality exceeds that of the Mannesmann Tally printer, but this machine, listed at $599, costs far less. The Okidata typeface is a partial "serif" style, which means the letters are similar to daisy wheel fonts using a pica typeface.

The correspondence quality prints at 40 characters per second, while the normal draft mode zips away at 160.

It is fairly simple to make the printer do very large type which would be good either for headings in reports, or for correspondence to someone with poor eyesight

This Okidata does excellent graphics, and can use Reportmaker. It also takes simple, old-fashioned, typewriter-like reel to reel ribbons. They are cheaper than most printer ribbons, but they are a mess to change.

Since the printer has a built-in pin-feed, you don't need a tractor for 8½ x 11" paper. It handles single sheets nicely, but envelopes can be a problem since they get caught in the pins.

My one complaint is that there isn't just a button on the front of the printer allowing you to switch to correspondence quality. Once you've set it up it's great, but you do have to know how to set it up. Okidata now offers step-by-step instructions for many word-processing programs.

Here is an economical printer which can give you both speed and quality. Unless you're absolutely set on a daisy wheel printer, I'd check this one out.

```
Here we have a sample of the OKIDATA
"Draft Quality."
```

Here we have a sample of the OKIDATA "Correspondence Quality."

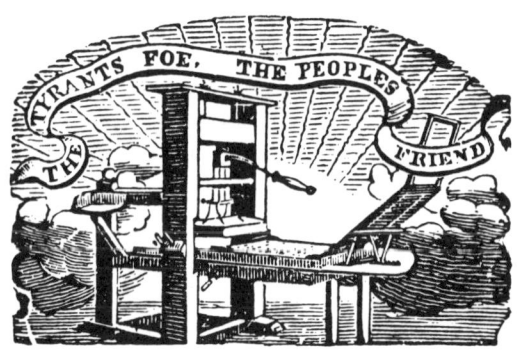

PERSONAL COMPUTERS AND THE DISABLED

Texas Instruments Model 855

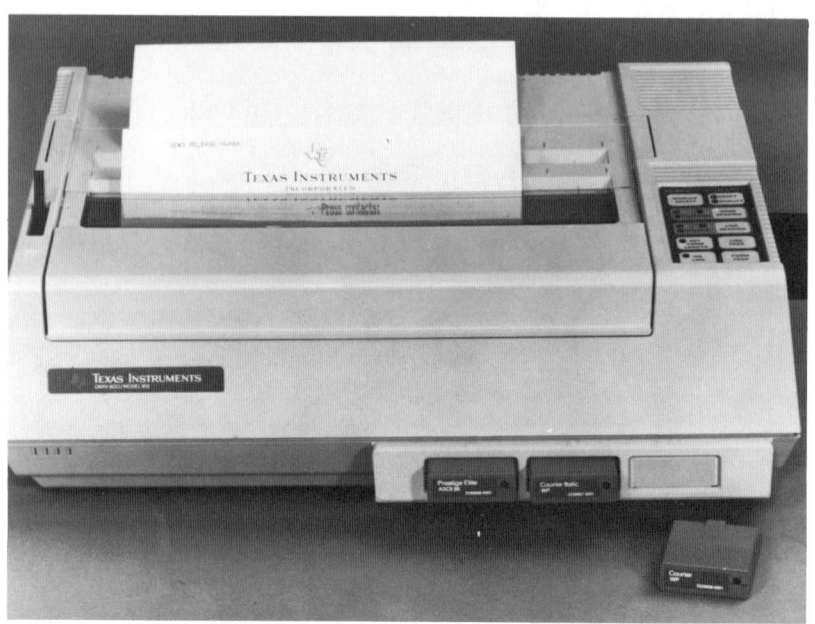

This is an innovative—and more expensive—dot matrix printer. What makes it innovative are its font modules, which look like palm-sized 8-track cartridges Instead of Barry Manilow songs, however, the font modules give the printer information concerning the type style (fonts). You can buy modules for such styles as Gothic, Courier, and Prestige. These modules are to dot-matrix printing as daisy wheels are to letter-quality printing. Three module sockets allow you to intermix three type styles at once.

Also handy with this printer are the command buttons on the top. If you want to change from 10 pitch to 12 pitch, or switch from draft quality to letter, you press a button. There is no need to imbed commands within your text. Of course, this kind of convenience is what helps make it more expensive.

The printing quality on the 855 impresses—the finest I've seen yet from a dot matrix. The print head uses 9 pins, and passes over each line twice. Upon close scrutiny, the larger letters still have a somewhat boxy look

Brand Name Buying Guide

to them, but most people won't notice. The speed is 35 characters per second, or, using the draft quality mode (which is horrible in comparison—not even good enough for notes) 150 characters per second.

```
Texas Instrument's Draft Quality
Using the 10-pitch Gothic Font.
```

```
Texas Instrument's Letter Quality
Using the 10-pitch Gothic Font.
```

Texas Instrument's Draft Quality
Using the 12-pitch Courier Italic Font.

Texas Instrument's Letter Quality
Using the 12-pitch Courier Italic Font.

Texas Instrument's Draft Quality
Using the Porportional Spaced Modern Font.

Texas Instrument's Letter Quality
Using the Porportional Spaced Modern Font.

There are (at press time) ten modules available, as well as a tractor feed.

I've had one problem with this machine. Inserting paper can be difficult. The front edge of my paper can't get by the print head without my loosening the platen and sort of tangoing the paper through. Each page, therefore, requires alignment, and I'm spending almost as much time loading paper as the machine does printing on it. Texas Instruments says they have fixed this problem, but check it out before you buy it.

The Model 855 lists at $935; $995 with a tractor feed. Modules are $40 each.

PERSONAL COMPUTERS AND THE DISABLED

Hewlett Packard Think Jet Printer

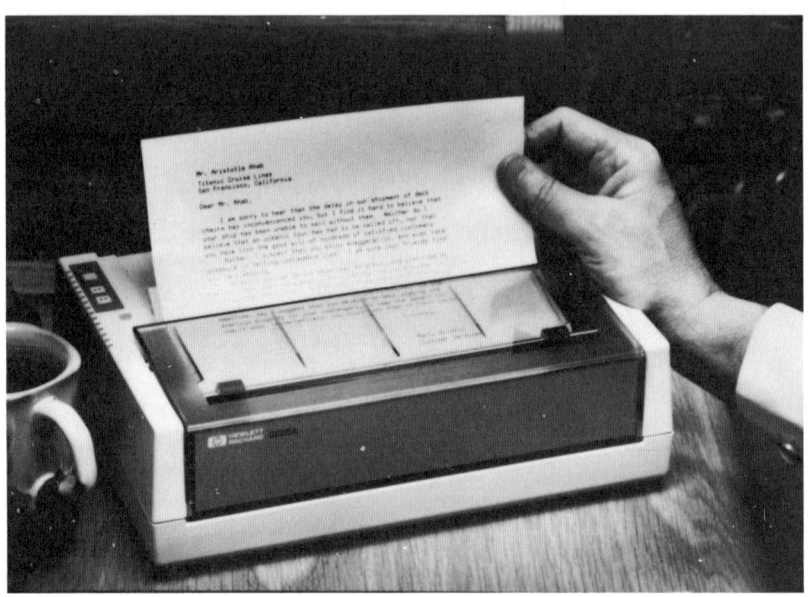

Ink jet printers are getting cheaper and better. They are not the panacea in the war between dot matrix and letter quality printers, but they're working on it.

The Think Jet Printer is a step in the right direction. Instead of hammering a character onto paper as does a daisy wheel or thimble printer, or instead of pushing pinfuls of ink at the page as does a dot matrix printer, the Think Jet Printer silently sprays micro-spots of ink. The finished product looks like high quality dot matrix printing.

The first few times I used the printer, I had to open the cover and stare at it in awe. It doesn't make any of the noises I'm used to hearing. There's only a small whir of the print head going back and forth and the ticks when the paper advances.

Near letter-quality can be had by double printing. While you can still see that the characters are made up of dots, the print is very clear, and certainly sharper than most dot-matrix printers. This high-quality whispers out at 75 characters per second. Draft quality comes at 150 cps.

Brand Name Buying Guide

Graphics are printed with an exceptional 192 x 96 dots per inch resolution.

All this is accomplished by a tiny replaceable ink cartridge about the size of a thumb. The cartridge lasts for about 500 pages and sells for around $7. Hewlett Packard has simplified the electronics and mechanics of this system so it should be extremely reliable. There are fewer moving parts compared to other printers.

Not all is perfect, however. It prints in a 12 pitch (elite), while standard business and manuscript work is in 10 pitch (pica). If you use this for your own drafts, it shouldn't matter.

```
Hewlett Packard Think-Jet Printer
This is a sample of draft quality 12 pitch
This is double-strike 12 pitch
This is the Compressed-expanded
This   is   Expanded   Expanded
```

Special paper comes with the printer, but "normal" paper can be used. Be careful, however: our letterhead, which is textured paper, did not work well, and inexpensive, thin form-feed paper tended to soak up the ink and look blotchy.

The printer's size impresses. At six pounds, it's only a little larger than a standard college dictionary, and could easily fit into a briefcase. This makes the best travelling printer I've seen.

The last but certainly not least amazing fact—the printer sells for $495. The sleeping giant named Hewlett Packard just woke up.

PERSONAL COMPUTERS AND THE DISABLED

Comrex CR-II/Brother HR-15/Dynax DX-15

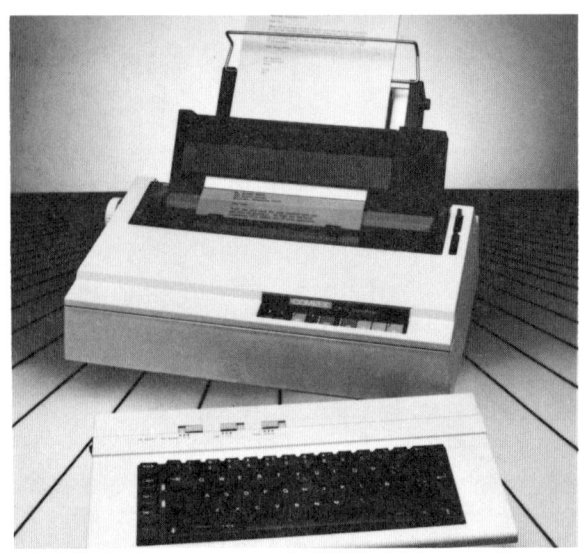

Though there are a variety of names, these printers are all the same—manufactured by Brother International. For a low-cost letter-quality printer (it lists at $599), it has many advanced features.

(For purposes of review, I'll call it the Comrex—the Comrex people were the most eager to help, and they sent the machine, while the Brother people were secretive and unresponsive. Brother wouldn't even give out the list price of their printer without a written request.)

The Comrex CR-II is a bi-directional printer rated at 13 characters per second. It's quiet, with a daisy wheel that is easier to remove than any I've seen. Its automatic paper feed does not scrunch paper.

Two features amaze me. First of all, there's an inexpensive cut-sheet feeder. Not only does it work well, feeding stationery sheet by sheet and depositing the printed pages on top, but also the price astounds: the feeder lists for $259 (and is usually discounted). IBM's cut sheet feeder for the Displaywriter is on sale for $1,095, and NEC's is $1,400. To pay a little over $200 is a bargain. To have one that works as well or better than its bigger brothers is a miracle.

Brand Name Buying Guide

For this price, you can avoid the expense of tipping stationery onto continuous paper, and you can avoid having the rough edges of tractor-fed bond. If you want a tractor feed, though, the Comrex has one: only $120.

The second feature that's new is a keyboard. If you want both a typewriter and a printer, then the keyboard, at $199, may be for you. It converts the CR-II into an electronic typewriter. You can even erase with it—the printer has the same erasing flypaper that the IBM Selectrics have. The advantages of a keyboard are not great unless you need a typewriter now and a printer later (after you buy a computer). You'll use your computer for most writing, but you'll still use the keyboard to type a quick envelope or to make small corrections without having to print out a new page.

The Comrex II has a 4K buffer, which works out to roughly two double-spaced pages. The "Copy" feature on the printer allows you to make multiple copies of a letter without tying up your computer.

The printer allows for 10, 12, and 15 pitch typestyles and will do proportional spacing, sub- and superscripting.

The only weakness to the machine is its speed. It's slightly faster than the Morrow MD-100 and the Smith-Corona L-1000, but slower than most higher-priced printers. With the cut-sheet feeder, though, just pack the machine with a load of paper and go do your shopping. For an inexpensive, letter quality printer that rates high in excellence, don't miss seeing the Comrex CR-II.

Brother HR-1 (also **Comrex CR-1**)

The Brother HR-1 (also sold as the Comrex CR-1) is a bit faster than the Smith-Corona L-1000 (17 vs. 12 characters per second) a bit quieter in operation, and naturally, costs a bit more. ($995, although like the Smith-Corona, tends to be discounted.)

The Brother and the Comrex will do double strike, bold, and underlining. They will not do proportional printing, sub- or superscripting.

PERSONAL COMPUTERS AND THE DISABLED

Bytewriter

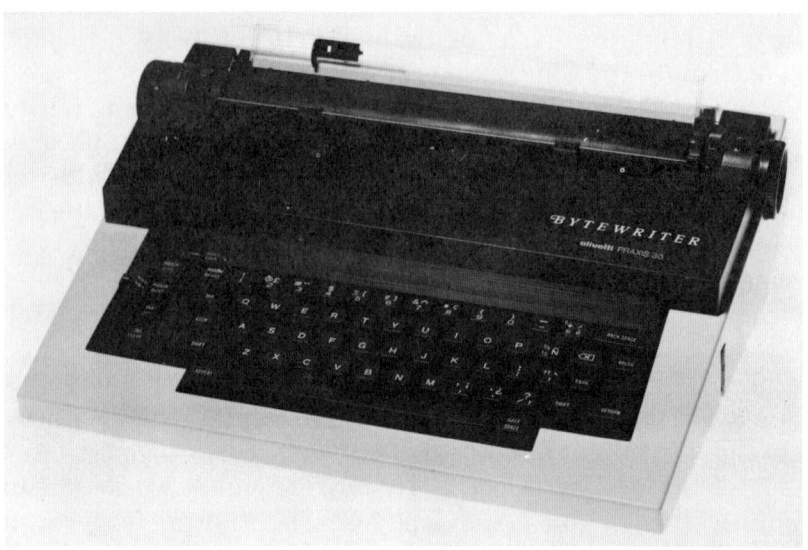

The Bytewriter is a converted Olivetti Praxis 40 electric typewriter with an interface that makes it a computer printer. It prints at about 10 characters per second. If you want a more portable version, the company offers a converted Praxis 35. Either model lists for $495. If you already own a Praxis typewriter, you can simply buy the interface for $165.

If you need a typewriter *and* a printer *and* you're on a budget, this would be the printer to get.

Diablo and Qume

While Diablo and Qume both make fine printers, if you're going to spend that much money, my suggestion is to buy an NEC. This is based upon the superior reliability of NECs over the years. The NEC is a workhorse.

If, however, you need a special feature offered by Diablo or Qume, or if you can get it for a special price, you will not be displeased with either printer.

Brand Name Buying Guide

Daisywriter

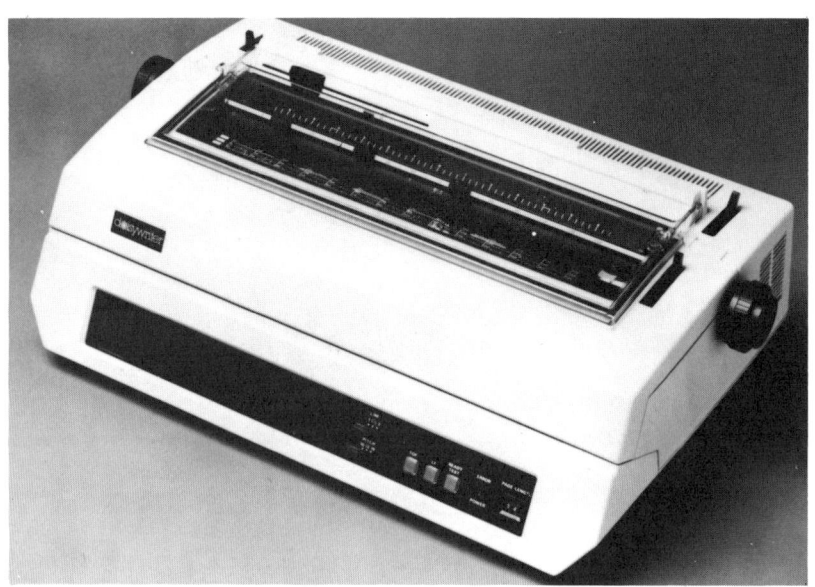

The Daisywriter will do true proportional printing, microspacing, superscripts and subscripts. The machine features a 48k buffer, which allows you to enter the file into the *printer's* memory. While the printer prints from its memory, your computer is free for other tasks. It lists at $1,495.

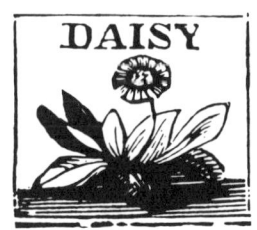

PERSONAL COMPUTERS AND THE DISABLED

NEC

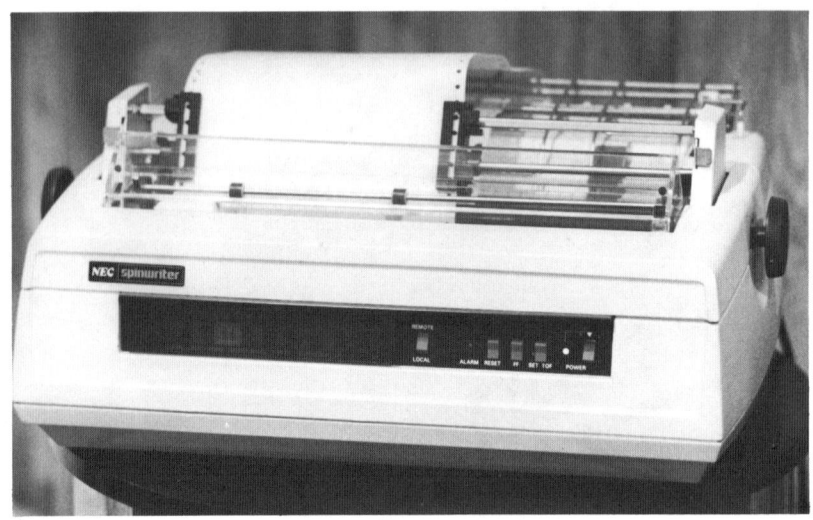

The NEC Spinwriter is a letter quality printer with an excellent reputation for print quality and durability. Time and time again I have heard unsolicited praise for the Spinwriter from people who know printers and have no vested interest in NEC or any other computer printer.

The Spinwriters print at a top speed of 55 characters per second, he fastest rated speed of any letter quality printer in its price range (around $3,000). A 35 cps model is available that has all the Spinwriter features except speed, and this retails for about $1,900.

Printers and software are the most frequently discounted part of any personal computer system. Even if a dealer does not give discounts on the computer he or she will frequently take something off the printer.

All the above NEC prices include a device known as a tractor. A tractor pulls the paper through the printer by little pins on the left and right sides of the page. This special perforated paper is known as **tractor paper** or **continuous form feed paper**. It's relatively endless so that page after page can be printed without stopping. It's good for rough drafts and for printing invoices, checks, and so forth.

Tractor paper is usually not of the best quality, but high-quality stationery can be glued or tipped onto standard tractor paper. This allows letter after letter to be printed without stopping to change paper after each sheet. This tipping process costs about $50 per thousand sheets and will work with envelopes, too. It's a good compromise between hand feeding and the expense of an automatic sheet feeder (about $1,500-$3,500).

If you don't mind feeding the sheets you print one at a time, rather like loading a standard typewriter, you can get the Spinwriter without the tractor and save about $200. If you're planning to use the printer for business applications right away, a tractor is recommended. If you might or might not use one eventually, the tractor can easily be added later.

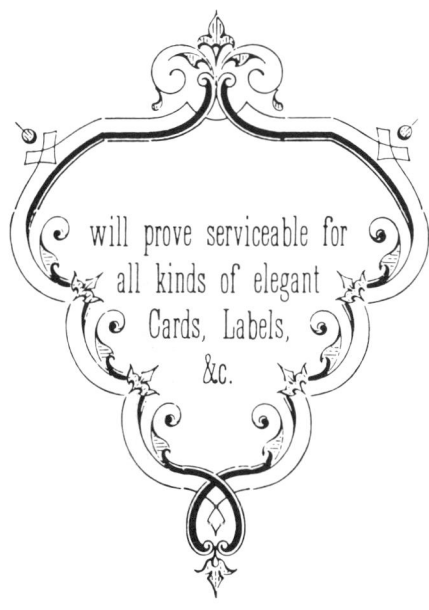

will prove serviceable for all kinds of elegant Cards, Labels, &c.

PERSONAL COMPUTERS AND THE DISABLED

Smith-Corona L-1000

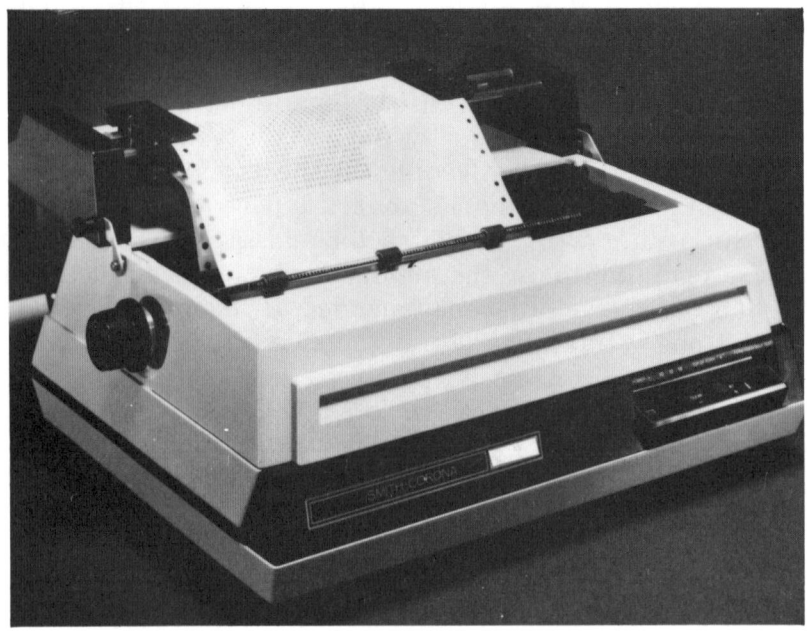

Those of you out there who are in serious need of a truly inexpensive letter quality printer should look at the new Smith-Corona L-1000. This is a solid little printer that weighs only 20 pounds. The print quality is good, with both underlining and boldface, and there is triple pitch spacing: 10, 12 and 15 characters per inch. The printing speed, unfortunately, is still a slow 12 cps using a bi-directional carriage.

The carriage and frame are very sturdy, and there's every reason to expect that this printer can stand up to a lot of form letters. The ribbon cartridges and print wheels are inexpensive and easy to replace. (It's all those years of making portable electric typewriters that's paying off.) The L-1000 also has both serial and parallel interface ports and an optional tractor feed attachment. There's also an input buffer of 570 characters.

The biggest drawback of the L-1000 is noise. It's hard to believe something so small can make such a racket, and this printer will shake whatever it is resting on without mercy—but it could be worse, and, the noise can be a small inconvenience if you need letter quality printing at a dot matrix price. The suggested list price is $545. Worth looking at.

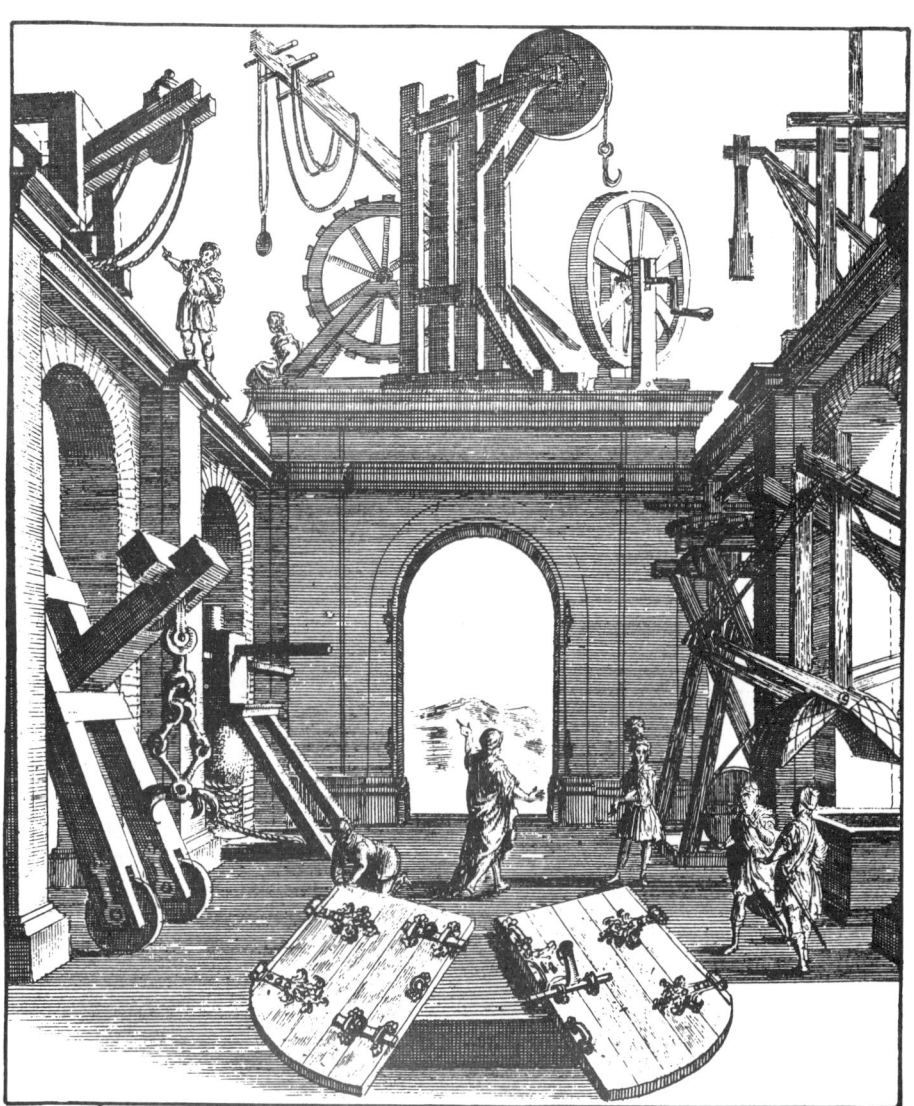

"And then we're going to put the printer over there in that building. Would you like to see?"

PERSONAL COMPUTERS AND THE DISABLED

Transtar 130

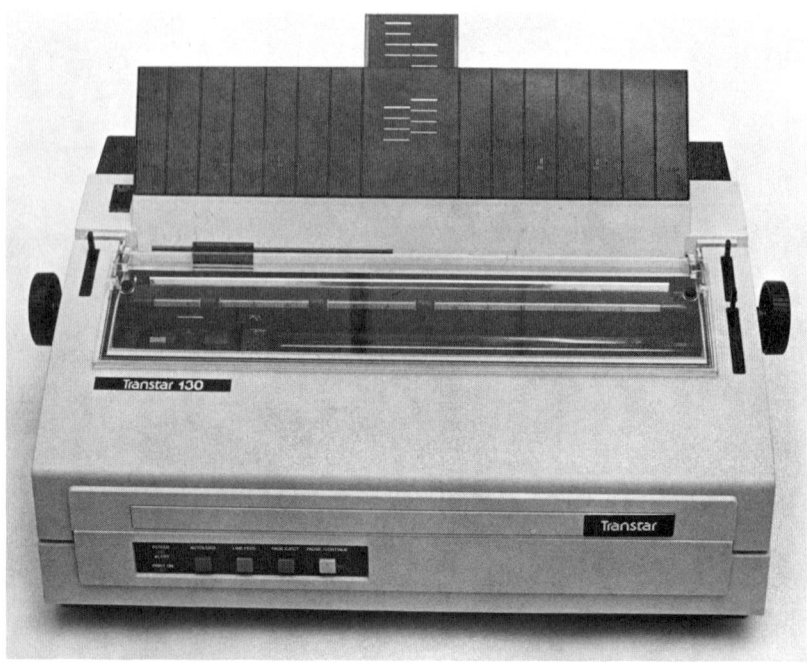

At $699 (list price though frequently discounted), you get an extremely sturdy machine with a wide carriage that will give sharp characters and prints at 18 cps. It is also one of the quietest printers around. The platen turns with silence, and, while typing, the machine sounds like a fast bird pecking rather than a Mack Truck trying to get in gear. The Transtar has features all good printers should have: automatic paper loading, pause, line feed and page eject. It does not have, however, a print buffer or bi-directional printing. A tractor feed is available for $149.

The printer supports proportional spacing, sub- and super-scripting. The platen knob turns when you turn it—no mickey mouse need for having to pull the knob out first as on the Comrex CR-1, et al.

The only problem I've had with it is that sometimes, when loading paper in with the autoload, a corner of the paper gets caught in a little horseshoe-shaped piece by the printer hammer. The autoload is adjustable, so I now have it stop before the paper reaches the horseshoe.

Brand Name Buying Guide

The Transtar printers are manufactured by Silver-Seiko of Japan, the parent company to Silver-Reed of America. Silver-Reed offers a similar printer to the Transtar 130 called the EXP-550. If you want letter quality at a medium speed and affordable price, check these out.

You should also know that Morrow Designs' MP-100 is the same printer as the Transtar 120 (and the MP-200 is really the Transtar 130).

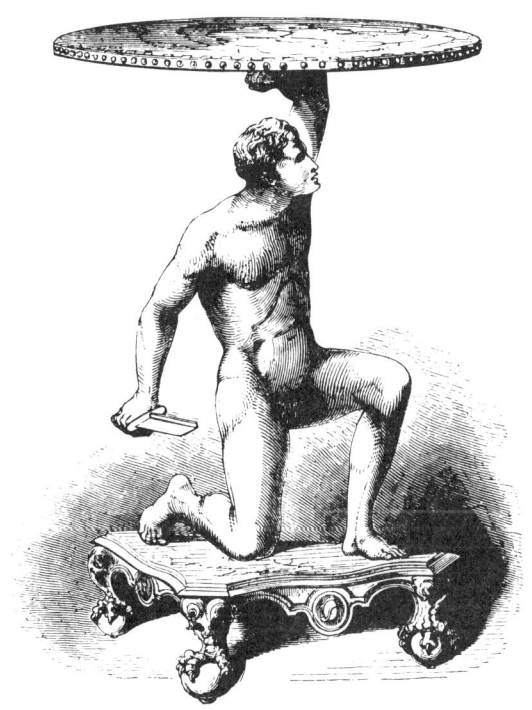

A printer stand.

PERSONAL COMPUTERS AND THE DISABLED

Hardware, Software, and Computer Services

This section is a glimpse at some of the hundreds of computer, computer-service, and software offerings designed especially for disabled individuals. For another good source on this subject, may I recommend the *Trace Center International Software/Hardware Registry—* **Programs and Modifications Created or Adapted for Use by Handicapped Individuals.** The registry is a notebook-sized, constantly updated listing of software and hardware items. The Trace Center is part of the University of Wisconsin, and can be reached at:

Trace Research and Development Center
University of Wisconsin
314 Waisman Center
1500 Highland Avenue
Madison, WI 53706
(608) 262-6966

Brand Name Buying Guide

For the Deaf and Hearing Impaired:

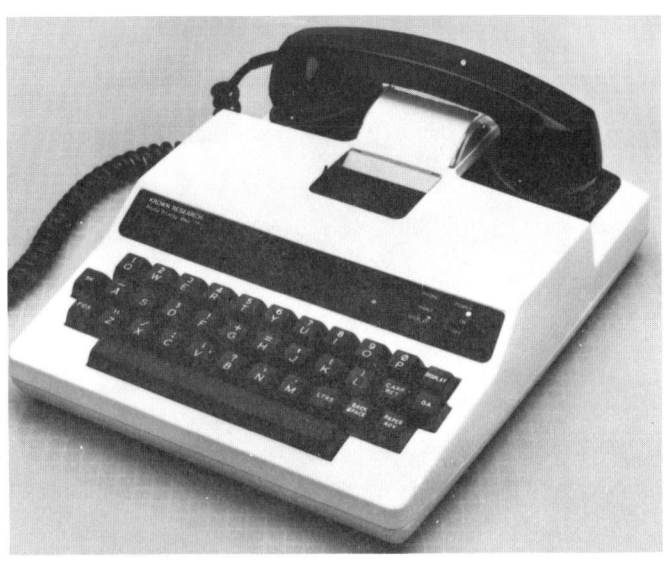

Product name: Baudot/ASCII Porta Printer Plus
Description: Telecommunications terminal for the deaf
Application: It allows a deaf person to communicate with computers or other terminals over the telephone. A one-line screen shows the user what is typed, and a built-in printer can be switched on to record the conversation.
Price: Baudot only/$599; Baudot and ASCII/$699

Manufacturer's Address:
Krown Research, Inc.
6300 Arizona Circle
Los Angeles, CA 90045
(213) 641-4306

PERSONAL COMPUTERS AND THE DISABLED

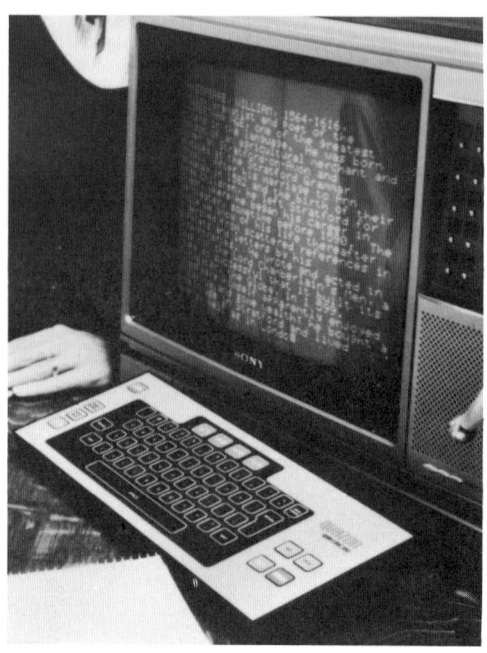

Product name: Quik-Link 600 Terminal
Description: A full-travel keyboard/modem
Application: A keyboard that will connect to a telephone in one port, and a television or printer in another port, allowing for communication on the road.
Price: $249.95

Comments: In development is the 600D terminal, which will send out in Baudot code as well as ASCII.

Manufacturer's Address:
Quazon Corporation
3330 Keller Springs Road
Carrollton, TX 75006
(214) 385-9200

Brand Name Buying Guide

For People with Learning Disabilities:

Product name: Academics with Scanning — MATH
Description: Writing Aid for the Apple II+
Application: Designed for severely disabled students unable to use a pencil and paper to do schoolwork. Problems and worksheets are first typed-in by the teacher/helper. The student then uses one or two switches to produce video and paper output similar to that produced by their able-bodied classmates. Appropriate for grades 3-7.
Price: $10

Manufacturer's Address:
Computers to Help People, Inc.
1221 West Johnson Street
Madison, WI 53715
(608) 257-5917

Product name: Math Disk
Description: Writing aide for math students
Application: Through the keyboard or other input device, the user can use an Apple II+ computer as a writing aid for doing math problems. A program within called "Math Drill" calls up preselected math facts for practice. The program has editing capabilities specifically to work on math.
Price: $10

Manufacturer's Address:
Computers to Help People, Inc.
1221 West Johnson Street
Madison, WI 53715
(608) 257-5917

PERSONAL COMPUTERS AND THE DISABLED

Product name: TutoMath
Description: Random math problems generator software
Application: This program generates and prints out random math problems quickly and efficiently.
Price: $20

Comments: A unique feature of this program is that an unlimited number of problems can be generated, no two of them the same. The type of problem and degree of difficulty can be chosen. Learning disabled children using this program will benefit from having a different math worksheet everytime, as well as becoming familiar with the computer.

Manufacturer's Address:
Parwane Paarsa
19 Fairland Street
Lexington, MA 02173
(617) 862-4141

Product name: The World of Counting
Description: Special Education courseware that teaches counting on an Apple II+ computer.
Application: This program is designed to interact with the student. It demonstrates, reviews, and reinforces with music and sound effects. Scores and response time are automatically recorded.
Price: $26.50

Manufacturer's Address:
Educomp Enterprises
Dept. 110
191 North 650 East
Bountiful, UT 84010

Brand Name Buying Guide

For People with Muscular, Motor, and Movement Disabilities:

Product name: The Communicator
Description: Single-switch text editor for an Apple II
Application: Allows a person who uses a single-switch input device to write.
Price: $130

Manufacturer's Address:
Prometheus Software
5 Devon Street
Lynbrook, NY 11563
(516) 599-1416

❦❦❦❦❦

Product name: Compudapter
Description: Offers a variety of alternate input to the Apple II computer.
Application: A special keyboard allows input to the computer through several types of touch switches, mechanical switches and sip and puff switches. Any combination can operate the system.
Price: $1,500 to $1,700

Comments: Installation is simple, takes about 20 minutes, and requires only a screwdriver. It does not interfere with the normal operation of the Apple or auxiliary pieces of equipment.

Manufacturer's Address:
R/M Systems
22903 Fern Avenue
Torrance, CA 90505
(213) 534-1880

❦❦❦❦❦

PERSONAL COMPUTERS AND THE DISABLED

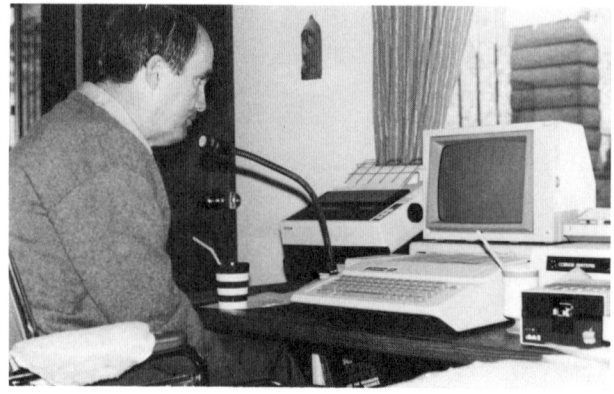

Product name: Computer Aided System for the Handicapped (CASH)
Description: Full-function voice-controlled work station
Application: Allows a person to operate an Apple IIe computer to full advantage by voice alone. The system includes word processing, electronic spreadsheets, data base management, programming, computer-aided drawing and 3-D modeling. In addition, CASH can control the environment, such as the telephone (dialing, answering, hanging up), lights (on, off, dimmer and brighter), and such electric devices as a page turner, window opener, electric bed, and television.
Price: $3,980 to $15,190, depending on optional accessories.

Comments: The environmental controls can work while you are within a program. For instance, you could be working with word processing when the phone rings. You would say "toggle interrupt" and then say "answer telephone," then when you're finished talking, say "hang-up" and "reenter," and you return to word processing, exactly where you left off.

Manufacturer's Address:
Voice Machine Communications
1000 South Grand Avenue
Santa Ana, CA 92705
(800) 821-2226
(714) 541-0454

Brand Name Buying Guide

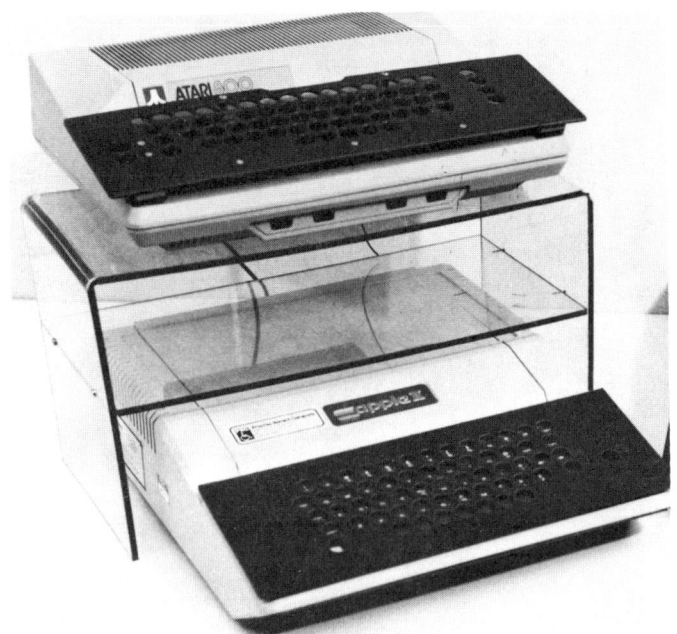

Product name: Computer Keyguards
Description: Keyboard guards for Apple, Franklin Ace, Texas Instruments, Epson, IBM-PC and PCjr computers.
Application: The keyguards fit over the keyboard allowing improved typing accuracy for individuals with difficulties in motor-control. A bi-stable mechanical rocker over the shift and control keys allows the computer to be operated by one hand, a mouthstick, or head pointer.
Price: $100

Manufacturer's Address:
Prentke Romich Company
8769 Township Road 513
Shreve, OH 44676-9421
(216) 567-2906

PERSONAL COMPUTERS AND THE DISABLED

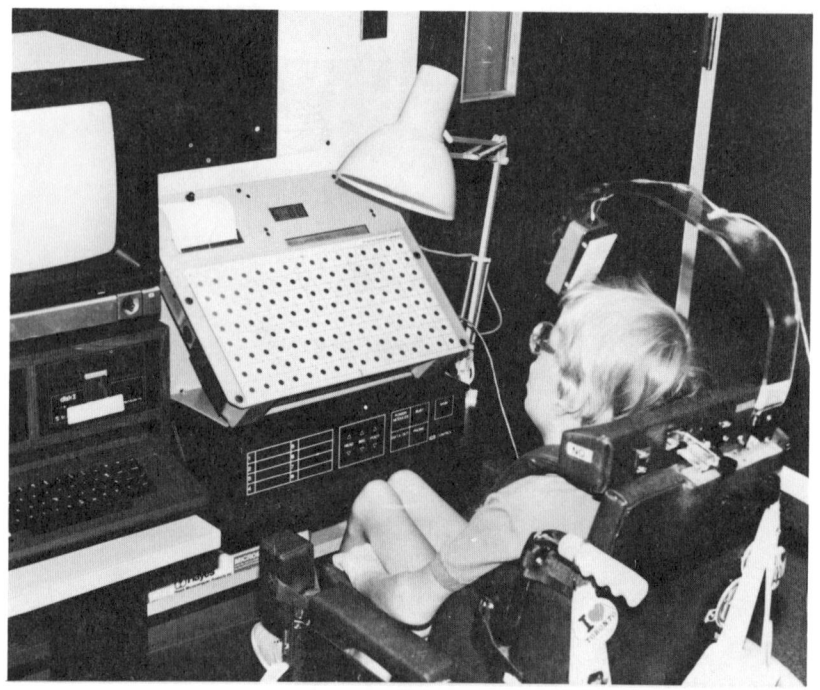

Product name: Control 1
Description: Environment controller
Application: This is a unit, operated through a computer, that permits people with severe physical impairment to operate various electrical devices in their surroundings. It provides for control of appliances, telephone, electric bed and other fuuctions such as television channel selection, door opening, intercom, power drapery control, nurse call, and more.
Price: $1,250

Manufacturer's Address:
Prentke Romich Company
8769 Township Road 513
Shreve, OH 44676
(216) 567-2001

Product name: COPH Computer Keyguards
Description: Apple and TRS-80 keyguards
Application: These well-designed, and easily removable keyguards are available from COPH-2 for the TRS-80 Models I and II and the Apple II computers. One finger, mouthstick, or headpointer typists are enabled to access the shift key function through a software program rather than a mechanical switch.
Price: $25

Comments: Software works with the TRS-80 Model I only. However, hardware or software adaptations allowing single digit operation of Apple keys that normally require depression of two keys are forthcoming.

Manufacturer's Address:
COPH-2
2030 West Irving Park Road
Chicago, IL 60618
(312) 477-1813

❦❦❦❦❦

Product name: Expanded Keyboard for Apple
Description: This expanded keyboard was designed to accommodate persons with a variety of physical disabilities, including cerebral palsy, motor or limb dysfunction, visual impairment, or learning difficulties.
Application: The keyboard simply replaces the standard one—installs in seconds.
Price: $695

Manufacturer's Address:
EKEG Electronics Co., Ltd.
P.O. Box 46199, Station G
Vancover, BC
Canada V6R-4G5
(604) 685-7817

PERSONAL COMPUTERS AND THE DISABLED

Product name: Handicapped Typewriter
Description: Single-switch typewriter
Application: Designed for severely disabled persons unable to use a regular keyboard. The Apple II+ computer together with a Silentype printer becomes a dedicated typewriter controlled by a single switch. Control of a scanning cursor selects characters from a screen-displayed picture of a keyboard. Includes a user definable word and phrase dictionary, a calculator, a telephone answering/dialing/directory service, and an environmental control system. All controlled by a simple, single-switch closure.
Price: $200

Manufacturer's Address:
Rocky Mountain Software, Inc.
214-131 Water Street; #210
Vancouver, BC
Canada V6B-4M3
(604) 681-3371

Product name: I-COM
Description: Single-switch control for computers
Application: This plugs into the serial port of most computers, and allows severely disabled users to control their computers with just a single switch. There is a built-in speech synthesizer.
Price: $2,500

Manufacturer's Address:
Intex Micro Systems Corporation
755 West Big Beaver Road
Suite 1717
Troy, MI 48084
(313) 540-7601

Brand Name Buying Guide

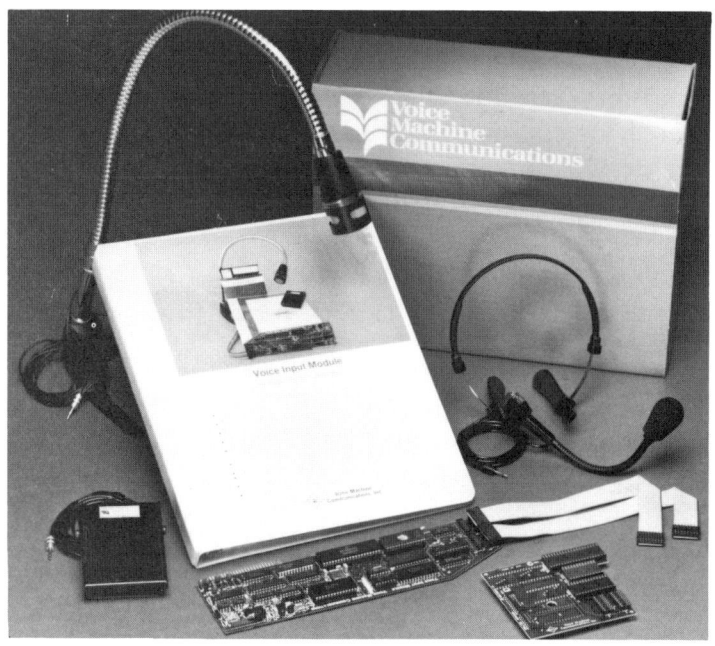

Product name: IntroVoice I & II
Description: Voice input system
Application: Allows user to command an Apple II, IIe, or Franklin Computer by voice. System allows a vocabulary of 80 words per application with 98% accuracy.
Price: $460 to $1,225

Manufacturer's Address:
Voice Machine Communications
1000 South Grand Avenue
Santa Ana, CA 92705
(800) 821-2226
(714) 541-0454 (California)

PERSONAL COMPUTERS AND THE DISABLED

Product name: John's Program
Description: Hello program for a joystick and the Apple II
Application: Developed for a C/P child who was able to use both joystick and buttons. Cursor points to program name and moves one step for each full up and down movement of the stick. Programs are selected by pressing button "O". Included are: modified Apple games, easier math, breakout, etc.
Price: $10

Manufacturer's Address:
Computers to Help People, Inc.
1221 West Johnson Street
Madison, WI 53715
(608) 257-5917

Product name: Micro Communicator
Description: Stationary communication aid program for the Apple II or II+
Application: A single keystroke by finger or mouthstick will display any sentence chosen from 60 or more programmed sentences which can be changed at anytime by the user for individuality. Messages of up to 100 words and phrases can be constructed for display or printout (optional) by double keystroke selections of built-in vocabulary which exceeds 1600 sentence-building words, phrase suffixes, and a 50-word list of user-changeable words and phrases.
Price: $48

Manufacturer's Address:
Grover and Associates
7 Mt.Lassen Dr. D116
San Rafael, CA 94903
(415) 479-5906

Brand Name Buying Guide

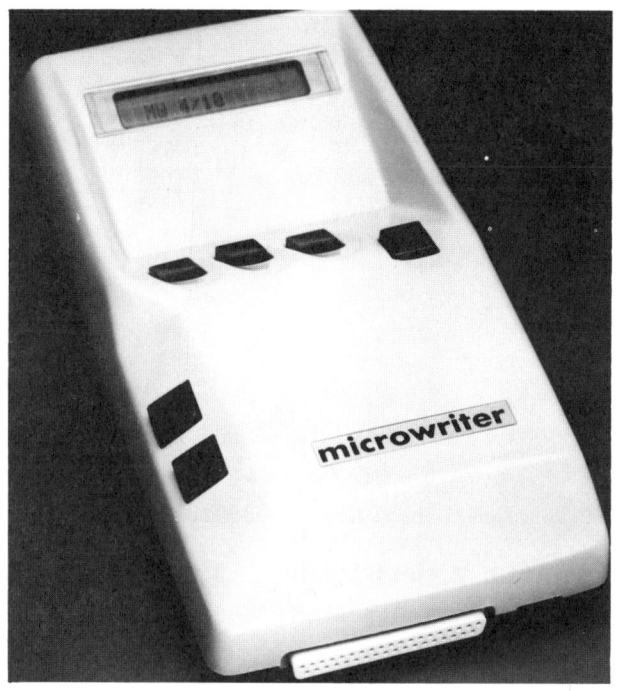

Product name: Microwriter
Description: A hand-held word processor with a six button keyboard.
Application: Weighing under two pounds and slightly larger than a hand, the Microwriter permits one-handed word processing. Can be linked to computers for a printout.
Price: $499

Manufacturer's Address:
Microwriter, Inc.
251 East 61st Street
New York, NY 10021
(212) 319-8602

PERSONAL COMPUTERS AND THE DISABLED

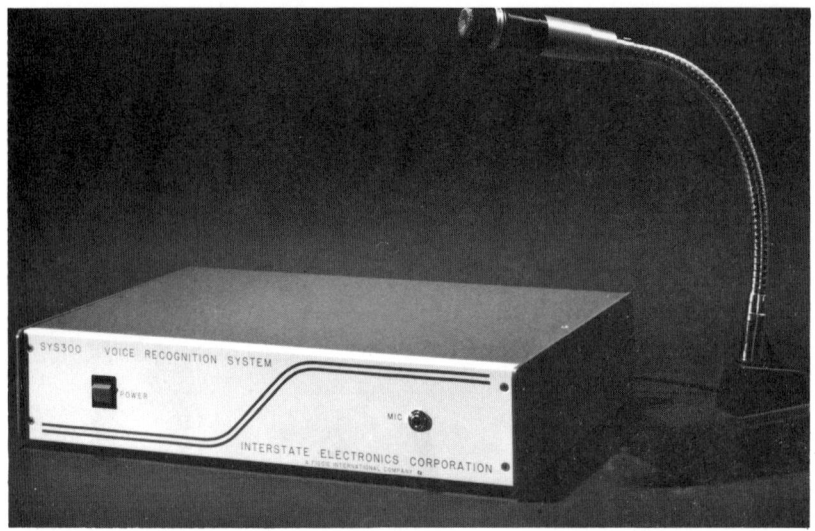

Product name: Model SYS300
Description: A self-contained, user-trained, speech recognition system.
Application: Allows user to command by voice most computers which have an RS232 serial port, utilizing a 200 word/short-phrase vocabulary with 99% accuracy.
Price: $1,995

Manufacturer's Address:
Interstate Electronics Corporation
1001 East Ball Road
Anaheim, CA 92803
(800) 854-6979
(800) 422-4580 (California)

Brand Name Buying Guide

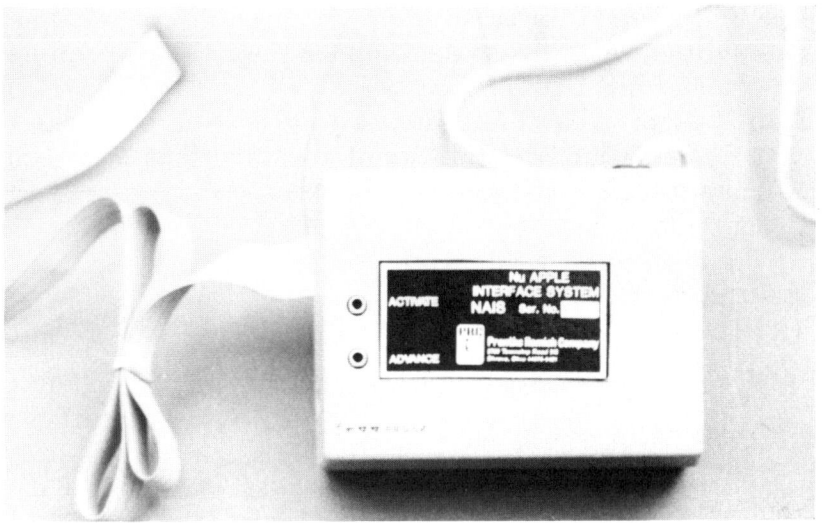

Product name: NU Apple Interface (NAIS)
Description: Text generation and device control
Application: Allows the user to build text one line at a time and assemble the lines into pages that are stored in memory. Pages may be saved on disk and loaded from disk. Two switches are used—one switch advances the selection cursor, while the other switch is used to activate the current selection. A telephone with modular cable connectors or a speakerphone permit telephone access.
Price: $468

Comments: An optional BSR Interface Card allows for environmental control functions.

Manufacturer's Address:
Prentke Romich Company
8769 Township Road 513
Shreve, OH 44676-9421
(216) 567-2906

PERSONAL COMPUTERS AND THE DISABLED

Product name: PC-Orator
Description: A software package for the IBM PC running under MS-DOS 2.0 or 2.1.
Application: Allows all input from PC to be spoken. Punctuation, capitalization, and other material can be spoken or silenced by the user.
Price: $495

Manufacturer's Address:
ARTS Computer Products
145 Tremont Street; #407
Boston, MA 02111
(617) 482-8248

Product name: Porta Micro Mate
Description: Computer stand
Application: The stand was originally designed for Kaypro computers, but works for many. Its best feature is that it has two large buttons on the front. One button turns the computer on and off, the other, the printer. Thus, for people without a great deal of mobility, it simplifies what should be a simple process of starting and stopping.
Price: $99.95

Manufacturer's Address:
SOS Computers
362 South LaBrea Avenue
Los Angeles, CA 90036
(213) 857-0371

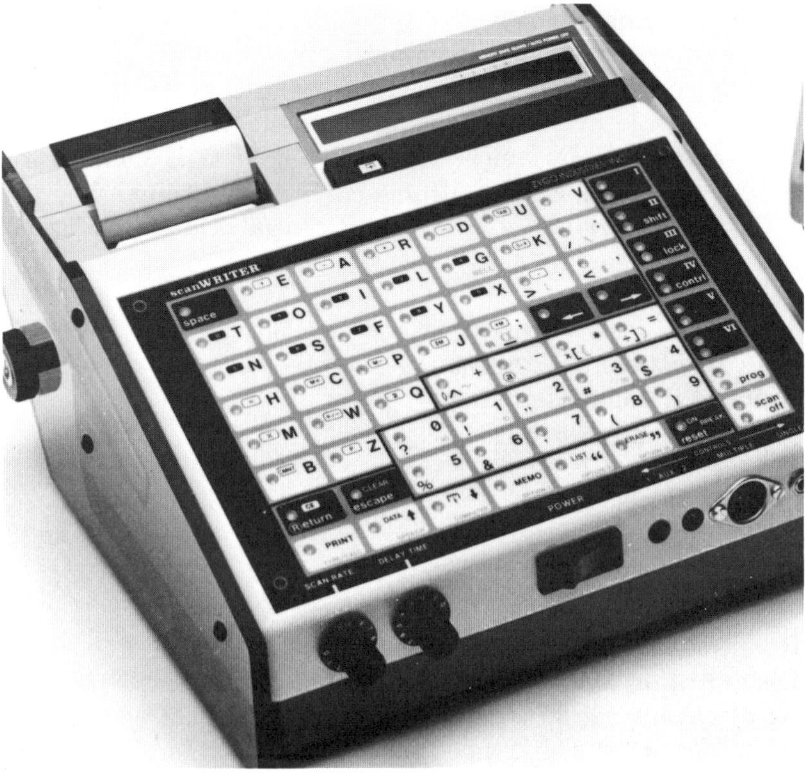

Brand Name Buying Guide

Product name: scanWRITER
Description: A miniature typewriter and calculator for the non-speaking, profoundly physically disabled.
Application: Word processing and calculating. When the scanWRITER is connected to a computer, it allows the user to do anything that can normally be done on a computer's keyboard.
Price: $3,800

Manufacturer's Address:
Zygo Industries, Inc.
P.O. Box 1008
Portland, OR 92707
(503) 297-1724

PERSONAL COMPUTERS AND THE DISABLED

Product name: Shadow Vet
Description: Voice entry terminal
Application: Allows a severely handicapped person to control his or her environment and program a computer by voice. Accurate to 98%, it holds a 40-word vocabulary with overlays of additional 40-word vocabularies available. Compatible with most languages.
Price: $599

Manufacturer's Address:
Prentke Romich Company
8769 Township Road 513
Shreve, OH 44676
(216) 567-2936

Product name: Target (no.2410)
Description: Mouth-Operated Keyboard
Application: Designed to operate the Apple II+ computer. Features a balanced mouthstick which is used to point to any one of 49 "keys" on a Target matrix (the most commonly used keys are located near the center). A slight puff is all that's required to activate a corresponding key on the typewriter or computer.
Price: $1,229

Comments: The operating height and angle of the matrix are adjustable.

Manufacturer's Address:
TASH Inc
70 Gibson Drive; #1
Markham, Ontario
Canada L3R-2Z3
(416) 475-2212

Brand Name Buying Guide

Product name: Technical Aids & Systems for the Handicapped (TASH)
Description: Ability switches, keyguards, keyboards, Adaptive Firmware Cards, environmental controls, communication aids, and software for the handicapped.
Application: Many applications—free catalog available
Price: $160 to $250

Manufacturer's Address:
Executive Distributors of America
15055 32 Mile Road
Romeo, MI 48065
(800) 521-5902
(800) 732-0617 (Michigan)

Product name: TETRAscan II
Description: Computer interface (electronic keyboard) for the Apple II computer.
Application: An auxiliary or alternate keyboard, designed for use by quadriplegics who cannot, under any circumstances, manipulate a standard keyboard. Allows for single-switch operation for immediate recall of words, phrases, and other strings of data.
Price: $1,950

Comments: Computer interface cards extra $200 to $400.

Manufacturer's Address:
Zygo Industries, Inc.
P.O. Box 1008
Portland, OR 92707
(503) 297-1724

PERSONAL COMPUTERS AND THE DISABLED

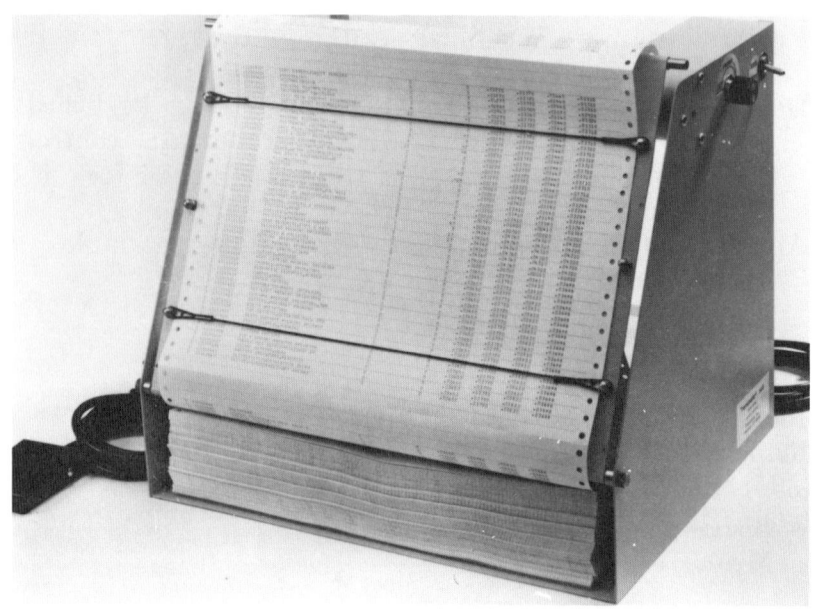

Product name: Transmatic Model 14.8 Printout Displayer
Description: A device for reading continuous form paper that will unfold, display for reading, and refold the paper.
Application: Where a person cannot hold a page up for reading, this device handily displays what has been printed. A single switch controls forward and backward paper movement.
Price: $398

Comments: Transmatic will modify the single switch to individual needs.

Manufacturer's Address:
Transmatic, Inc.
Box 186
Roxbury, CT 06783
(203) 354-3170

Brand Name Buying Guide

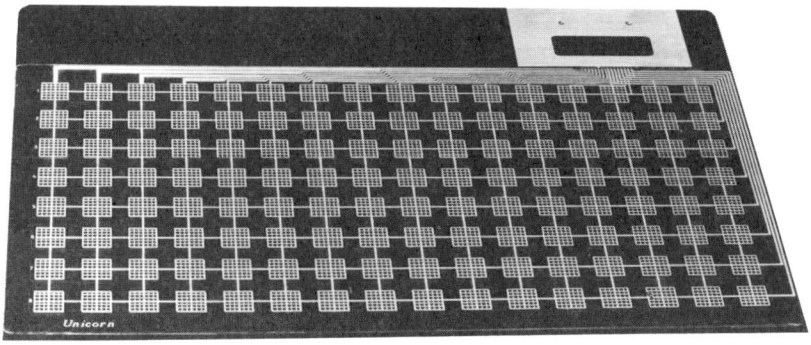

Product name: Unicorn Expanded Keyboards
Description: The keyboards permit disabled children and adults to use the Apple II, II+, and IIe computers.
Application: The 128 sensitive keys are large and widely spaced. Customization is performed easily. The keys can be programmed to hold up to forty characters each.
Price: $160 - $250

Manufacturer's Address:
Unicorn Engineering Company
6201 Harwood Avenue
Oakland, CA 94618
(415) 428-1626

❦❦❦❦❦

Product name: VARIETY
Description: Environmental controls, voice entry units, wireless data transmitters, keyguards, and more. Ask for their catalog for complete descriptions.

Comments: Prentke Romich is one of the leaders in computer accessory supplies for the disabled.

Manufacturer's Address:
Prentke Romich Company
8769 Twp. Road 513
Shreve, OH 44676
(216) 567-2906

PERSONAL COMPUTERS AND THE DISABLED

Product name: Voice Input Module
Description: Speech command for Apple II, IIe and Franklin computers (IBM compatibility scheduled by publication date of this book).
Application: Allows user to command an Apple (or compatible) computer by voice, with 98% accuracy. It operates with any existing Apple software.
Price: $920 to $1,095

Manufacturer's Address:
Personal Computer Supply
157 South Kalamazoo Mall
Kalamazoo, MI 49007
(800) 421-4157
(616) 345-8681 (Michigan)

Product name: Waldo
Description: Environmental control through speech command for Apple II
Application: Simple environmental actions, such as turning on or off lights, a television, etc., can be programmed into an Apple II computer and implemented by voice. It comes with a speech synthesizer—your computer can be used as an alarm clock or an electronic calendar, reminding you of whatever you need to be reminded of.
Price: $599—for handicapped individuals, $450

Manufacturer's Address:
Artra, Inc.
P.O. Box 653
Arlington, VA 22216
(703) 527-0455

Brand Name Buying Guide

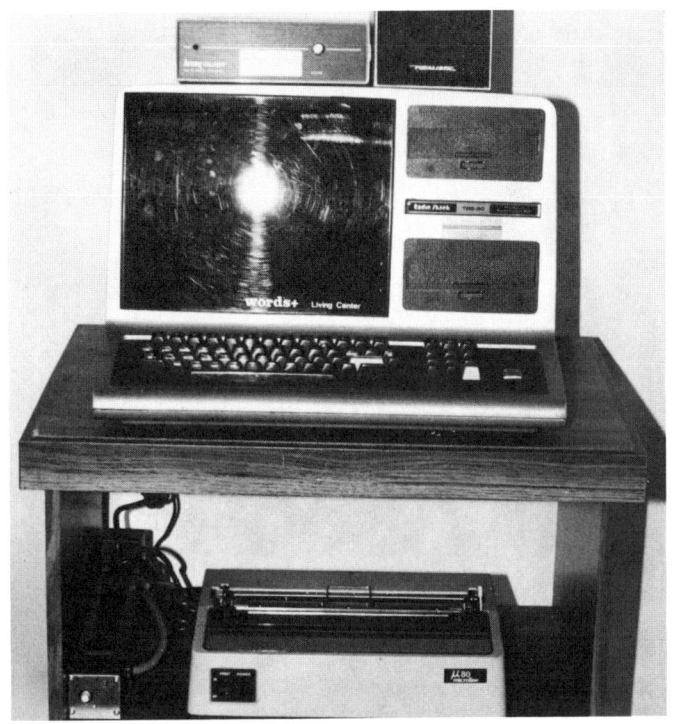

Product name: Words+ Living Center

Description: A combination of computer hardware and software that enables a severely physically handicapped person to perform a variety of functions with as little as a single switch.

Application: The Words+ Living Center can be divided into four categories of functions: 1) communication, 2) drawing, 3) entertainment, and 4) control. It comes with a Radio Shack computer, a printer, voice synthesizer, software, stand, and appropriate input devices.

Price: $2,900 to $3,500

Manufacturer's Address:
Words+, Inc.
Suite D 1125 Stewart Court
Sunnyvale, CA 94086
(408) 730-9588

PERSONAL COMPUTERS AND THE DISABLED

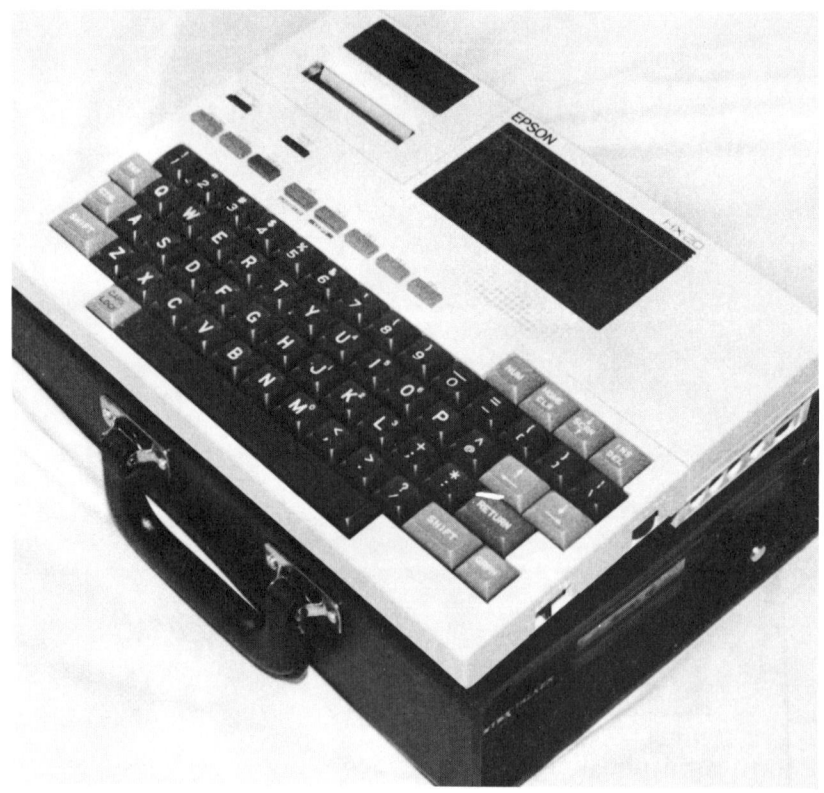

Product name: Words+ Portable Voice

Description: A specially outfitted Epson HX-20 computer that enables a non-vocal handicapped person to produce speech and/or printed output.

Application: Input to the Portable Voice can be from the keyboard, through a single switch using Morse code or scanning, or through an external switch/keyboard. Frequently used words, phrases, and sentences can be recalled by user-defined, numbered abbreviations.

Price: $1,675

Manufacturer's Address:
Words+, Inc.
Suite D 1125 Stewart Court
Sunnyvale, CA 94086
(408) 730-9588

Brand Name Buying Guide

For the Speech Impaired, and for the Blind and Visually Impaired:

(Many of the items particularly designed for the blind and visually impaired can be used by the speech impaired, and vice versa.)

Product name: The AVOS System
Description: Complete computer system for the visually impaired
Application: The AVOS system is an integrated hardware and software package, designed to allow a blind or visually impaired person to access personal and small business computing. It comes with WordStar, CalcStar, CP/M, a voice driver module, special word processing software, data base manager, checkbook manager, and games. The software will be updated for a year at no charge.
Price: $2,975

Comments: If you have a Zorba computer, the software to run a synthesizer can be bought separately.

Manufacturer's Address:
AVOS Inc.
1485 Energy Park Drive
St. Paul, MN 55108
(612) 646-1515

PERSONAL COMPUTERS AND THE DISABLED

Product name: BASIC Interpreter
Description: Software
Application: Menu driven, each section gives verbal commands and checks when needed. Affords the blind programmer the ability to proofread, correct, and edit their own programs. A new version using the Type-N-Talk synthesizer made by Votrax—now in the works—will have higher quality speech, and will be usable with any RS-232 computer.
Price: $15

Comments: Regional Winner in the Johns Hopkins 1st National for Applications of Personal Computing to Aid the Handicapped.

Manufacturer's Address:
James S. Schaefer
33 Jackson Road
Berlin, NJ 08009
(609) 767-2751

Product name: Braille-Edit
Description: A sophisticated word processing program which translates print into Grade Two (contracted) Braille, and vice versa.
Application: Enables blind people and sighted people unfamiliar with Braille to work together.
Price: $250

Comments: Compatible only with an Apple II+ computer.

Manufacturer's Address:
Raised Dot Computing
408 South Baldwin
Madison, WI 53703
(717) 523-6739

Brand Name Buying Guide

Product name: BTS-2
Description: A micro-based system that translates printed materials into Grade Two Braille.
Price: $7,995

Manufacturer's Address:
Triformation Systems, Inc.
3132 S.E. Jay Street
Stuart, FL 33497
(305) 283-4817

Product name: Cranmer Modified Perkins Brailler (CMPB)
Description: Braille computer terminal/printer
Application: Connects to many microcomputers, allowing a person using a conventional keyboard to print Braille. Capable of producing tactile graphics and maps.
Price: $2,750

Comments: One advantage to this system is that a sighted person who is unfamiliar with Braille could type in on a regular keyboard and produce Braille. Also, information from a database could be turned into Braille.
Manufacturer's Address:
Maryland Computer Services, Inc.
2010 Rock Spring Road
Forest Hill, MD 21050
(301) 879-3366

PERSONAL COMPUTERS AND THE DISABLED

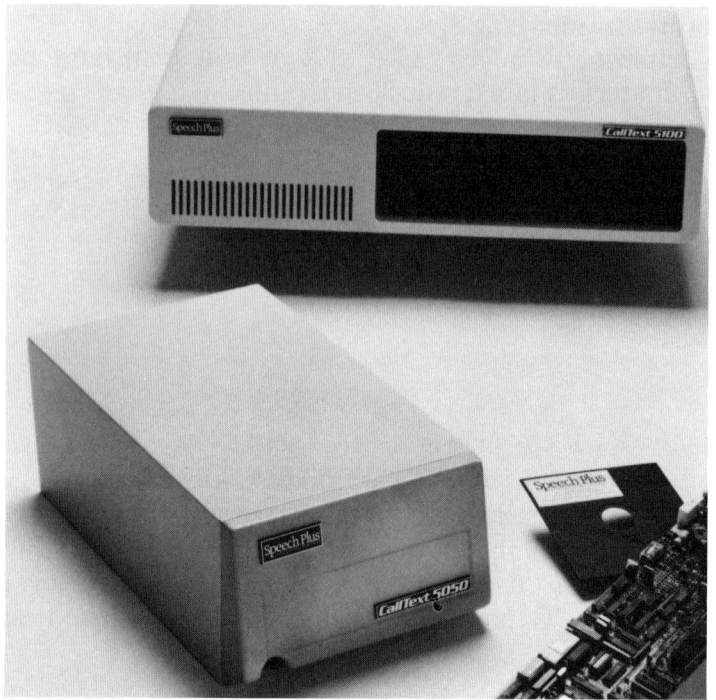

Product name: Call Text 5050

Description: Device for translating input from data bases into voice.

Application: Data bases can be automatically converted to voice for access by any touch-tone telephone. The Call Text can be programmed to answer the telephone, obtain text data from a host data base in response to touch-tone inputs, and supply the text data to the caller. Therefore, you could be at another site, call your computer, and pick up electronic mail or data base information.

Price: $2,975

Manufacturer's Address:
Speech Plus, Inc.
461 North Bernardo Avenue
Mountain View, CA 94043
(415) 964-7023

Brand Name Buying Guide

Product name: Cybertalker 2
Description: Speech synthesizer
Application: A text-to-speech device with a 4,000-character internal memory (expandable to 20,000 characters).
Price: $5,000

Manufacturer's Address:
Cyberon Corporation
1175 Wendy Road
Ann Arbor, MI 48103
(313) 994-0326

Product name: Deafsign
Description: Sign Language tutor
Application: Teaches finger spelling using video graphics on a Radio Shack TRS-80 Model III computer.
Price: $69.95/disk; $49.95/cassette

Comments: Allows student to interact a great deal; will give tests and interpret a typed word.

Manufacturer's Address:
Advanced Computer Services
Daniel K. Johnston
14 Lynne Lane
Frostproof, FL 33843

PERSONAL COMPUTERS AND THE DISABLED

Product name: DECtalk
Description: Text-to-speech system
Application: Enables computers to read text back to user by converting standard ASCII text into natural, human-quality speech. DECtalk has an unlimited vocabulary with pronunciation precision of over 20,000 words. Also allows input from touch-tone telephones.
Price: $4,000

Comments: DECtalk connects to computers via the serial port, just like a printer. (Naturally, DEC would be happy if you connected it to a DEC Rainbow or a DECmate word processor.) The DECtalk is the most sophisticated of all synthesizers. For one, it has many voices: men's, women's, and children's. What makes the DECtalk different from everything else on the market is that it contains a massive amount of linguistic rules in its electronic brain. This means that inflections are added automatically from punctuation such as periods, commas and question marks. "Gag me with a spoon!" sounds different from "Gag me with a spoon?"

DEC has recently developed word processing software for the blind to go with this unit. The software is called the "Talking Word Processor."

Manufacturer's Address:
Digital Equipment Corporation
146 Main Street
Maynard, MA 01754
(617) 493-6788

Product name: Echo II, PC, and GP speech synthesizers
Description: Text-to-talk device
Application: Converts ASCII text into speech
Price: $129.95

Comments: This is probably the least expensive synthesizer on the market. It is also the most difficult to understand (sounds like a robot with Wiener schnitzel stuck in its throat). Used often, I'm told, the synthesizer's voice soon makes sense. There are several companies making software for these units. The software will then allow specific machines to run a variety of programs, programs which send out more than just standard ASCII characters.

Manufacturer's Address:
Street Electronics Corporation
1140 Mark Avenue
Carpinteria, CA 93013
(805) 684-4593

❦❦❦❦❦

Product name: ED-IT Text Editor
Description: A line-oriented Braille text editor for the Apple II+ computer.
Application: The user enters Braille into the system from the computer's own keyboard which functions as a standard 6-Key Brailler, and the screen displays the Braille dot patterns. The system enables Braille transcribers to enter any Braille code, edit the material, and prepare complete 25-line pages for embossing. The program will drive a Braille printer with an appropriate interface card.
Price: $100

Manufacturer's Address:
Robert E. Stepp III
Station A, P.O. Box 5002
Champaign, IL 61820
(217) 359-7933

PERSONAL COMPUTERS AND THE DISABLED

Product name: Electronic Blackboard
Description: Braille translator which interprets Grade Two Braille or the Nemeth Braille math code to a TV monitor display.
Application: Intended for use by blind persons who need to present material to a sighted audience. This system was designed primarily for use by blind instructors/lecturers in a classroom situation where large ceiling mounted monitors are available. Operates on an Apple II+.
Price: $87

Manufacturer's Address:
David Holladay
Raised Dot Computing
408 South Baldwin
Madison, WI 53703

Product name: Grade Two Translator
Description: Software for formatting text on an Apple II into Braille
Application: A fast and simple program for high-grade translation into Braille. For a sample, you can send Raised Dot Computing a text file, and Raised Dot will process it using their program.
Price: $150

Manufacturer's Address:
Raised Dot Computing
408 South Baldwin
Madison, WI 53703

Brand Name Buying Guide

Product name: Intex Talker
Description: Text-to-speech system
Price: $295

Manufacturer's Address:
Intex Micro Systems Corporation
755 West Big Beaver Road
Suite 1717
Troy, MI 48084
(313) 540-7601

Product name: K Talker
Description: Speech synthesizer software for Kaypro computers
Application: Allows user to use a wide variety of programs which normally would be usable with speech synthesizers. Has a good review function which allows for easy review of what is on screen.
Price: $250

Comments: Demo tape available for $3.50

Manufacturer's Address:
K Talker Sales
P.O. 81082
Seattle, WA 98108
(206) 722-8599

PERSONAL COMPUTERS AND THE DISABLED

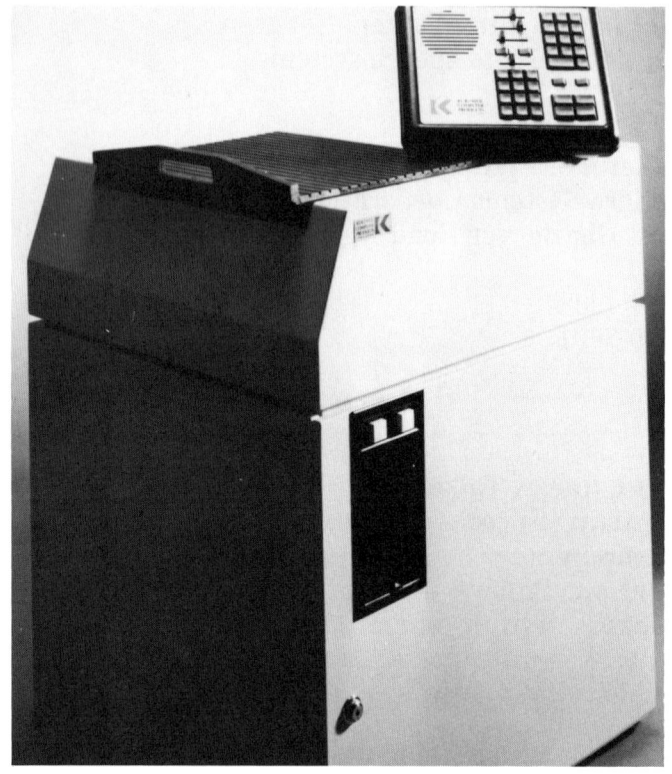

Product name: Kurzweil Reading Machine
Description: A compact system for converting ordinary printed material into high quality, full-word synthetic English speech.
Application: Allows for rapid access to the printed word. It also has a talking calculator within it.
Price: $29,800

Manufacturer's Address:
Kurzweil Computer Products
185 Albany Street
Cambridge, MA 02139
(617) 864-4700

Product name: Large Type

Description: A Special Typewriter program for any computer which has 4K of RAM and uses Level II or Model III Basic (such as, TRS-80 Models I or III, PM-80, PMC-81, LNW).

Application: Useful for poorly sighted individuals who have need of a simple, low-cost way to type in large print. Normal-sized print is also available. Displays keyboard entries on the screen in large format (double-width, 32 characters per line). When a line has been typed in, it can be edited or reformatted directly from the keyboard before printing. Since the program is not stored in memory, unlimited amounts of text can be generated without the need for more than a 4K computer.

Price: $19.95

Manufacturer's Address:
N.I.R.E. — Mr. Don Selwyn
97 Decker Road
Butler, NJ 07405
(201) 838-2500

Product name: LED-120

Description: A high-speed braille printer which can produce braille from a keyboard, from a computer, from magnetic cassettes or from almost any source of coded information.

Price: $14,500

Manufacturer's Address:
Triformation Systems, Inc.
3132 S.E. Jay Street
Stuart, FL 33497
(305) 283-4817

PERSONAL COMPUTERS AND THE DISABLED

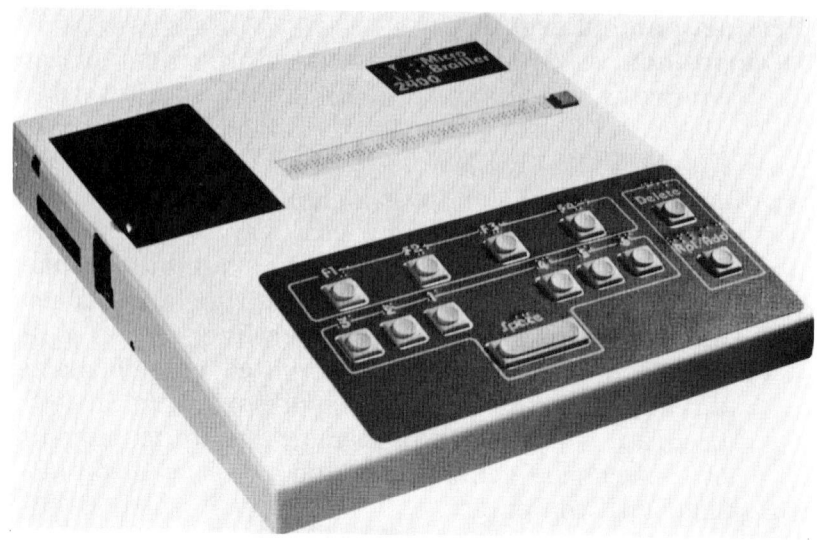

Product name: MicroBrailler-2400 Paperless Braille Display Device

Description: A portable word processor and computer terminal with a 24-character braille display.

Application: It can be used as a notebook, audio recorder, data processor and computer terminal. Specifically, you can use the MicroBrailler to drive a printer in creating Braille or standard print. You can use it as a terminal to contact data bases. It uses standard cassette tapes on which it stores data—roughly 1,000 pages of Braille on a 90-minute tape. This works as a lap-sized computer, but with a Braille input device.

Price: $4,850

Manufacturer's Address:
Triformation Systems, Inc.
3132 S.E. Jay Street
Stuart, FL 33497
(305) 283-4817

Brand Name Buying Guide

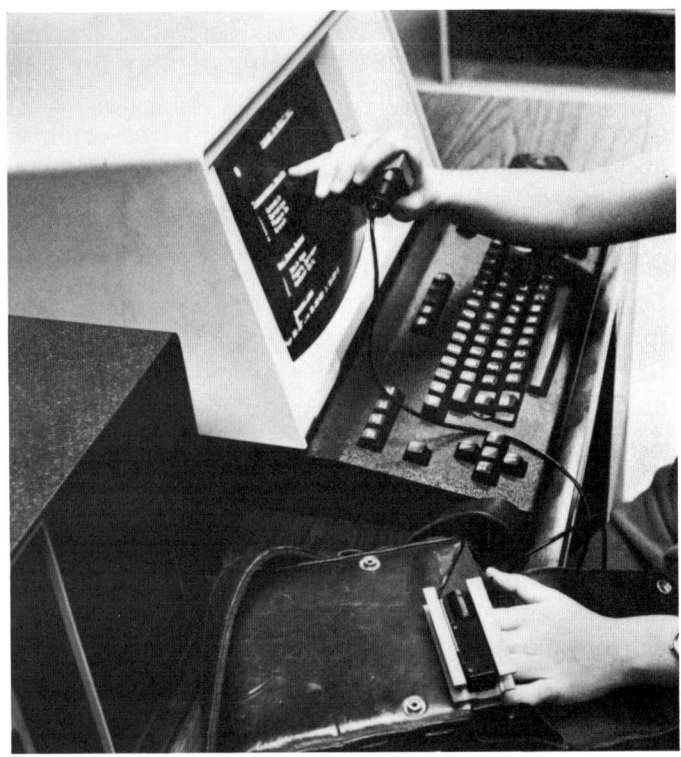

Product name: Optacon Print Reading System
Description: Unit which converts regular print into an enlarged vibrating tactile form.
Application: The blind person moves a miniature camera across a line of print, using the right hand. The index finger of the left hand is placed on the Optacon's tactile array. The user then feels the shape of the letters which the camera passes over.
Price: $4,495

Manufacturer's Address:
Telesensory Systems, Inc.
455 North Bernardo Avenue
Mountain View, CA 94043
(415) 960-0920

PERSONAL COMPUTERS AND THE DISABLED

Product name: PC-LENS

Description: Variable size character display for IBM and compatible computers which use MS-DOS 2.0 or 2.1 operating systems. Works with all line-oriented and screen-oriented software including spreadsheets and full screen editing programs. Uses the monochrome screen for output.

Application: Allows the standard screen of the IBM PC to be viewed at various magnifications. The user can move a "window" over the monochrome screen and have the selected area displayed in large characters on a colored graphics display. Updates the colored display as application programs update the monochrome display.

Price: $495

Comments: Runs on any IBM PC or XT that has both monochrome and color graphics display adapters. Any monitor can be used with the color graphics adapter.

Manufacturer's Address:
ARTS Computer Products, Inc.
145 Tremont Street
Boston, MA 02111
(617) 482-8248

❦❦❦❦❦

Product name: PC-SPEAK

Description: Allows a voice synthesizer to work with an IBM PC (with or without display)

Application: Most IBM software works on it, including Lotus' 123, and WordStar.

Price: $400

Comments: You may not want to use WordStar as a text editor. The what-you-see-is-what-you-get feature is great for sighted people, but a hindrance to those less sighted. A word processor that is format oriented is suggested.

Manufacturer's Address:
Solutions by Example
P.O. Box 307
New Town Place
Boston, MA 02258
(617) 244-5880

❧❧❧❧❧

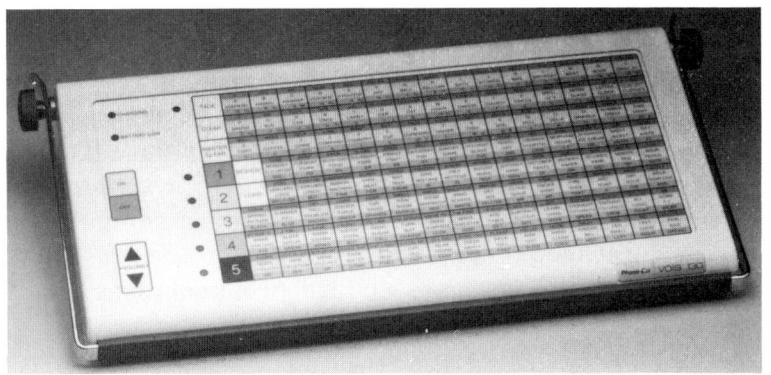

Product name: Phonic Ear Vois
Description: Speech output instrument that speaks for the non-oral person
Application: A portable device where the user strings together words and phonic phrases to make sentences.
Price: $2,995

Manufacturer's Address:
Phonic Ear, Inc.
250 Camino Alto
Mill Valley, CA 94941
(415) 383-4000

❧❧❧❧❧

PERSONAL COMPUTERS AND THE DISABLED

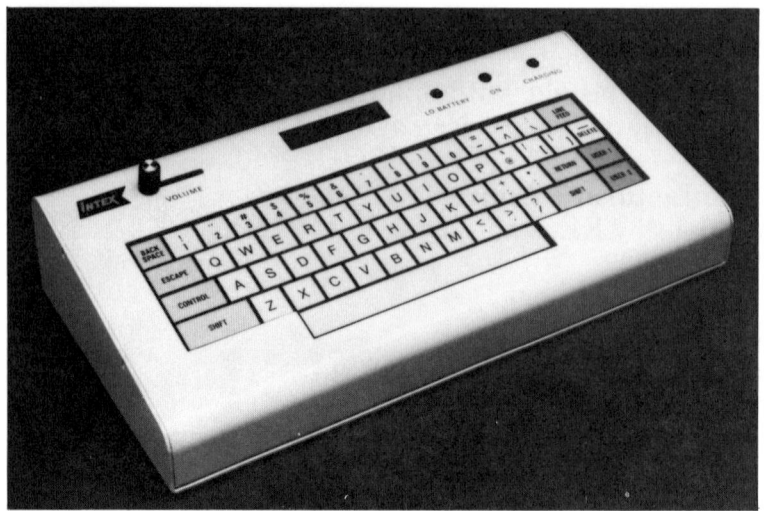

Product name: Speech Aid
Description: Talking keyboard for the non-vocal
Application: This portable, three-pound keyboard speaks whatever is typed into it, displaying the text on its LCD screen. The Speech Aid's vocabulary is unlimited. A unique feature to the machine is that its built-in memory stores the pronunciation of 5,000 words that have non-standard pronunciations, making for more correct sentences.
Price: $1,595

Manufacturer's Address:
Intex Micro Systems Corporation
755 West Big Beaver Road
Suite 1717
Troy, MI 48084
(313) 540-7601

Product name: Talk II
Description: Stationary Communication Aid for the Apple II+
Application: Talk II turns the Apple II into a highly versatile and flexible speech output system for non-vocal communication. It holds between 500 and 750 words and phrases, and from 60 to 200 sentences. Vocabulary is user-programmed. Outputs can be in the form of synthesized speech, monitor display, and printout. Messages can be saved while using the program for future use.
Price: $90

Manufacturer's Address:
G.Evan Rushakoff
Box 3W, Dept. of Speech
University of New Mexico
Las Cruces, NM 88003
(505) 646-2801

Product name: TextTalker
Description: Text-to-speech software
Application: This turns an ordinary Apple II into a full-function talking computer. It requires the Echo II speech synthesizer.
Price: $25

Manufacturer's Address:
Street Electronics
1140 Mark Avenue
Carpinteria, CA 93013
(805) 684-4593

PERSONAL COMPUTERS AND THE DISABLED

Product name: Total Talk II

Description: A talking Hewlett-Packard 125 computer terminal.

Application: Whatever appears on the screen will then be spoken. It easily switches from full word to spelled speech (one letter at a time), enabling word and character verification. It features an unlimited vocabulary, and the pitch, tone, volume, and rate of speech can be adjusted.

Price: $5,995

Comments: This is a terminal, with no disk drives. For disk drives (i.e. a complete computer), Maryland Computer Services offers a stand-alone machine called the ITS. It is a complete Hewlett-Packard 125 computer outfitted so it can talk.

Manufacturer's Address:
Maryland Computer Services, Inc.
2010 Rock Spring Road
Forest Hill, MD 21050
(301) 879-3366

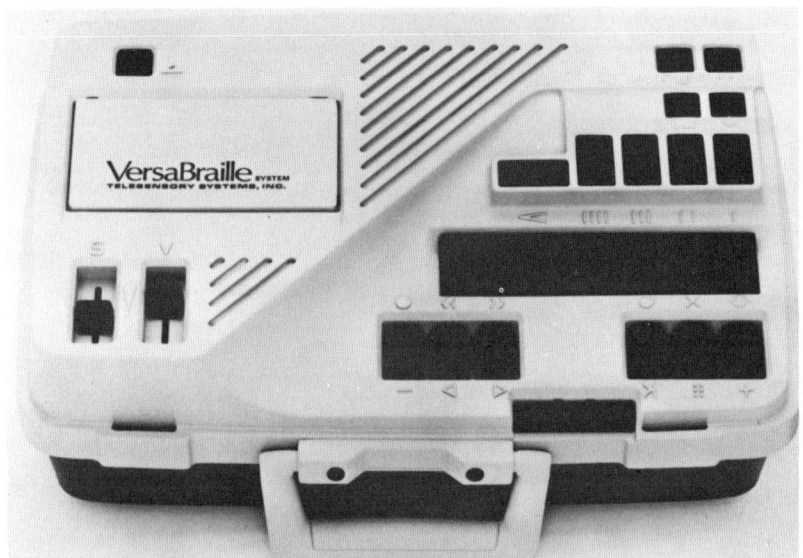

Product name: VersaBraille System
Description: Word processor/computer terminal
Application: A Braille information center that combines the functions of word processor, computer terminal, and read-write notetaker all in one. It's battery powered and portable. The VersaBraille controls are designed so that a minimum of keys performs all necessary functions, arranged into two functional groups—Braille reading, writing and editing; and text retrieval. Four hundred pages of Braille information will fit on one C-60 cassette.
Price: $6,750

Manufacturer's Address:
Telesensory Systems, Inc.
455 North Bernardo Avenue
Mountain View, CA 94043
(415) 960-0920

PERSONAL COMPUTERS AND THE DISABLED

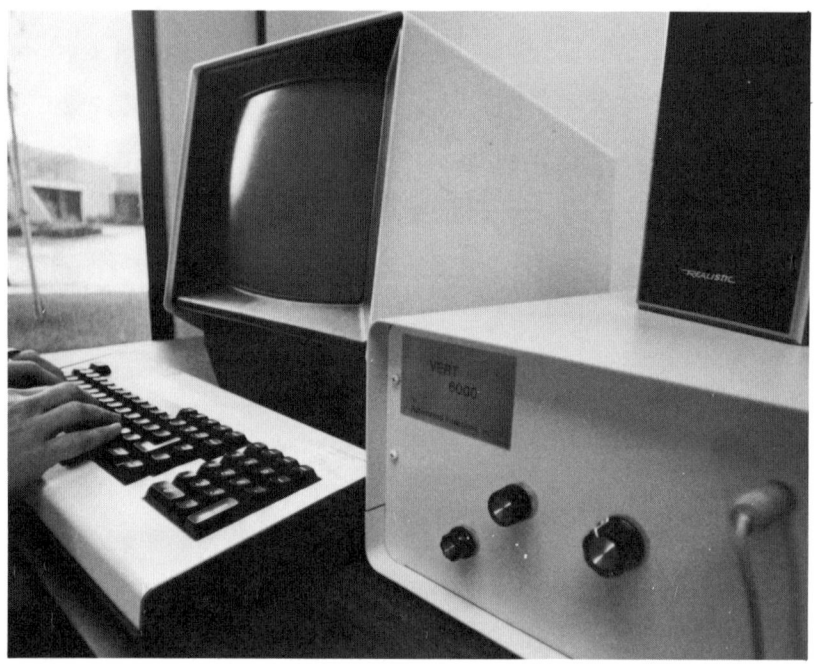

Product name: VERT 6000
Description: A speech device that gives verbal access to computers for visually impaired people.
Application: This is a device that sits between the host computer and the existing terminal, allowing the user to listen to what has been written.
Price: $5,995

Manufacturer's Address:
Telesensory Systems, Inc.
455 North Bernardo Avenue
Mountain View, CA 94043
(415) 960-0920

Brand Name Buying Guide

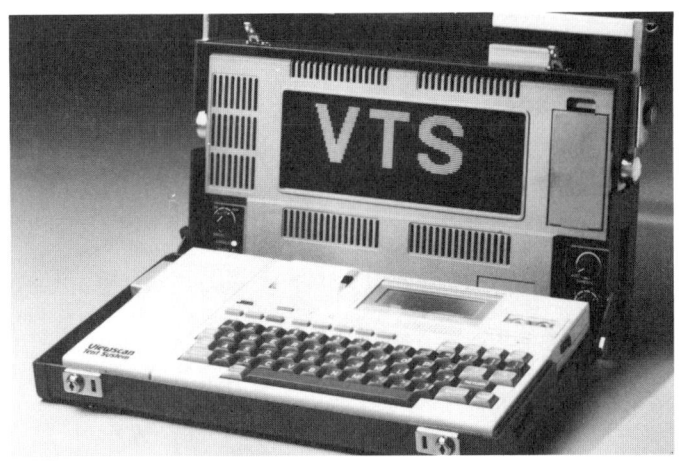

Product name: Viewscan

Description: Portable electronic computer and reading aid for the partially sighted.

Application: A miniature fiber optic camera on roller-guides scans text and magnifies it on a display screen. Viewscan can glide across any page and handle handwriting, typing, numerals, and different languages.

Price: $3,675

Comments: The heart of the device is an Epson HX-20 lap-sized computer. Its one-line screen gives an extra large display. The system seems to work well when used as a terminal or as an on-the-road computer whose information you download later. The camera part of it, though, seems to give some people problems. If the camera is not perfectly aligned at all times, the resulting distortion renders it nearly useless. The built-in software is powerful, and, being well-documented, easy to learn.

Manufacturer's Address:
Sensory Aids Corporation
Suite 110
White Pines Office Centre
205 West Grand Avenue
Bensenville, IL 60106
(312) 766-3935

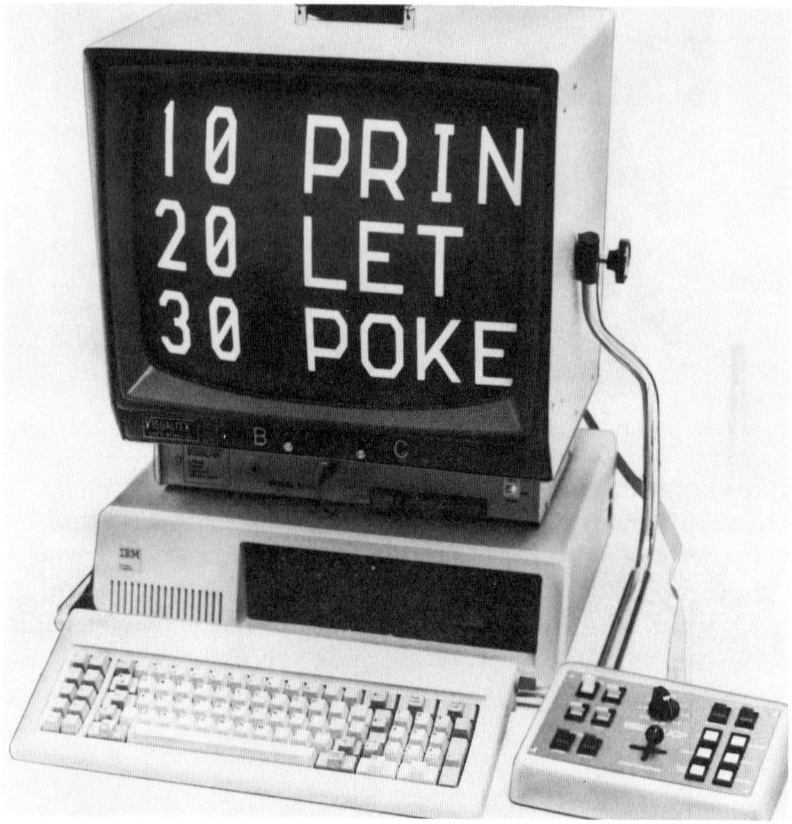

PERSONAL COMPUTERS AND THE DISABLED

Product name: Visualtek DP-10/DP-11
Description: Large print display processor
Application: Enlarges displayed words and data from two to sixteen times normal size
Price: $2,470

Manufacturer's Address:
Visualtek
Dept. MS-3
1610 26th Street
Santa Monica, CA 90404
(213) 829-6841

Brand Name Buying Guide

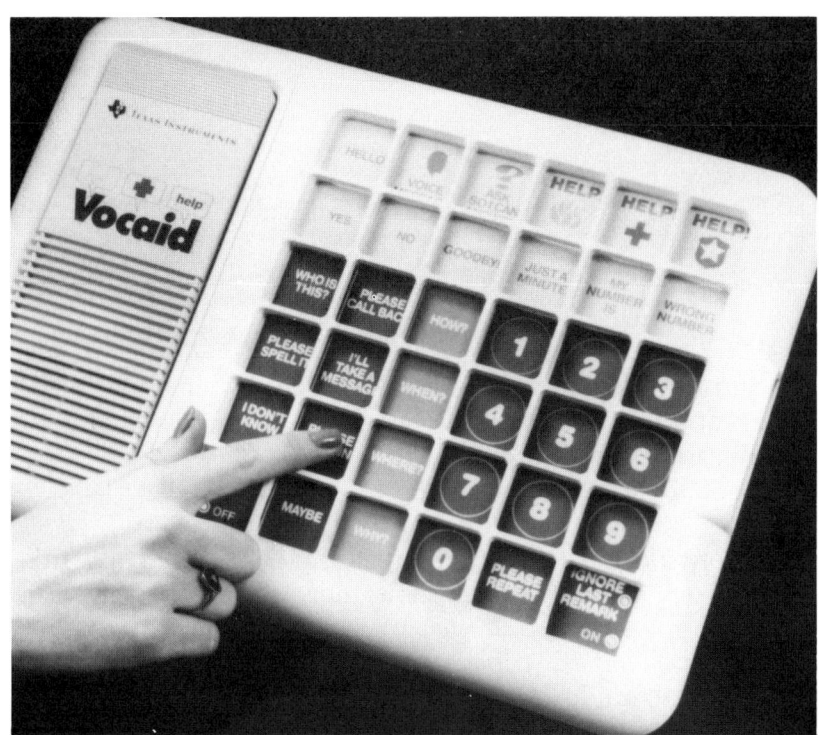

Product name: Vocaid
Description: Device for the speech impaired
Application: The user can type and store common phrases that need to be spoken, over the telephone or otherwise. "I am speech impaired and am using this device to talk," might be one phrase, or "I need a doctor," is another. This will also spell words out.
Price: $150

Manufacturer's Address:
Texas Instruments
P.O. Box 225012, MS84
Dallas, TX 75265
(214) 995-2011
(214) 995-5020

PERSONAL COMPUTERS AND THE DISABLED

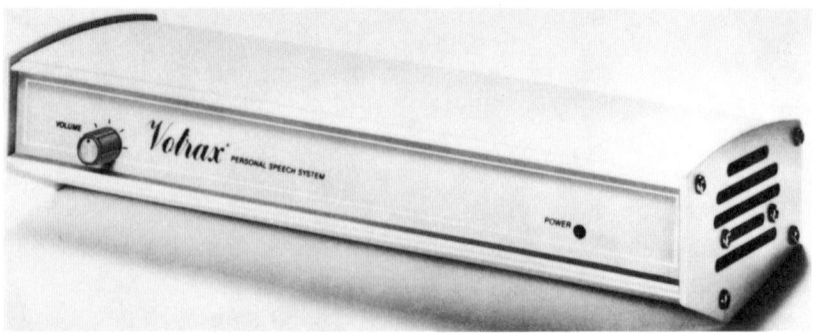

Product name: Votrax Personal Speech System
Description: Speech synthesizer
Application: Text-to-speech
Price: $295

Comments: There is much good to be said about this synthesizer. Though it is a little more expensive than the Echo-PC speech synthesizer, its pronunciations are a bit more crisp. That is, it is a step up in speech quality—it's a bit easier to understand than the other. Be sure of one thing before you get this or any synthesizer: Be sure there is software to run it for your particular computer. Software is being developed for many computers (Apples, IBMs, Kaypros, Commodores, etc.) but they are designed to then run specific voice synthesizers. Therefore, you have to match software to both computer and synthesizer.

Manufacturer's Address:
Votrax Inc.
1394 Rankin
Troy, MI 48083
(313) 588-2050

Brand Name Buying Guide

Computers

Here are special items or discounts offered by a few computer companies for the disabled. Their addresses are included in the Addresses section.

Apple:
Apple has a free pamphlet entitled "Personal Computers and the Disabled" (of all things!) which lists third party software and hardware which disabled people might use. They also have two grant programs for qualified organizations: The Education Foundation Grants and the Community Affairs Grants. These are not for disabled people per se, but disabled people can qualify. Contact Apple for more information.

Atari:
Many types of controllers are made for Ataris by KY Enterprises, whose address is in the Addresses section.

Commodore:
Their instruction manuals are available on audio tape for the blind or the motor disabled through: Recording for the Blind, 20 Roszel Road, Princeton, NJ 08540 (609-452-0606). Also, Commodore publishes a magazine called "Commodore: The Microcomputer Magazine," and within the magazine there have been articles detailing Commodore computers and the disabled. The articles have covered such subjects as special keyboards and light pens. For more information, contact the magazine at: 1200 Wilson Drive, West Chester, PA, 19380 (215-431-9100).

Digital Equipment Corporation:
Digital, as has been noted, manufactures the DECtalk speech synthesizer. Not only does it work on the DEC Rainbow and DECmate word processor, but on many other computers. This is the state-of-the-art machine, incorporating several choices of voices. $4,000.

PERSONAL COMPUTERS AND THE DISABLED

Lanier:
Lanier and the American Express Company have combined forces to create *Project Homebound,* a special operation which employs people at home to type dictation and sort data. (See the Resources section under "Business.")

Radio Shack:
Radio Shack offers a special model of the Model 100 where the shift and control keys stay down after being pressed. This makes it easy for one-finger or mouthstick typing.

Texas Instruments:
With Speech Command, the Texas Instruments Professional Computer may be useful for people who cannot use a keyboard.

Victor Business Machines:
Victor accepts requests for discounts, but only from institutions (hospitals, etc.) For the blind individual, Victor sells a read-out voice capability package that plugs into the Victor 9000. It is called the "Audio Tool Kit," and sells for $345.

Brand Name Buying Guide

Computer Services

This is a small but special group of people I've found who specialize in adapting various computers to individualized needs. Many of the companies already listed will also adapt their particular product to individual needs.

Adapt-a-Computer
17057 Adlon Road
Encino, CA 91436
(818) 906-0349
(Adapts Apples and IBMs to individual's needs—peripheral allows use of all software)

Legacy Computers
26356 Carmel Rancho Lane
Carmel, CA 93923
(408) 625-6562
(Customizes keyboards for disabled individuals)

Chapter Thirteen

Resources

rganized support is what this chapter is all about. No matter what the impairment, there are others in the community ready to offer information, rehabilitative services and advocacy.

Major groups with extensive networks of local chapters are listed by the type of impairment under "Associations." Smaller membership societies that focus on computers and disability are also included. Federal agencies are huge, and that may mean form letter replies or endless telephone transferring. Section II lists Federal agencies and programs in Washington, D.C., with key contacts specializing in funding and services for the disabled.

"Business" suggests major corporate programs for computer training and employment on a national scale. For details about university-affiliated research programs and courses of study, turn to "Higher Education." Section IV also includes a regional listing of colleges with substantial populations of disabled students. The next three headings deal with information: data banks; magazines, newsletters and newspapers; and books and book-related services, such as the National Library Service. For those with story ideas, "Media" will assist you. Contact the newspaper editors who write on health and/or computers. The last group of addresses lists state agencies specializing in government programs for the disabled community.

PERSONAL COMPUTERS AND THE DISABLED

I. ASSOCIATIONS
All Disabilities

AAAS=American Association for Advancement of Science
Projects on the Handicapped in Science
1515 Massachusetts Ave NW
Washington, DC 20005
Martha Ross Redden, Director
202-467-4400

Division of the professional association for disabled scientists and engineers. Advocacy and information services on education and employment in the sciences. Publishes *Resource Directory of Handicapped Scientists* and others.

American Coalition of Citizens with Disabilities
1200 15th St NW
Suite 201
Washington, DC 20005
Dr. Phyllis Rubenfeld, President
202-785-4265

Leading advocacy group with 143 member agencies and a quarterly newsletter.

ARPDP=Assoc. of Rehab. Programs in Data Processing
c/o Federal Systems Division
IBM
18100 Frederick Pike
Gaithersburg, MD 20879

Consortium of training programs for IBM/PWI projects meets twice yearly.

Boy Scouts of America
Handicapped Division
Box 61030
Dallas, TX 75261
214-659-2000

Local Boy Scout Councils in major cities provide information about computer programs for disabled youth.

CACHE=Chicago Area Computer Hobbyist Exchange
Micros & Disability Group
Box C-176
Chicago, IL 60606

User group for disabled computer aficionados.

COPH-2=Committee on Personal Computers & the Handicapped
2030 W. Irving Park Rd
Chicago, IL 60618
Tom Shworles, Chairman
312-866-8195

Nationwide membership and advocacy organization offering
free technical aid, computer adaptations, networking, hardware loans. and a library. Publisher of *Link-and-Go* (see MEDIA, Section VI).

DIGSIG=Disabled Interest Group of the San Diego Computer Society
1301 Dell Crest Lane
La Jolla, CA 92037
Milton Blackstone
619-459-8255

Resources

Goodwill Industries
9200 Wisconsin Ave
Bethesda, MD 20814
Steven Snyderman
301-530-6500

Over 160 autonomous Goodwill Industries nationwide involved in training, employment and rehabilitation of the disabled. Headquarters offers full range of legal, financial and management services to member Industries.

National Committee, Arts for the Handicapped (NCAH)
1825 Connecticut Ave NW
Suite 417
Washington, DC 20009
Tracy Quinn
202-332-6960

Teacher training and visiting artist workshops at 220 sites nationwide. Model arts programs funded by Dept. of Education.

National Council on the Aging
600 Maryland Ave SW
West Wing 100
Washington, DC 20024
202-479-1200

Regional offices in New York, LA, San Francisco and Atlanta with more than 200 membership organizations involved in Independent Living for the Aging (NVIOLA). NVIOLA publishes newsletter and national directory on member organizations. Other branches include National Institute on Adult Daycare (NIAD), National Institute of Senior Centers (NISC), and National Center on Rural Aging. Library facilities open to the public. Catalog of publications available.

National Easter Seal Society
2023 W. Ogden Ave
Chicago, IL 60612
Contact: Janice Minton
312-243-8400

Largest and oldest voluntary health agency offering rehabilitation services to disabled persons. 870 member groups and 2000 programs. Publishes the venerable *Rehabilitation Literature* and many others. For more information, contact the Communication Dept. These Easter Seal projects offer computer training for the disabled:

> **Crossroads Rehab Center of Central Indiana**
> 3242 Sutherland Ave
> Indianapolis, IN 46205
> James Vento, Pres.
> 317-924-3251
>
> Ten month training program for 8-12 students annually. 75% go on to full employment at an average income of $14,000 per year.
>
> **Du Page Easter Seal Treatment Center Inc**
> 706 E. Park Blvd
> Villa Park, IL 60181
> James W. Arrant, Jr.
> 312-832-2270
>
> Personal computers used in therapy.

PERSONAL COMPUTERS AND THE DISABLED

Easter Seal Goodwill Industries Rehab Center
20 Brookside Ave
New Haven, CT 06515
Malcolm H. Gill
203-389-4561

One year training program in computer programming on Yale University mainframes. 46 graduates since 1976. Applicants must have either management or supervisory experience, or college degree for admission. All disabilities served. 90% job placement ratio.

These Easter Seal summer camps have computer programs:

Camp Fair Lee Manor
Easter Seal Society of Del Mar
2705 Baynard Blvd
Wilmington, DE 19802
Sandra Kother
302-658-6417

IBM donated 20 computers for these two-week sessions at the residential camp.

Camp Sunnyside
Iowa Easter Seal Society
Box 4002
Des Moines, IA 50333
Ed Stracke
515-298-1933

Easter Seal Handicamp
Colorado Easter Seal Society
609 W. Littleton Blvd
Littleton, CO 80120
Todd Lowthar
303-795-2016

Hemlocks Outdoor Education Center
Jones St
Amston, CT 06231
Carl Larson
203-228-9496

NOD=National Organization on Disability
2100 Pennsylvania Ave NW
Suite 232
Washington, DC 20037
Jean Fitzgerald
202-293-5960

Major information service linking up 400 organizations and 1200 community projects nationwide. Helps form local committees to encourage public awareness, develop job programs, etc. Publications: *Report*, quarterly newsletter for the public; *Update*, newsletter designed for participants in community partnership programs; *Liaison Manual*, guide for community organizers in the disability field.

Parents' Campaign for Handicapped Children & Youth
1201 16th St NW
Washington, DC 20036

Resources

Visual, Hearing and Speech Impairments

Alexander Graham Bell Association for the Deaf
3417 Volta Place NW
Washington, DC 20007
202-337-5220

Involved primarily with hearing-impaired children since 1890. Deaf adults also served. Publisher of *Volta Review*. Lending library available.

American Council of the Blind
1211 Connecticut Ave NW
Suite 506
Washington, DC 20036
800-424-8666

Advocacy and information services. Special interest affiliate:

Visually Impaired Data Processors International
Lee Brown, Director
16205 Fantasia Dr
Tampa, FL 33624

American Foundation for the Blind
15 West 16th St
New York, NY 10011
212-620-2000

Manufacture and sales of more than 400 devices to aid the blind. Social and technology research for the visually impaired. Produces 400+ talking books for National Library Service for the Blind. Many publications including *Journal of Visual Impairment and Blindness*. Film rentals. 30,000+ library collection.

American Speech-Language-Hearing Association
10801 Rockville Pike
Rockville, MD 20852
301-897-5700

Professional association that certifies therapists. 46 state affiliates offer extensive information services on employment and education. Publications include monthly magazine, *Asha*.

Blinded Veterans Association
1735 De Sales St NW
Washington, DC 20036
202-347-4010

Blind vets offer rehabilitation services to other blind veterans thru Field Service Program. Job development programs, advocacy and recorded newsletter available to members in 35 regional units.

Braille Institute
741 N. Vermont Ave
Los Angeles, CA 90029
Francis Daniels
213-663-1111

Sensory Aids Demonstration Center and extensive publications program includes *Braille Mirror*.

PERSONAL COMPUTERS AND THE DISABLED

Convention of American Instructors of the Deaf
Conference of Executives of American Schools for the Deaf
5034 Wisconsin Ave NW
Washington, DC 20016

Professional associations of the deaf community and publisher of *American Annals of the Deaf*. Instructional certification, media captioning, regional workshops.

Helen Keller National Center
111 Middle Neck Rd
Sands Point, NY 11050
516-944-8900

Nine regional offices funded by Congress serve the deaf-blind. Residential training in life and job skills. Design of sensory aids, training for professionals and demographic research. *NAT CENT NEWS* is their newsletter and "Raising the Curtain", a captioned film.

International Association of Laryngectomees
c/o American Cancer Society
777 Third Avenue
New York, NY 10017
212-371-2900

300 clubs sponsored by American Cancer Society publish bimonthly newsletter, registry of instructors, annual directory and a resource book for rehabilitation.

International Association of Parents of the Deaf
814 Thayer Avenue
Silver Spring, MD 20910
301-585-5400

Clearinghouse on information exchange through 77 affiliates nationwide.

Junior National Association of the Deaf
814 Thayer Avenue
Silver Spring, MD 20910
301-587-1788

Encourages leadership among deaf youth with 107 school programs nationwide, summer camps, awards and quarterly magazine.

NAVH=National Association for Visually Handicapped
305 East 24th Street, 17-C
New York, NY 10010
212-889-3141

Information clearinghouse also with office in San Francisco. Free loaner library, sale and display of visual aids, newsletter for children. Discussion groups, advocacy and counseling.

National Association of the Deaf
814 Thayer Avenue
Silver Spring, MD 20910
301-587-1788

Full service consumer organization with 49 state affiliates. Extensive information resources: 15,000 book library, legal and statistical research, and direct services referral. Educational programs include sign language instruction, curriculum development, professional certification, and media captioning. Publishes wide

Resources

variety of books, including *Sign for Computer Technology* handbook. Journals: *The Deaf American*, monthly magazine; *The Broadcaster*, monthly legal newspaper; and a newsletter on state issues.

National Federation for the Blind
Committee on Evaluation of Technology
1800 Johnston Street
Baltimore, MD 21230
301-659-9314

400 chapters nationwide active in legislative advocacy. National Blindness Information Center offers assistance by phone or mail. Publishes *Braille Monitor* and 50 other publications.

Sensory Aids Foundation
399 Sherman Avenue, Suite 12
Palo Alto, CA 94306
415-329-0430

Encourages companies to hire the disabled by offering employer orientations to sensory aids equipment. Training programs for rehabilitation professionals. Research on communication aids for the deaf. Publisher of *Sensory Aids for Employment of Blind and Visually Impaired Persons*, resource guide with 130 devices.

Telecommunications for the Deaf
7108 27th Road North
Arlington, VA 22213

Publisher of *International Telephone Directory of the Deaf*.

Learning and Emotional Disabilities

AAMD=American Association on Mental Deficiency
1719 Kalorama Road NW
Washington, DC 20009
Al Berkowitz, Director

1984 convention in Minneapolis will feature, in part, computer applications.

Association for Children & Adults with Learning Disabilities
4156 Library Rd
Pittsburgh, PA 15234
412-341-1515
Jean Petersen

Professional and lay organization with 60,000 members in 800 chapters. Advocacy and research at national level; state affiliates work with school systems; and local units offer direct services. Upcoming conference will feature computer-related themes. Publications include biography of 400+ publications on learning disabilities, scientific reprints, national listing of educational facilities, and a newsletter.

ARC=Association for Retarded Children
2501 Avenue J
Arlington, TX 76011
817-640-0204

Resource center with 1700 local units serving the mentally retarded. Publishes bimonthly magazine, *The ARC*.

PERSONAL COMPUTERS AND THE DISABLED

Council for Exceptional Children
1920 Association Drive
Reston, VA 22091
703-620-3660

Organization for Special Educators with 46,000 members. Magazine publications include: *Exceptional Children* and *Teaching Exceptional Children*. Offers computer data base with printouts or machine search available through DIALOG and BRS, data base vendors listed in Section V, INFORMATION. Also publishes: *Microcomputer Resource Book, Microcomputers & Special Education—Selection & Decision Making Process*, Proceedings from 1983 Conference on Use of Microcomputers in Special Education. Distributor of *Specialware Directory*, published by LINC. See READING LIST, Section VII, for publication details.

Down's Syndrome Congress
1640 W. Roosevelt Rd
Chicago, IL 60608
312-226-0416

Referrals for 450 local chapters. Publishes two newsletters and a bibliography on the disabled.

Joseph P. Kennedy Foundation
1701 K Street NW
Suite 205
Washington, DC 20006
202-331-1731

Foundation for the mentally retarded established in 1946. Supports research, treatment centers, and recreational programs including the Special Olympics. Literature and film rentals available.

Mental Health Association
1800 N. Kent St
Arlington, VA 22209
703-526-6405

Advocacy and public education thru 850 local chapters. Extensive publications list, film rentals and bimonthly newsletter.

NASDSE=National Association of State Directors of Special Education
1201 16th St
Suite 404E
Washington, DC 20036
James Galloway
202-822-7933

Offers "Special Net", computer data network for educators (see INFORMATION, Section V).

NSAC=National Society for Children and Adults with Autism
1234 Massachusetts Ave NW
Suite 1017
Washington, DC 20005
202-783-0125

157 chapters involved in Special Education advocacy and information. Professional job and referral services. Book store and publications, including bimonthly newsletter for professionals, *The Advocate*.

Resources

Recovery
116 South Michigan Avenue
Chicago, IL 60603
312-263-2292

1000 chapters serve nervous disorders and former mental patients.

Young People's LOGO Association
1208 Hillsdale Drive
Richardson, TX 75081
214-783-7548

Computer club for users of LOGO, a computer language for learning.

Motor and Medical Impairments

American Cancer Society
777 Third Ave
New York, NY 10017
212-371-2900

ACS has state, major city and 3000 county units offering a full range of programs and services.

American Diabetes Association
2 Park Ave
New York, NY 10016
212-683-7444

American Heart Association
7320 Greenville Ave
Dallas, TX 75231
214-750-5300

2000 affiliates with extensive information services.

American Lung Association
1740 Broadway
New York, NY 10019
212-245-8000

AMVETS=American Veterans of World War II, Korea and Vietnam
4647 Forbes Blvd
Lanham, MD 20706
301-459-9600

Education, rehabilitation, employment and advocacy for disabled vets thru 1400 local units. Individual litigation available at regional offices of the VA.

Arthritis Foundation
3400 Peachtree Rd NE
Suite 1101
Atlanta, GA 30326
404-872-7100

Information services and community outreach programs staffed by volunteers from 70 chapters. Supports 42 research centers.

PERSONAL COMPUTERS AND THE DISABLED

Cystic Fibrosis Foundation
6000 Executive Blvd
Suite 309
Rockville, MD 20852
301-881-9130

Funds 125 treatment centers and research grants. Annual professional conference. *Commitment* is their quarterly and *Focus*, their newsletter.

Disabled American Veterans
Box 14301
Cincinnati, OH 45214
606-441-7300

> DAV National Service Headquarters
> 807 Maine Ave SW
> Washington, DC 20024

Counseling and advocacy for veterans since 1920. Full range of services from employment, training and scholarships to removal of barriers for disabled vets. Extensive outreach programs into rural areas. 700,000 members. 300 National Service Officers in 67 cities represent vets as *de facto* attorneys before government agencies. Publishes monthly magazine. The Ohio address is for information. For benefit claim assistance, contact the Washington office.

March of Dimes Birth Defects Foundation
1275 Mamaroneck Ave
White Plains, NY 10605
914-428-7100

Extensive medical education and publications program, including *International Directory of Genetic Services*. Funds BDIS, computerized data base listed under INFORMATION, Section V.

Muscular Dystrophy Association
810 7th Ave
New York, NY 10019
212-586-0808

200 local chapters and 240 clinics provide everything from diagnostic aids to recreational activities. Offers some subsidies for personal services. Bimonthly newsletter, A/V materials, and quarterly available. Excellent referral sources.

National Association for Sickle Cell Disease
3460 Wilshire Blvd
Suite 1012
Los Angeles, CA 90010

75 community programs nationwide. Newsletter is *Viewpoint*.

National Institute for Rehabilitative Engineering
97 Decker Rd
Butler, NJ 07405
Donald Selwyn
201-838-2500

Resources

National Multiple Sclerosis Society
205 East 42 St
New York, NY 10017
212-986-3240

Active in full range of programs from counseling to recreational support thru 130 local chapters. Home care courses offered with aid of Red Cross.

National Spinal Cord Injury Association
369 Elliot St
Newton Upper Falls, MA 02164
617-964-0521

Information clearinghouse founded by Paralyzed Vets of America in 1948, now with 40 chapters that either make referrals or provide direct care to para- and quadriplegics. Sponsors independent living projects.

Paralyzed Veterans of America
4350 East West Hwy
Suite 900
Washington, DC 20814
301-652-2135

Advocacy and information dissemination thru offices in 48 VA centers and 35 local chapters. Publishes monthly magazine.

Parkinson's Disease Foundation
William Black Medical Research Bldg
Columbia Univ. Medical Center
640 W. 168th St
New York, NY 10032
212-923-4700

Primarily involved in research. Some publications and a film are available.

RESNA=Rehabilitation Engineering Society of North America
Suite 402
4405 East West Highway
Bethesda, MD 20814
301-657-4142
Director, Patricia Horner

Membership society, interest group and information center for the applications of technology to rehabilitation. Newsletter and annual conference: June, 1984, Ottawa; Microcomputers for Physically Handicapped Individuals.

SIGCAPH=Special Interest Group for Computers and Physically Handicapped
c/o Association for Computing Machinery
11 West 42 St
New York, NY 10036
Karen Anderson, Director lives in Rochester, NY. 716-427-1834

Dr. Ross Lambert, Newsletter Editor lives in Hines, IL.
312-261-6700 x 2240

Promotes professional interests of disabled computing personnel since 1970. Open to non-disabled professionals as well.

PERSONAL COMPUTERS AND THE DISABLED

Spina Bifida Association
343 S. Dearborn St
Suite 319
Chicago, IL 60604
312-663-1562

An outgrowth of National Easter Seals, SBA also works closely with March of Dimes Birth Defects. 100 chapters active in parent and patient support. Publications include bimonthly newsletter, directory of chapters and publicity for use in media presentations.

United Cerebral Palsy Associations
66 East 34 St
New York, NY 10016
Rosemary Addanich
212-481-6300

A leader in funding research and in public education, rehabilitation and advocacy for the disabled. 241 affiliates offer full range of services including employment, education, access, etc. Extensive information network for professional and lay person, including two journals, telephone support, and cartoon booklet for children.

Advocacy

American Bar Association
Commission on the Mentally Disabled
1800 M St NW
Washington, DC 20036
202-331-2240
Bruce J. Ennis, Chairman

Information clearinghouse on the law and mentally disabled. Publishes *Mental & Physical Disability Law Reporter.*

Mental Health Law Project
2021 L St NW
Suite 800
Washington, DC 20036
Norman S. Rosenberg, Director
202-467-5730

Public interest group involved in law reform advocacy on a national level, primarily group actions. A small referral list available.

National Center for Law and the Deaf
Gallaudet College
800 Florida Ave NE
Washington, DC 20002
202-447-0445

Information collection, legal representation and educational workshops.

Resources

II. FEDERAL GOVERNMENT

Administration on Developmental Disabilities
Division, Office of Human Development Services
200 Independence Ave SW
Washington, DC 20201
Dr. Jean Elder, Director
202-245-2910

Public Law 95-602, enacted in 1978, defines developmentally disabled as having major functional limitations that began prior to age 22. $51 million DD grant program available to states for basic services and advocacy. Administered by State DD Councils, 50% of whose members must be disabled individuals. Additional $7 million to 36 University facilities (UAF's) for research and training of personnel.

Employment Initiative, ADD
Michael Fishman, Director
202-245-2888

Works to encourage employment of the developmentally disabled by corporate leaders, media, volunteer organizations, placement services and government agencies. Its 1984 goal is to place 25,000 in jobs.

EEOC=Equal Employment Opportunities Commission
Handicapped Individuals Program Division
2401 E St NW
Room 424
Washington, DC 20506
Clayton Boyd, Director
202-634-6753

Monitors and offers guidance to federal agencies in regard to Section 501 of the 1973 Rehab. Act, training and employment of disabled workers in government. Included are student programs and executive development.

Interagency Committee on Handicapped Employees
EEOC/Office of Secretariat
2401 E St NW Room 4294
Washington, DC 20506

Cabinet-level support committee to spur government employment of the disabled, headed by EEOC Chairman.

Federal Communications Commission
2025 M St
Room 6216
Washington, DC 20554
Gregg Vogt
202-632-4890

Telecommunications regulations regarding the disabled.

House of Representatives
Committee on Education & Labor
2181 Rayburn House Office Bldg
Washington, DC 20515
Rep. Carl D. Perkins, Chairman
Donald M. Baker, Staff Director
Jane Von Knorring, staff member for Vocational Rehab
202-225-4527

PERSONAL COMPUTERS AND THE DISABLED

House Subcommittee on Select Education
Committee on Education & Labor
Rep. Austin J. Murphy, Chairman
Rose Anne Tulley, staff member on educational technology
202-226-7532

NASA Technology Utilization Program
Maryland Ave at 4th
Bldg 6, Room 7109
Washington, DC 20546
Ronald J. Philips, Director
202-453-8430

Adapts aerospace technologies to aid the disabled. Available products listed in their brochure, *Technologies for the Handicapped and the Aged*. Publishes quarterly, *NASA Tech Briefs*. Offers NASA-developed computer programs to non-governmental researchers thru COSMIC (Computer Software & Management Information Center). The STAC Program applies technology to specific state needs.

National Institute of Handicapped Research
U.S. Dept of Education
Switzer Bldg Room 3060
330 C St NW
Washington, DC 20202
Dr. Douglas Fenderson, Director
202-732-1146

Leading government contact for educational institutions involved with rehabilitative technologies. Instrumental in organizing 1984 White House Conference on computers and the disabled. Conference papers prepared by Larry Scadden (NSF), Frank Bowe (ACCD) and Greg Vanderheiden (Trace Center) are in the Congressional Record. Proceedings also available.

National Institutes of Health
Computer Research and Technology Division
9000 Rockville Pike
Bethesda, MD 20205
Director: Dr. A.W. Pratt
Information Officer: Patricia Miller
                    Room 3027 Bldg 12A
                    301-496-6203

    Computer Systems Laboratory at NIH
    David Songco and Perry Plexico
    Engineers active in development of computers for use in voice response systems for the blind.

National Science Foundation
Electric, Computer & Systems Engineering Division
1800 G St NW
Room 1151
Washington, DC 20550
Lawrence Scadden, Program Director
202-357-9618

Federal agency minimally involved in computer education for the disabled. Mr. Scadden, a leader in the field of rehabilitative technology, was instrumental in setting up 1984 White House Conference on computers and disabled. Writes for *Journal of Rehabilitation, Journal of Visual Impairment*, et al. His independent consulting firm is Rehabilitative Technology Inc., 3122 N. Nottingham St, Arlington, VA 22207. 703-241-8035.

Resources

Office for Civil Rights
Dept. of Health & Human Services
300 Independence Ave SW
Washington, DC 20201
Jim Bennett, Voluntary Compliance Section
202-472-6674

Where to file Section 504 complaints of discrimination against disabled individuals by institutions securing federal funding.

Office of Federal Contract Compliance Programs
Veterans & Handicapped Branch
Dept. of Labor
200 Constitution Ave NW
Washington, DC 20210
James Warren
202-523-9410

Where to file Section 503 complaints of discrimination against disabled individuals by companies securing federal contracts.

Presidential Committee on Employment of the Handicapped
1111 20th St NW
Washington, DC 20036
Bernard Posner, Exec. Director
202-653-5079

Computer-related subdivisions:

Employers Committee
Jay Rochlin, Director.

Development of JAN=Job Accommodation Network, employer-oriented computerized data bank. Information on how worksites can be accommodated for the disabled, including anything from adjustment of hours to removal of physical barriers. Start-up date: Sept 1, 1984. Free to employers for three years. Companies are encouraged to submit information on how accommodations have been handled. Funded by NIHR.

Worksite Committee
Ed Leonard, Director
202-653-5079

Studies how worksites can be improved to remove the barriers to employing the disabled. Deals with unions, ergonomics, physical barriers, etc. About 25 volunteers include doctors, rehabilitation engineers, employers.

Library & Information Service
Dale Brown, Director

Information on how libraries are working with computers to assist the disabled.

PERSONAL COMPUTERS AND THE DISABLED

President's Committee on Mental Retardation
330 Independence Ave SW
4057 North Bldg
Washington, DC 20201
Linda L. Tarr, Director
George Bouthilet, data base specialist
202-245-7634

Writes annual reports to the President on human services and employment, and advises Dept. of Health & Human Services.

PWI=Projects with Industry
Dept. of Education/RSA
Switzer Bldg., Room 3318
400 Maryland Ave SW
Washington, DC 20202
Wes Geigle, Director
202-732-1335

Major grant program for over a decade with about $13 million allocated for 1983. Applying companies and agencies compete for funds and must put up 20% matching services, facilities or other. Local communities establish an Advisory Council composed of business leaders with potential job offerings. PWI projects can be actual training, referral services or other. State Vocational Rehab agencies may act as applicants or interested parties. IBM, Control Data Corp, Minneapolis, and Electronics Industries Foundation, Washington, DC, have sponsored major PWI projects. (See BUSINESS, Section III for details.) PWI has a newsletter, *PWI Pioneer* (see MEDIA, Section VI).

RSA=Rehabilitation Services Administration
Dept. of Education
330 C St SW
Switzer Bldg
Washington, DC 20202
George A. Conn, Commissioner
202-732-1282

> Fred Windbeck, Assoc. Commissioner on Developmental Programs
> 732-1353
> John Chapman, computer affairs
> 732-1290

RSA, a major division of the Dept. of Education along with SERS, is involved in administering services to the disabled. Regional offices are:

New England: JFK Bldg, Room E-400, Government Center, Boston, MA 02203. 617-223-6820. John Szufnarowski, Commissioner.

NY, NJ, Puerto Rico: 26 Federal Plaza, Room 410, NYC 10278. 212-264-4016. Richard Engelhardt, Commissioner.

Mid-Atlantic (includes WV): 3535 Market St, Room 3350, Philadelphia, PA 19101. 215-596-1327. Ralph Pacinelli, Commissioner.

Midwest: 300 S. Wacker Dr, 15th floor, Chicago, IL 60606. 312-886-5372. Ralph Church, Commissioner.

IA,KS,MO,NE: 324 East 11 St, 11 Oak Bldg, 10th floor West, Kansas City, MO 64106. 816-374-2381. Isaac Johnson, Commissioner.

Resources

Southeast: 101 Marietta St NW, Suite 821, Atlanta, GA 30323. 404-221-2352. Stephen Cornett, Jr., Commissioner.

TX,OK,LA,NM,AR: 1200 Main Tower Bldg, Room 1400, Dallas, TX 75202. 214-767-2961. Robert L. Davis, Commissioner.

West Central (includes Dakotas): 19th & Scout Sts, Federal Office Bldg, Room 7415, Denver, CO 80202. 303-837-2135. James Ballantyne, Commissioner.

CA,NV,AZ,HI: 50 UN Plaza, Federal Bldg, Room 480, San Francisco 94102. 415-556-7333. Anthony DeSimone, Commissioner.

AL,WA,OR,ID: 2901 Third Ave, Room 120, Seattle, WA 98121. 206-442-5331. William Bean, Commissioner.

Senate Subcommittee on the Handicapped
113 Hart Senate Office Bldg
Washington, DC 20510
Lowell Weicker, Chairman
Jennings Randolph, Ranking Member
John Doyle, Staff Director
202-224-6265

Other Senate members: Robert Stafford, Strom Thurmond, Donald Nickles, Thomas Eagleton, Spark Matsunaga.

Involved with all legislation and budget recommendations pertaining to the disabled, including the Vocational Rehabilitation Act and the Education For All Handicapped Children Act.

SERS=Office of Special Education and Rehabilitation Services
Dept. of Education
330 C St SW
3006 Switzer Bldg
Washington, DC 20202
202-245-8492

Subdivision of Dept. of Education in charge of Special Education Programs. 462 employees and $1.5 billion budget for the disabled. Divisions include:

Educational Services
Marty Kaufman
202 732 1106

Operates 15-20 programs each year relating to disabilities, as formulated by Secretary of Education.

Innovation and Development
Tom Behrens
202-732-1157

Research and model demonstration programs include, but are not limited to, the severely disabled.

Assistance to States
David Rostetter
202-732-1014

Personnel Preparation
Max Mueller
202-732-1070

PERSONAL COMPUTERS AND THE DISABLED

Veterans Administration
810 Vermont Ave NW
Washington, DC 20420
Dorothy Starbuck, Director of Veterans Benefits
202-393-4120

Provides full range of services from vocational training to specially adapted cars and homes for severely disabled vets. Unpublished statistical data collected by the VA available thru its Office of Reports and Statistics.

Office of Technology Transfer
252 Seventh Ave
New York, NY 10001
212-620-6659

Reference library on rehabilitation engineering for public use. Publishes *Bulletin of Prosthetic Research* available thru U.S. Government Printing Office.

U.S. GOVERNMENT STATISTICS ON DISABILITIES

Bureau of the Census
Washington, DC 20233
301-763-4100

Provides information on published reports:

Demographic, Social and Economic Profile of States, 1976 detailed survey includes work disability status of persons aged 18-64 by state.

Provisional Estimates of Social, Economic and Housing Characteristics, Stock #003-024-03626-6, 1980 census data to be published on a state-by-state basis.

For detailed, unpublished survey data on the disabled from the Bureau of the Census, contact Jack MacNeil at 301-763-7946.

ERIC Reference Facility
Box 190
Arlington, VA 22210
703-841-1212

Fourth Annual Report to Congress on the Implementation of Public Law 94-142: Education of All Handicapped Children Act. 1982 educational statistics on disabled children. Document #215-553. Cost: $14.40

National Center for Educational Statistics
Dept. of Education
Room 1001
400 Maryland Ave SW
Washington, DC 20202
202-436-7900

Statistics on disabled students in higher education.

Resources

National Center for Health Statistics
Dept. of Health and Human Services
3700 East West Hwy
Room 1-57
Hyattsville, MD 20782
301-436-8500

    Prevalence of Selected Impairments, 1977 general study.

    Use of Special Aids, 1977 survey.

Social Security Administration
Office of Disability Studies
2223 Annex
6401 Security Blvd
Baltimore, MD 21235
Kathryn Allan
301-594-0599

    Survey of Disabled and Work Data Book, 1978 study based on work age population 18-64.

PERSONAL COMPUTERS AND THE DISABLED

III. BUSINESS: Training and Employment

AFL-CIO
Human Resources Development Institute
815 16th St NW
Washington, DC 20006
Larry Glantz, Placement Specialist
202-638-3912

Assists in job development, training and placement for the disabled. List of local Coordinators available.

American Express International Banking Corp
125 Broad St
New York, NY 10004
Warren Gotto, Technical Director
212-323-2621
Human Resources, 323-4706

"Homebound" involves ten disabled employees, working for the company from their homes. Computer operations primarily for the International Banking Division. Private Industry Council, a business consortium in New York, initiated the project in 1983. Employees have severe medical or motor impairments. "Project Homebound", 15 min. VHS tape, is available from Human Resources.

Arkansas Enterprises for the Blind
2811 Fair Park Blvd
Little Rock, AR 72204
James Cordell, Director
501-664-7100

Pioneer in the training of the blind to be computer programmers. 100 students from all over the U.S. have graduated in last five years. 80%-85% placement ratio. Rigorous nine-month program requires 8-hour days and 20 hours overtime per week. Recruitment from state offices of Vocational Rehabilitation. Funding sources include state agencies, Lions Clubs and Levi-Strauss.

Control Data Corporation
8100 34th Ave South
Bloomington, MN 55440
Steve Wastvedt, Director PWI Project
612-853-7551

Hiring program within Control Data to encourage employment of disabled. Clerical training programs in Minneapolis and New York City branches. (See also PWI under FEDERAL GOVERNMENT, Section II.)

Disabled Programmers
1 West Campbell Ave
Suite 36
Campbell, CA 95008
408-866-5818

Computer programmer training for the disabled. Graduates often hired to work in their contract programming business.

Resources

Electronic Industries Foundation (EIF)
2001 Eye St NW
Washington, DC 20006
Carol Dunlap, National Director
Daniel Sheehey, Program Director
202-457-4995

Non-profit social service arm of the electronics industry. Acts as clearinghouse for Projects With Industry, helping to match over 2400 disabled individuals with high tech employers since 1977. More than 300 companies participate nationwide. Marketing strategies utilized in job placement. Staff of about 30 work with all rehabilitation agencies, from whom prospective employees come. Current programs include:

Multi Resource Centers
1900 Chicago Ave
Minneapolis, MN 55404
612-871-2402

Rehabilitation Institute of Chicago
345 E. Superior
Chicago, IL 60611
312-649-6000

Adept
260 Sheridan Ave
Suite 312
Palo Alto, CA 94306
Lisa Ervin
415-327-0575

15643 Sherman Way
Suite 410
Van Nuys, CA 91406
Lark Galloway-Gilliam
213-873-1614

Southwest PWI
4410 N. Saddleback Trail
Suite B
Scottsdale, AZ 85251
Kevin Gregor, Project Director
602-949-0135
Information on Tucson project also.

Delaware Valley PWI
6 Franklin Plaza
Philadelphia, PA 19102
Dan Sullivan, Project Director
215-665-5080
Information on Wilmington, DE, project also.

Massachusetts PWI
20 Park Plaza Room 1140
Boston, MA 02116
Marty Kennedy, Project Director
617-890-2698

Hewlett-Packard
3000 Hanover St
Palo Alto, CA 94304
Dick Farr, Personnel Affirmative Action
415-857-3930

Liaison for disabled employees. Publishes *Achiever* newsletter and distributes "Just Three People", a tape about three disabled HP employees, available in all VCR formats.

PERSONAL COMPUTERS AND THE DISABLED

IBM Project to Train the Disabled
Rehabilitation Training Programs
Federal Systems Division
18100 Frederick Pike
Gaithersburg, MD 20879
Irwin Kaplan, Director
301-840-4980

A comprehensive program to train the disabled as computer programmers throughout the U.S. Started in 1972 as part of Projects With Industry. April, 1984, marked 1000th graduate with 81% placement ratio. Aptitude tests required. Applicants usually come thru state offices of Vocational Rehabilitation. Training sessions generally nine months long. Director and staff of four give two years of close attention to new projects. Here are details on two projects:

Center for Independent Living
Computer Training Project
2020 Milvia, Suite 470
Berkeley, CA 94704
415-849-2911
Joan Breves, Director
Deborah Meehan, Job Placement

Nine-month intensive training to become entry-level programmers. Students recruited mainly from State Dept. of Rehabilitation, though some also from VA and private facilities. Serves wide range of disabilities. About 16 students per session. Recruitment from June to September and December thru February. 92% placement ratio since inception eight yrs ago. Last part of training includes actual work experience on the job site.

Maryland Rehabilitation Center
2301 Argon Drive
Baltimore, MD 21218
301-366-8800
Richard Conroy, Director

Computer training for the visually and physically impaired. One-year program to develop job skills includes daily eight-hour classes.

The 29 IBM-sponsored centers currently operating are:

ALABAMA	Augusta Cash Lakeshore Rehab Facility 3800 Ridgeway Dr Birmingham 35209	205-939-6600
CALIFORNIA	Joan Breves CIL 2020 Milvia St Berkeley 94704	415-849-2911
	Jack Grubbs Westside CIL 5760 W. Arbor Vitae St Los Angeles 90045	213-670-4413
	Georganne Yarger Dayle McIntosh Center 2050 W. Chapman Orange 92668	714-385-1701

Resources

COLORADO	Lil Hunsaker Community College of Denver 1111 W. Colfax, Box 400 Denver 80204	303-629-3300
CONNECTICUT	Ceil Brown Easter Seal/Goodwill Rehab Ctr 20 Brookside Ave New Haven 06515	203-389-4561
	Joe LaMaine BIPED Corp Easter Seal Rehab Ctr 26 Palmer's Hill Rd Stamford 06902	203-324-3935
FLORIDA	Bruce Cole Vocational Rehab 1150 SW First St Miami 33130	305-547-2544
	Diann Schultz Abilities Rehab Ctr 2735 Whitney Rd Clearwater 33520	813-535-6526
	Beverly Chapman Valencia Community College Box 3028 Orlando 32802	305-299-5000 x72383
GEORGIA	Joy Kniskern Goodwill Evaluation Ctr 2201 Glenwood Ave SE Atlanta 30316	404-894-3972
INDIANA	Gregg Nussbaum Crossroads Rehab Ctr 3242 Sutherland Ave Indianapolis 46205	317-924-3251
LOUISIANA	Linda Holliday CRT Program East 123 Pleasant Hall Louisiana State Univ. Baton Rouge 70803	504-388-1965
MAINE	Robert Cormier 135 Eastport Hall Bangor Community College Bangor 04401	207-581-6121
MARYLAND	Richard Conroy Maryland Rehab Ctr 2301 Argonne Dr Baltimore 21218	301-366-8800
MICHIGAN	Jim Moore State Technical Inst. & Rehab Ctr Plainwell 49080	616-664-4461

PERSONAL COMPUTERS AND THE DISABLED

MISSOURI	Dr. Ronald Wilson Severely Handicapped Training Program Univ. Extension Division Univ. of Missouri Rt 4 Box 199 Columbia 65201	314-449-3481
NEW JERSEY	Doreen W. Cevasco Goodwill Industries 400 Worthington Ave Harrison 07029	201-481-2300
NEW YORK	Mark Lasky United Cerebral Palsy 122 East 23 St New York 10010	212-677-7400
	Joe LaMaine BIPED Burke Rehab Ctr 785 Mamaroneck Ave White Plains 10605	914-949-5656
	Jim Diffley Human Resources Ctr I.U. Willetts Rd Albertson 11507	516-747-5400
OHIO	Jo Ann Decker Goodwill Industries 10600 Springfield Pike Cincinnati 45215	513-771-4800
	James Cunningham Computer Programmer Training for the Disabled CORC 1331 Edgehill Rd Columbus 43212	614-294-5181
	Madeline Rosenschein College of Business Kent State Univ. Kent 44242	216-672-2755
PENNSYLVANIA	James Vagnoni Physically Handicapped Training Ctr 4025 Chestnut St Philadelphia 19104	215-898-8108
UTAH	Susan Besser Salt Lake Skills Ctr 431 S. 600 East Salt Lake City 84102	801-531-9310
VIRGINIA	Wayne Olive Woodrow Wilson Rehab Ctr Fishersville 22939	703-885-9735

Resources

WASHINGTON	Ruth Walsh Project Entry Resource Ctr for the Handicapped 20150 45th Ave NE Seattle 98155	206-362-2273
CANADA	Margo Byrd Alternative Computer Training for the Disabled 250 The Esplanade Suite 203 Toronto, Ontario ON M5A 1J2	416-365-3330

L.A. Unified School District
Government & Industry Sponsored Programs
Handicapped Adult Education
1320 W. 3rd
Room 824
Los Angeles, CA 90017
Holly Johnston
213-625-6668

Extensive city program to provide vocational and coping skills to individuals of all disabilities. Teacher training stations donated by Epson.

Lift
350 Pfingsten
Northbrook, IL 60062
Charles Schmidt, Director
Susan Dwyer, Administrator
312-564-9005

Non-profit organization training disabled people to become computer programmers since 1975. Prerequisite is a severe motor impairment. 75 graduates with 51 currently enrolled. 99% placement ratio. After six-month training at no charge, graduate is contracted out to sponsoring company for one year. Programmer then becomes employee of company. Active in New York, LA, Chicago, Dallas, Houston, Miami, Minneapolis, Milwaukee, et al.

Mainstream
1200 15th St NW
Washington, DC 20005
202-833-1160
Fritz Rumpel, Information Services and Newsletter Editor
Dallas office, 214- 969-0118

Job placement of the disabled, including computer employment. "Project Link" had 350 placements in metro Washington, DC, and Dallas during 1983.

Rehabilitation Center 191 Eighth St. San Francisco, CA 94103 415-431-9200 Louise Goeckel, Director	**Mt. Diablo Rehab Center** 490 Golf Club Rd Pleasant Hill, CA 94523 415-682-6330

Technical office training for the disabled, including word processing, accounting, secretarial. San Francisco center with 30 students opened eight years ago. Excellent job placement services—97% placement ratio. Partial funding thru PWI.

PERSONAL COMPUTERS AND THE DISABLED

IV. HIGHER EDUCATION

AHSSPPE=Association on Handicapped Student Service Programs in Post-Secondary Education
Box 21192
Columbus, OH 43221
Jane Jarrow, Director
614-488-4972

Membership organization of 575 academic institutions and individuals.

Baruch College
Computer Center for the Visually Impaired
17 Lexington Ave
Box 515
New York, NY 10010
212-725-7644
Dina Nath Bedi, Director
Randi Baker, Associate Director

Programs: 13-week intensive training sponsored by corporations who commit, in advance, to hire upon graduation; 2 to 5 week sessions to develop computer literacy; Bachelors and Masters degrees; research in employment and tactile graphics.

Education Turnkey
256 N. Washington St
Falls Church, VA 22046
703-536-2310
Charles Blashke
Al Morin, Director of MEAN

Educational consulting firm providing technical research assistance to 20 states and Federal Government. Microcomputer Education Application Network (MEAN) services 4500 Special Ed administrators. Recent study on technology's future in Special Education, including microcomputers and videodisc, prepared for Dept. of Education and available thru ERIC Clearinghouse system.

Electronic University
TeleLearning Systems
505 Beach St
San Francisco, CA 94133
415-928-2800

Home study using personal computers. More than 150 courses offered for the disabled and non-disabled student. Students can talk with instructors in more than 350 cities via computer. Set up by Ron Gordon, ex-Atari executive, in 1981.

Gallaudet College
800 Florida Ave NE
Washington, DC 20002
202-651-5000

Leading academic institution for the hearing-impaired established by Congress in 1864. 26 bachelor degree programs, 5 M.A.'s and a Ph.D in administration. Also runs elementary education model programs which accept students nationwide, pre-school to 12th grade. Research Institute publishes *Directions*. Other divisions include Demographic Studies and Law. Extension classes, interpreter training, extensive library holdings.

Resources

Computer Services Division
Kevin Casey, Director
202-651-5610

Staff of 35 involved in all phases of computer activities related to the student body.

ISAAC=Int'l Society for Augmentative & Alternative Communication
Convention Committee/Children's Hospital
300 Longwood Ave
Boston, MA 02115
Dr. Howard Shane

Convention at MIT on October 18-20, 1984.

National Home Study Council
1601 18th St NW
Washington, DC 20009
202-234-5100
Michael Lambert, Assistant Director

Information on college-level courses available nationwide thru home study.

National Technical Institute for the Deaf
Rochester Institute of Technology
1 Lomb Memorial Drive
Rochester, NY 14623
716-475-6400
Cathy Finks, Admissions

University offering 32 majors for the hearing-impaired, including Data Processing. Currently with 1295 students in undergraduate and graduate degree programs. NTID also has developed the David System, computer-assisted instruction program, and Real Time Graphics, a computer interpreter. Publishes *Eduational Resources for the Deaf* catalog.

Northwestern University
Rehabilitation Engineering Program
345 E. Superior
Room 1441
Chicago, IL 60611
Dr. Dudley Childress, Director
Craig Heckathorne, computer specialist

An early pioneer in the use of computers for the motor-impaired. Works both with referrals and patients at the Rehabilitation Institute.

Ohio State University
College of Medicine
700 Childrens Drive
Columbus, OH 43214
Dr. Jim Mulick, Associate Professor
614-461-2100

Regional Director of American Association on Mental Deficiency and Editor of *Transitions in Mental Retardation* series. Dr. Mulick is a research authority in computer applications for Special Ed.

PERSONAL COMPUTERS AND THE DISABLED

Rensselaer Polytechnic Institute
Human Interface Lab
Science & Technology Studies
Troy, NY 12181
518-266-6756
Dan Zuckerman

Research in personal computers for the blind and deaf.

SUNY at Binghamton
Childrens Units/Dept of Psychology
Binghamton, NY 13901
Raymond G. Romanczyk
607-798-2829

Research in computer applications for Special Ed, primarily autistic and severely emotionally-disturbed children. Studies comparing computer- and teacher-assisted instruction. Educational and administrative software developed for research can be purchased thru SUNY. On-going state funded project currently involves 24 students. Summary of recent findings published by Association for Advancement of Behavior Therapy, New York.

TLC=The Learning Center for Deaf Children
848 Central St
Framingham, MA 01701
Christopher Huggins, Curriculum Development
617-879-5110

> Paul Goldenberg, Faculty Member
> 36 Amherst Rd Waban,
> MA 02168
> 617-332-1491
>
> Author of several books on computer applications in Special Education (see BOOKS, Section VII). Also Director of Computer Education at Lincoln Sudbury High School and faculty member at Tufts School of Medicine, Boston.
>
> Bill Ash
> Bolt, Beranek & Newman
> 10 Molton St
> Cambridge, MA 02238
> 617-497-3677
>
> Research and development firm that does some computer-related studies. Mr. Ash, affiliated with TLC, is involved with new computer project for mentally retarded children.

Trace Center
University of Wisconsin
314 Waisman Center
1500 Highland Ave
Madison, WI 53706
Dr. Gregg Vanderheiden, Director
608-262-6966 or 263-5697

Major research and resource center for computer uses among the disabled. Evaluates and produces technical aids for all disabilities. Trains and consults with rehabilitative personnel who come to Trace and in the field. Publications: *International Software/Hardware Registry* revised annually; *Non-vocal Communication Resource Book*; and many other pamphlets. Prominent at most major conferences. Dr. Vanderheiden is a leading researcher in the field.

Resources

Tufts New England Medical Center
171 Harrison Ave
Box 75KR
Boston, MA 02111
Rick Foulds, Director of Rehab Engineering Center
617-956-5036

Ongoing projects using computers for motor impairments, particularly spinal injuries and cerebral palsy.

University of Arkansas
Rehabilitation Services
1401 Brookwood Drive
Little Rock, AR 72203
Vernon Gleen, Director
501-575-3656

Research to improve employability of disabled people. The college of Education, Fayetteville, is studying vocational rehabilitation for the hearing-impaired.

University of Wisconsin
Stout Vocational Rehab Institute
Menomonie, WI 54751
Daniel McAlees
715-232-1464

Research in all phases of employing the disabled, including those homebound.

Vanderbilt University
Peabody College
Box 45
Nashville, TN 37203
Ted Hasselbring, Associate Professor of Special Education and Director of Learning Technology Center
615-322-8070

A wide range of computer-related projects for the disabled include Multimedia Access of Microcomputers for Visually Impaired Students and Instructional Media Production Project for Severely Handicapped Students.

Wright State University
Dayton, OH 45435
Handicapped Student Services
Stephen Simon, Director
513-873-2140
Carol Siyahi, Newsletter Editor
873-3248

Serves about 500 handicapped students. Campus facilities offer excellent accessibility, plus off-campus apartments designed by disabled students. Dr. Jerold Petrofsky, bio-engineer researching computer-aided mobility, is developing portable computer walking systems for the disabled. HSS Director Simon is exploring the expansion of personal computers into everyday living skills, as well as job search. Their newsletter is *National Center for Rehabilitation Engineering.*

For a complete listing of Research Centers, most of which are University-affiliated, consult *Rehabilitation Literature,* November-December, 1983, pp. 338-340. The Institute of Handicapped Research in the U.S. government's Department of Education also maintains an updated list of nationwide research projects.

PERSONAL COMPUTERS AND THE DISABLED

Universities with large student populations and programs for the disabled:

EAST
Northeastern U, Boston, MA 02115
U Massachusetts Harbor Campus, Boston, MA 02135
Boston U, Boston, MA 02215
Ramapo College, Mahwah, NJ 07430
Long Island University, Brooklyn, NY 11201
Queens College, New York, NY 11367
Albany State U, Albany, NY 12210
National Technical Inst. for the Deaf, RIT, Rochester, NY 14623
Gallaudet College, Washington, DC 20002
George Washington U, Washington, DC 20052
U Maryland, College Park, MD 20783
Marshall U, Huntington, WV 25701
U So. Carolina, Columbia, SC 29208
Georgia State, Atlanta, GA 30303

CENTRAL
U Kentucky, Lexington, KY 40506
Ohio State, Columbus, OH 43210
Columbus Technical Institute, Columbus, OH 43215
Kent State, Kent, OH 44242
Wright State, Dayton, OH 45435
Ball State U, Muncie, IN 47306
U Michigan, Ann Arbor, MI 48109
Michigan State, E. Lansing, MI 48824
U Wisconsin, Whitewater, WI 53190
U Wisconsin, Madison, WI 53706
U Wisconsin at Stout, Menomonie, WI 54751
U Minnesota, Duluth, MN 55812
Southwest State, Marshall, MN 56208
U No. Dakota, Grand Forks, ND 58202
Northern Illinois U, DeKalb, IL 60115
Triton Community, River Grove, IL 60171
U Illinois Champagne-Urbana, Urbana, IL 61801
Southern Illinois Univ, Carbondale, IL 62901
U Missouri, Columbia, MO 65211

WEST
U Arizona, Tucson, AZ 85721
San Diego State, San Diego, CA 92182
San Diego City College, San Diego, CA 92123
U California, Berkeley, CA 94720
UCLA, Los Angeles, CA 90024
San Jose State, San Jose, CA 95162

Resources

V. INFORMATION: Data Banks and Bases

To access most data services via computer, subscription to one of these vendors is required:

Bibliographic Retrieval Services
1200 Rt 7
Latham, NY 12110
800-833-4707

DIALOG
Lockheed Information Systems
Dept 50-20 Bldg 201
3251 Hanover St
Palo Alto, CA 94304
415-858-3785 or 800-227-1960

SDC Search Service
System Development Corp
2500 Colorado Ave
Santa Monica, CA 90406
213-453-6194 or 800-421-7229

Accent on Information
Box 700
Bloomington, IL 61701
Raymond Cheever, Director
309-378-2961

Computerized information service with a data base mainly of assistive devices. Also publishes magazine and a series of pamphlets on everyday living skills.

BDIS
Center for Birth Defects Information Services
171 Harrison Ave
Boston, MA 02111
617-956-7400
Dr. Mary Lou Buyse, Director

Computerized data bases: 1000+ articles updated 3 times a year; diagnostic assistance for clinicians with over 2000 test cases and 600 conditions; undiagnosed birth defects registry. Subscription service wholly-funded by March of Dimes. Established in 1978. The Center publishes quarterly journal and newsletter (see MEDIA, Section VI).

CITH=Center for Innovation in Teaching the Handicapped
Indiana University
2805 East 10th St
Room 150
Bloomington, IN 47405
812-335-5847

Research and information center for new teaching materials in Special Education. Software packages available for reading and math skills. Also 300 research reports and A/V aids. Funded by National Institute of Education.

PERSONAL COMPUTERS AND THE DISABLED

CRISP=Computer Retrieval of Information on Scientific Projects
Research Documentation Section
National Institutes of Health
Westwood Bldg, Room 148
5333 Westbard Ave
Bethesda, MD 20205
301-496-7543

Scientific information base, developed from recent government health research, includes 500,000 entries. Specific or generic data searches available with printout. No charge to all but profit-making institutions.

Deaf-Net
SRI International
333 Ravenswood Ave
Menlo Park, CA 94025
Teresa Middleton, Program Mgr.
415-859-2236

Computer network designed for, but not limited to, the hearing impaired. Makes TDD's and computers compatible. Two year demonstration project funded by Dept. of Education with ten sites nationwide. 400 current users pay no fees. Training manual and telephone instruction available. Modem required. Network may continue to operate after 1985 expiration date.

ERIC=Educational Resources Information Center
National Institute of Education
1200 19th St NW
Washington, DC 20208
Charles W. Hoover, Director
202-254-5500

National data base with 400,000 educational documents available via computer or microfiche. NIE-funded since 1966 with $5 million allocated for 1983. A nationwide clearinghouse system with 16 centers mainly in universities, plus some professional associations. For microfiche holdings, consult their monthly journal, *Resources In Education*. Microfiche collections located in over 700 state and university libraries. To access via computer, subscribe to one of the three vendors listed above. Among the 16 ERIC clearinghouses these two are most relevant:

> **ERIC on Handicapped and Gifted Children**
> Council for Exceptional Children
> 1920 Association Dr
> Reston, VA 22091
> 703-620-3550
> Dr. Donald Erickson, Director

> **ERIC on Adult Career & Vocational Education**
> Ohio State University
> 1960 Kenny Rd
> Columbus, OH 43210
> 614-486-3650
> Dr. Juliet Miller, Director

Exceptional Child Educational Resources
Council for Exceptional Children
1920 Association Drive
Reston, VA 22091
703-620-3660

Computer data base in Special Education. Printout or machine search available through BRS and DIALOG listed above.

Resources

Institute for Scientific Research
3501 Market St
Philadelphia, PA 19104
215-386-0199 x 1371

Social Sciences Citation Index (SSCI) contains 115,000+ entries from 1400 magazines, 9% of which refer to disabilities and special education. Computer searches available thru DIALOG, BRS and ISI itself. *Index to Social Science & Humanities Proceedings* is a data base of over 20,000 new conference papers presented each year. *Current Contents* reproduces contents pages of 1300 magazines and 800 new books each week.

MDC=Materials Development Center
University of Wisconsin-Stout
School of Education & Human Services
Menomonie, WI 54751
715-232-1342

National center for information on vocational rehabilitation, including government rehab conferences. Fee-based data searches.

NARIC=National Rehab. Information Center
Catholic University
4407 8th St NE
Washington, DC 20017
202-635-5826

Abledata, 202-635-6090
Rehabdata, 202-635-5822

Computerized data bases for the disabled community. Abledata has 8000+ commercially available products; Rehabdata, 5000+ bibliographic documents on file. All users welcome. Access through BRS. Funded by Catholic University and National Institute of Handicapped Research since 1976.

National Clearinghouse of Rehab Training Materials
Oklahoma State University
115 Old USDA Bldg
Stillwater, OK 74078
405-624-7650
Paul Gaines, Director
Jean Hudder, Information Officer

Educational resources oriented toward professionals. Non-computerized service with some materials on computers in rehabilitation and Special Education. Funded by Rehabilitation Services Administration.

NICSEM
3716 S. Hope St
Suite 301
Los Angeles 90007
213-743-6681

Computerized data base of instructional materials for the disabled housed at USC, Los Angeles. Compiled between 1977-1980. Indexes available for purchase. Owned by Access Innovation, Albuquerque, NM, since April, 1984.

PERSONAL COMPUTERS AND THE DISABLED

NICHCY=National Info Center for Handicapped Children & Youth
InterAmerica
Box 1492
Washington, DC 20013
202-528-8480
Toni Haas

Federally funded information service for disabled children under 21. Answers 13,000 letters annually.

NTIS=National Technical Information Service
Dept. of Commerce
5285 Port Royal Rd
Springfield, VA 22161
703-487-4600

Computer searches, 487-4642
Documents, 487-4650

The leading source for government research and reports. Bibliographic Data File contains 850,000 documents, largely exclusive to NTIS. Total collection exceeds 1.3 million titles, 15% of which are foreign. Prior data searches on 2200 topics are published and available for order. Government research is indexed and summarized in 26 newsletters biweekly, including these relevant to disabilities: *Behavior & Society, Health Planning, Medicine & Biology,* and *Biomedical Technology & Human Factor Engineering.* Federally created computer programs are catalogued annually by their Federal Software Exchange Center. Subscription microfiche service (SRIM) offered bi-weekly. All three major data base vendors service NTIS. For a free listing of agency offerings, consult *NTIS Information Services.*

Special Net
NASDSE
1201 16th St NW
Washington, DC 20036
202-822-7933

Computer network for educators with primary emphasis on Special Education. Over 1500 users pay yearly fee.

Well-Net
CHIP=Community Health Information Project
222-C View St
Mountain View, CA 94141
Joel Yudkin, director
415-968-8798 or 968-1126 for modems.

Nationwide electronic bulletin board for the disabled. 50 to 100 users per week pay no membership fees. Requires 300 baud modem. Start up, 1982.

Resources

VI. MEDIA: Magazines, Newspapers and Newsletters

MAGAZINES

Accent on Living
Box 700
Bloomington, IN 61701
Raymond Cheever, Editor
309-378-2961
(Quarterly with 18,000 circulation. Published since 1952.)

American Annals of the Deaf
814 Thayer Avenue
Silver Spring, MD 20910
(September, 1983, issue includes "Sign Teachers: A microcomputer application for the teaching of sign language" by Kate Grosman, et al. (128:5:577-584))

American Journal of Occupational Therapy
1383 Piccard Dr
Rockville, MD 20850
Elaine Viseltear, Editor
301-948-9626
(Monthly with 38,000 circulation.)

American Rehabilitation
Dept of Education/RSA
Switzer Bldg
330 C St SW
Washington, DC 20201
Ron Bourgea, Editor
202-472-9120

Asha
American Speech Language Hearing Association
10801 Rockville Pike
Rockville, MD 20852
301-897-5700
Dr. Frederick T. Spahr, Editor
(Monthly house organ for the professional association.)

Braille Book Review and *Talking Book Topics*
Library of Congress
National Library Service for Blind & Physically Handicapped
1291 Taylor St
Washington, DC 20542
202-287-9281
George Thuronyi, Editor
(Bimonthly free to the blind.)

Braille Mirror
Braille Institute of America
741 N. Vermont Ave
Los Angeles, CA 90029
Jody Avery, Editor
213-663-1111

Bulletin of Science & Technology for the Handicapped
American Association for Advancement of Science
1515 Massachusetts Ave NW
Washington, DC 20005
Sue Forman, Editor
202-467-4400

PERSONAL COMPUTERS AND THE DISABLED

Closing the Gap
CTG Publications
Rt 2, Box 39
Henderson, MN 56004
Bud Hagen, Editor
(Newspaper on computers and the disabled.)

Computer-Disability News
National Easter Seal Society
2023 W. Ogden Ave.
Chicago, IL 60612
Jean Bartholomew, Editor
312-243-8400
(New quarterly focusing on computers for the disabled. Premiere issue May, 1984.)

Computers in Healthcare
6530 S. Yosemite St.
Englewood, CO 80111
303-694-1522
Don S. Peterson, Editor
(15,000 circulation)

Disabled USA
President's Committee on Employment of the Handicapped
1111 20th St NW
Washington, DC 20210
Robert Gorski, Editor
202-653-5044

International Rehabilitation Review
432 Park Ave South
New York, NY 10016
Barbara Duncan, Editor
212-869-0460
(Quarterly with 20,000 circulation.)

Journal of Applied Rehabilitation Counseling
National Rehabilitation Counseling Association
633 W. Washington St
Alexandria, VA 22314
703-836-6766

Journal of Learning Disabilities
5613 W. Cermak Rd
Cicero, IL 60650
(Includes new ongoing section, "Computers in the Schools".)

Journal of Rehabilitation
National Rehab Association
633 S. Washington St
Alexandria, VA 22314
Dick Dietl, Editor
703-836-0850
(Quarterly with 18,000 circulation.)

Link-and-Go
611 N. Humphrey
Oak Park, IL 60302
Karen Culliname, Editor
(Quarterly magazine of COPH-2, professional computer association.)

Resources

Mental & Physical Disability Law Reporter
American Bar Association
1800 M St NW
Washington, DC 20036
202-331-2240
John Parry, Editor
John Taylor, Research
(Published bimonthly by the ABA Commission on the Mentally Disabled. Deals primarily in legal issues of the mentally disabled.)

Mental Retardation
American Association on Mental Retardation
1719 Kalorama NW
Washington, DC 20009
(June, 1983, issue includes article on microcomputers in administering state DD facilities by David Smith. (21:3:111-115))

Newsounds
A.G. Bell Assoc. for the Deaf
3417 Volta Place NW
Washington, DC 20007
Gina Doggett, Editor
202-337-5220

Paraplegia News
5201 N. 19th Ave #111
Phoenix, AZ 85015
Cliff Crase, Editor
602-246-9426
(Monthly published by Paralyzed Veterans of America since 1946. 24,000 readership of which half are nonvets.)

Physical Therapy
American Physical Therapy Association
1111 N. Fairfax St
Alexandria, VA 22314
Marilyn Lister, Editor
703-684-2782
(Monthly with 38,000 circulation.)

Rehabilitation Gazette
Gazette International Networking Institute
4502 Maryland Ave
St. Louis, MO 63108
314-361-0475
(Annual begun in 1962.)

Rehabilitation Literature
National Easter Seal Society
2023 W. Ogden Ave
Chicago, IL 60612
Steve Regnier, Editor
312-243-8400
(Leading rehab journal for more than 40 years. March-April, 1983, and November-December, 1983, issues both focus on technology and disability.)

PERSONAL COMPUTERS AND THE DISABLED

Rehabilitation World
1123 Broadway
New York, NY 10010
John Moses, Editor
212-741-5160
(Quarterly with 5000 circulation.)

Volta Review
A.G. Bell Assoc. for the Deaf
3417 Volta Place NW
Washington, DC 20007
Gina Doggett, Editor
202-337-5220
(Professional journal for the hearing-impaired community with bimonthly section, "Software Review".)

NEWSLETTERS

Communication Outlook
Artificial Language Lab
Computer Science Dept
Michigan State University
East Lansing, MI 48824
517-353-0870
(Quarterly newsletter from important research center. $12.)

Computer Access to the Severely Handicapped
Prentke-Romich Co
8769 Township Rd #513
Shreve, OH 44676
216-567-2906
(Product-oriented newsletter from hardware/software manufacturer.)

Education of the Handicapped
Capitol Pubs.
1300 N. 17th St
Arlington, VA 22209
703-528-5400

Handicapped Rights And Regulations
Business Pubs.
951 Pershing Dr
Silver Spring, MD 20910
301-587-6300
Leonard Eiserer, Editor

In Focus (children)
Seeing Clearly
National Association for Visually Handicapped
305 East 24 St
New York, NY 10010
212-889-3141
(Biannual newsletters for visually impaired community. Writers may submit articles on new products, poems, crosswords.)

Resources

Kurzweil Update
185 Albany St
Cambridge, MA 02139
800-343-0311; in Mass, 617-864-4700
(New quarterly newsletter on manufacturer's products. No charge. Occasionally deals with computer interfaces.)

Links
Natl Assoc of Private Residential Facilities for Mentally Retarded
6269 Leesburg Pike
Suite B5
Falls Church, VA 22044
703-536-3311
Joan Fritz, Editor

Maryland Computer Services Newsletter
2010 Rock Spring Rd
Forest Hill, MD 21050
301-879-3366
(Bimonthly for visually impaired users of MCS software products, based on Hewlett-Packard hardware.)

National Federation of the Blind
Writers Division Newsletter
132 Beach Dr
Merrick, NY 11566
Contact: Loraine Stayer
(Two annual newsletters providing publishing information to visually impaired members and nonmembers. Writers Division evaluates writers' submissions and recruits contributors to NFB publications (*Braille Monitor, Future Reflections*).)

New Directions
Natl Assoc of State Mental Retardation Program Directors
113 Orinoco St
Alexandria, VA 22314
703-683-4202
Ruth Katz, Editor

PWI Pioneer
Multi Resource Centers
1900 Chicago Ave
Minneapolis, MN 55404
Margaret Howard, Coordinator
612-871-2402
(Newsletter on Projects With Industry, a joint grant program of business and Dept. of Education. (See FEDERAL GOVERNMENT, Section II.)

Raised Dot Computing Newsletter
310 S. 7th St
Lewisburg, PA 17837
717-523-6739
(Monthly on computer products for the visually impaired. Available in cassette or print for $12.)

Rehabilitation Technology Review
Rehab Engineering Society of North America (RESNA)
4405 East West Hwy
Bethesda, MD 20814
Dr. Michael Rosen, Editor
301-657-4142
(Professional newsletter of rehab engineering.)

PERSONAL COMPUTERS AND THE DISABLED

The Catalyst
Western Center for Microcomputers in Special Education
1259 el Camino Real
Suite 275
Menlo Park, CA 94025
Sue Sweezey
415-326-6997

Tielines Newsletter
Journal of Clinical Dysmorphology
Center for Birth Defects Information Services
171 Harrison Ave
Boston, MA 02111
617-956-7400
(Quarterly publications dealing with birth defects.)

GENERAL COMPUTER MAGAZINES

Byte
70 Main St
Peterborough, NH 03458
603-924-9281
Circulation: 402,000

Compute!
505 Edwardia Dr
Greensboro, NC 27409
919-275-9809
350,000

Computerworld
375 Cochituate Rd
Box 880
Framingham, MA 01701
617-879-0700
125,000

Creative Computing
39 E. Hanover Ave
Morris Plains, NJ 07950
201-540-0445
350,000

Family Computing
730 Broadway
New York, NY 10003
212-505-3000
200,000

InfoWorld
530 Lytton Ave
Palo Alto, CA 94301
415-328-4602
50,000

Interface Age
16704 Marquardt Ave
Box 1234
Cerritos, CA 90701
213-926-9544
93,000

Resources

PC
1 Park Ave
New York, NY 10016
212-725-4694
130,000

PC World
555 De Haro St
San Francisco, CA 94107
415-861-3861
180,000

Personal Computing
10 Mulholland Drive
Hasbrouck Heights, NJ 07604
201-788-7520
525,000

Popular Computing
70 Main St
Peterborough, NH 03458
603-924-9281
320,000

Teaching, Learning, Computing
1061 S. Melrose #d
Placentia, CA 92670
714-632-6924
60,000

MAJOR NEWSPAPERS

National:

Wall Street Journal
22 Cortlandt St
New York, NY 10007
212-285-5140
Medical: Michael Waldholz
    Jerry Bishop
Computers: Susan Chace
Circulation: 2,020,000

USA Today
1000 Wilson Blvd
Arlington, VA 22209
703-276-3671
Science: Marcie Ersoff
Medical: Joe Carey
Circulation: 1,000,000

Northeast:

Boston Globe
135 Morrissey Blvd
Boston, MA 02107
617-929-3000
Science: Gerry O'Neill
Medical: Loretta McLaughlin
Computers: Ron Rosenberg
500,000

Boston Herald
1 Herald Square
Boston, MA 02106
617-426-3000
309,000

New York Daily News
220 East 42 St
New York, NY 10017
212-949-1234
Health: Mary Ann Giordano
Science/Med: Edward Edelson
1,726,000

New York Post
210 South St
New York, NY 10002
212-349-5000
Science/Med: Joe Nicholson
Computers: Mark Kalech
962,000

PERSONAL COMPUTERS AND THE DISABLED

Northeast (Continued):

New York Times
229 West 43 St
New York, NY 10036
212-556-1234
Science: Richard Flaste
Computers: Eric Stanberg-Diment
Circulation: 963,000

Newark Star Ledger
Newark, NJ 07101
Computers: Betty Ebron
Science/Med: Joan Whitlow
415,000

Philadelphia Inquirer
400 N. Broad St
Box 8263
Philadelphia, PA 19101
215-854-2000
Science: Jim Detjen
Medical: Donald C. Drake
Computers: Andrea Knox
560,000

Pittsburgh Press
34 Blvd. of the Allies
Box 566
Pittsburgh, PA 15230
412-263-1100
Science: Lee Holtz
270,000

Washington Post
1150 15th St
Washington, DC 20071
202-334-6000
Science: Philip Hilts
Computers: Michael Schrage
747,000

Newsday
235 Pinelawn Rd
Long Island, NY 11747
516-454-2020
Science: David Zinman
Computers: Phil Mintz
525,000

Philadelphia Daily News
400 N. Broad
Box 7788
Philadelphia 19101
215-854-2600
Medical: Pat McKeown
Computers: Robert Swabach
305,000

Baltimore Sun
Calvert & Centre Sts.
Box 1377
Baltimore, MD 21278
301-332-6000
Computers: Ann Cooper
Science: Albert Sehlstedt
Medical: Mary Knudson
345,000

Mid-West:

Chicago Tribune
435 N. Michigan Ave
Chicago, IL 60611
312-222-3232
Science/Med: Ronald Kotulak
Computers: Clarence Petersen
757,000

Detroit News
615 Lafayette Blvd
Detroit, MI 48231
313-222-2000
Science: Hugh McCann
Computers: Erick Wujcik
651,000

Chicago Sun-Times
401 N. Wabash
Chicago, IL 60611
312-321-3000
Computers: Dan Rosenheim
655,000

Detroit Free Press
321 W. Lafayette
Detroit, MI 48231
313-222-6400
Science: David McKay
Computers: Colin Covert
Medical: Delores Katz
636,000

Resources

Cleveland Plain Dealer
1801 Superior Ave NE
Cleveland, OH 44114
216-344-4500
Medical: Robert Becker
497,000

Minneapolis Star & Tribune
425 Portland Ave
Minneapolis, MN 55488
612-372-4141
Science: Lewis Cope
Medical: Gordon Slovut
Computers: Zeke Wigglesworth
360,000

St. Louis Post-Dispatch
900 N. Tucker Blvd
St. Louis, MO 63101
314-622-7000
Science/Med: Roger Signor
240,000

Milwaukee Journal
333 W. State St
Box 661
Milwaukee, WI 53201
414-224-2000
Medical: Neil Rosenberg
325,000

Kansas City Star
1729 Grand Ave
Kansas City, MO 64108
816-234-4300
Science/Med: Ann Hellmuth
243,000

South:

Atlanta Constitution/Journal
72 Marietta St NW
Box 4689
Atlanta, GA 30302
404-526-5151
Technology: Robert Jones
Science/Med: Charles Seabrook
210,000

Houston Chronicle
801 Texas Ave
Box 4260
Houston, TX 77210
713-220-7171
Medical: Ruth Sorelle
439,000

Dallas Morning News
Box 225237
Communications Center
Dallas, TX 75265
214-745-8222
Science: Larry Rose
Medical: Joann Schulte
328,000

Miami Herald
1 Herald Plaza
Miami, FL 33101
305-350-2111
Science: Mike Toner
Medical: Steve Sternberg
Computers: Melissa Davis
412,000

Houston Post
4747 SW Freeway
Houston, TX 77001
713-621-7000
Science/Med: Mary Jane Schier
377,000

Dallas Times Herald
1101 Pacific Ave
Box 225445
Dallas, TX 75265
214-744-6111
Medical: Linda Little
Computers: Scott Ticer
273,000

West:

Los Angeles Times
Times Mirror Square
Los Angeles, CA 90053
213-972-7000
Medical: Harry Nelson
Computers: Paul Richter
Science: George Alexander
1,043,000

Los Angeles Herald-Examiner
1111 S. Broadway
Los Angeles, CA 90015
213-744-8000
Medical: Rich Nordwind
285,000

PERSONAL COMPUTERS AND THE DISABLED

West (Continued):

San Francisco Chronicle
901 Mission Street
San Francisco, CA 94103
415-777-1111
Science: David Perlman
Medical: Charles Petit
Computers: Tim Gartner
538,000

Sunday Examiner/Chronicle
110 5th Street
San Francisco, CA 94120
415-777-2424
Science/Med: Richard Saltus
Computers: John Eckhouse
690,000

Rocky Mountain News
400 W. Colfax Ave
Box 719
Denver, CO 80204
303-892-5000
Science: Sandy Graham
Medical: Pam Avery
271,000

Denver Post
650 15th St
Box 1709
Denver, CO 80201
303-820-1010
Computers: Dan Buecke
Science/Med: Bill Symons
260,000

Seattle Times
Fairview Ave No. & John St.
Box 70
Seattle, WA 98111
206-464-2111
Science: Hill Williams
Medical: Warren King
Computers: Richard Buck
250,000

NEWS SERVICES AND SYNDICATES

These news services and syndicates do features on medicine and science:

Associated Press
50 Rockefeller Plaza
New York, NY 10020
212-621-1500
Science: Paul Raeburn

Associated Press
1111 South Hill St
Room 263
Los Angeles, CA 90015
Science: Lee Siegel

The leading wire service. One interview can put you in 500 newspapers.

Copley News Service
Science & Medicine
Box 190
San Diego, CA 92112
619-293-1818

Chronicle Features
Exploring the Universe
870 Market St
San Francisco, CA 94102

Field Newspaper Syndicate
1703 Kaiser Ave
Irvine, CA 92714

International Medical Tribune Syndicate
600 New Hampshire Ave NW
Suite 700
Washington, DC 20037

Resources

King Features
235 East 45 St
New York, NY 10017
212-682-5600

Los Angeles Times Syndicate
Science For You
Bob Brown
Times Mirror Square
Los Angeles, CA 90053

LUI Associates
26135 Telegraph Rd
Southfield, MI 48075

Mid Continent Feature Syndicate
Dorothy Sayres
Box 1662
Pittsburgh, PA 15230

New York Times Syndicate
Michael Halberstam
200 Park Ave
New York, NY 10017

Press Associates
Work & Health
806 15th St NW
Suite 632
Washington, DC 20005

Science News
1719 N St NW
Washington, DC 20036
202-785-2255
News service

SIPA News Service
Science Today
Anthony Shelley
59 East 54 St
New York, NY 10022
212-759-5571

Smithsonian News Service
Arts & Industries Bldg Room 2410
900 Jefferson Drive
Washington, DC 20560
202-357-1300
Madeleine Jacobs

United Press International
220 East 42 Street
New York, NY 10017
212-850-8600
Health &
 Education: Patricia McCormack

UPI
316 West 2nd St
Los Angeles, CA 90012
213-620-1230
Mgr: Douglas Dowie

PERSONAL COMPUTERS AND THE DISABLED

VII. READING LIST

A Beginner's Guide to Personal Computers for the Blind & Visually Impaired, D.L. Croft, Editor. National Braille Press, 88 St. Stephen St, Boston, MA 02115. 617-266-6160. November 1983.

Aids & Appliance Review, Summer-Fall 1983 issue, Carroll Ctr for the Blind, 770 Centre St, Newton, MA 02158. 617-969-6200. Speech output computers, software and speech devices. Spring 1984 issue covers Braille computer aids.

Computers, Education and Special Needs, Paul Goldenberg, Susan Jo Russell & Cynthia Carter. Addison-Wesley, Boston. 1984. Non-tutorial uses of computers for research in special education. Focus on instructional issues.

Directory of National Information Sources on Handicapping Conditions and Related Services, Dept of Education, Clearinghouse on the Handicapped. August 1982. Publication E-82-22007, U.S. Government Printing Office.

Discovery '83: Computers for the Disabled. University of Wisconsin Press, Menomonie, WI. Conference proceedings.

Handicapping America, Frank Bowe. Harper & Row, New York. 1978.

High Technology Aids for the Disabled, W.J. Perkins, Editor. Computer Science Lab Director for National Inst. for Medical Research, London, England. Published by Butterworths, London, New York and Toronto. Reduction of handicaps using computers.

IEEE Computer Society Workshop on Computing to Aid the Handicapped. Proceedings of November 4, 1982 conference. IEEE Computer Society Press, Charlotte, VA. 1983.

IEEE Computer Society Workshop on Using Computers in the Employment & Education of the Handicapped. Proceedings of Minneapolis conference. IEEE Computer Society Press, Charlotte, VA. 1983.

International Software/Hardware Registry, Gregg Vanderheiden. Trace Center, Univ. of Wisconsin, Madison. 1983. $15.

Learning Technology & the Hearing Impaired, Frank B. Withrow, A.G. Bell Association for the Deaf, Washington, DC. 1981.

Microcomputer Resource Book For Special Education, Delores Hagen. Council for Exceptional Children, 1920 Association Dr, Reston, VA 22091. 1984. $16.

Microcomputers & Special Education: Selection & Decision Making Process, Florence M. Tabor. Council for Exceptional Children, Reston, VA 22091. 1983. $8.

"New Voices: Communication through Technology", Stanley D. Klein. *The Exceptional Parent*, June 1983. 13:3:18-25. Computer systems and learning disabilities.

1983 Revised Non-Vocal Communication Resource Book, Gregg Vanderheiden. Trace Center, Univ. of Wisconsin, Madison.

Remmes, Hal, 41 Woodglen Rd, Hyde Park, MA 02136. 617-361-8523. Author on computers and disabilities.

Signs for Computing Technology, Steven Jamison. National Association of the Deaf, 814 Thayer Ave, Silver Spring, MD 20910. 1983.

Resources

Sourcebook of Aid for the Mentally & Physically Handicapped, Dr. Judith Norback, Editor. Van Nostrand Reinhold Co, 135 West 50 St, New York 10020. 1983. Comprehensive resource book.

Special Technology for Special Children, Paul Goldenberg, University Park Press, Baltimore, MD, 1979. Uses of computers to study communication impairments in children. Focus on psychology.

Specialware Directory, LINC Resources. Distributed by Council for Exceptional Children, Reston, VA. Software directory for special education.

Speech Systems for Your Microcomputer, Gary Shade. Wayne Green Publications, New Hampshire. 603-924-9471. 1984.

Technology & Handicapped People, Congressional Office of Technology Assessment. Springer Press, New York. 1983. $29.50.

Transitions in Mental Retardation series, Vol I: *Advocacy, Technology & Science*, Dr. Jim Mulick, Editor. Ablex Press, Norwood, NJ.

Use of Microcomputers in Special Education. Proceedings from 1983 Conference in Hartford, CT. Distributed by Council for Exceptional Children, Reston, VA. $20.

Use of Technology in the Care of the Elderly & the Disabled, Jean Bray, Editor. Clinical Research Centre, Harrow, England. Published by Greenwood Press, Westport, CT, 1980. Disabilities in EEC countries; some statistics.

Uses of Computers in Aiding the Disabled, Josef Raviv, Editor. No. Holland Publishing Co, New York, 1982. Distributed by Elsevier Science Publishing, 52 Vanderbilt Ave, New York, NY 10017. Proceedings of the 1981 UN Conference on Computers to Aid the Disabled held at Technion, Israeli Institute of Technology, Haifa, November, 1981.

NATIONAL DIRECTORIES

American Annals of the Deaf: Reference Issue, American Annals of the Deaf, Silver Spring, MD. Published annually in April.

Directory for Exceptional Children, Porter-Sargent Publishers, Boston.

Directory of Agencies Serving the Deaf-Blind, Helen Keller National Center, Sands Point, NY.

Directory of Agencies Serving the Visually Handicapped in the United States, American Foundation for the Blind, New York City.

Directory of Educational Facilities for the Learning Disabled, Association for Children & Adults with Learning Disabilities, Pittsburgh, PA.

Directory of Learning Resources for the Handicapped and *Directory of Learning Resources for Learning Disabilities*, Croft-Nei Pub., Waterford, CT.

International Directory of Services for the Deaf, Gallaudet College, Washington, DC.

International Telephone Directory of the Deaf, Telecommunications for the Deaf, Arlington, VA.

National Directory of Children and Youth Service, CPR Directory Service, Washington, DC.

PERSONAL COMPUTERS AND THE DISABLED

National Directory of 4-Year Colleges, 2-Year Colleges, and Post High School Training Programs for Young People with Learning Disabilities, Partners in Publishing, Tulsa, OK. 918-584-5906.

National Resource Handbook: A Guide to Vocational Rehabilitation Services in the United States, Vocational Rehab Ctr, Pittsburgh, PA.

Resource Directory of Handicapped Scientists, American Association for Advancement of Science, Washington, DC.

Volunteers Who Produce Books, National Library Service for the Blind & Physically Handicapped, Washington, DC., Consumer Relations Section.

BOOK CLUBS

Children's Braille Book of the Month Club
National Braille Press
88 St. Stephens St
Boston, MA 02115
Information: Diane Croft

Generally books priced in the $7 to $8 range. Free membership with no obligation to buy monthly selections.

Macmillian Book Club
Library of Special Education
Front & Brown Streets
Riverside, NJ 08370
609-461-9100

LIBRARY SERVICES

Canadian National Institute for the Blind
National Library Division
1929 Bayview Ave
Toronto, Ontario
Canada M4G 3E8
Francoise Hebert, Director
416-486-2576.

Books in Braille and on cassette produced for the disabled. Offers talking books thru National Lending Library and public libraries at no cost to disabled readers.

Library of Congress
National Library Service for Blind & Physically Handicapped
1291 Taylor St NW
Washington, DC 20542
202-287-5104
Frank Cylke, Director

A network of 56 regional and 100 local libraries. (See STATES, Section VIII for addresses.) Books and magazines available in braille and on cassette. Mailed to borrowers at no charge, along with playback equipment, if required. The following books on computers are available through the NLS library system:

Adler, Irving, *Thinking Machines; A Layman's Introduction to Logic, Boolean Algebra and Computers*. John Day, New York, 1974.

Resources

Barden, William, *How to Program Microcomputers*. Howard Sams, Indianapolis, 1977.

Cohn, Daniel, *The Human Side of Computers*. McGraw-Hill, New York, 1975.

DeKen, Joseph, *The Electronic Cottage*. Morrow, New York, 1981.

Evans, Christopher, *The Micro Millennium*. Viking Press, New York, 1980.

Hyde, Margaret O., *Computers That Think; The Search for Artificial Intelligence*. Enslow Pubs, Hillside, NJ. 1982.

Jacobsen, Karen, *Computers*. Children's Press, Chicago, 1982.

Kleinberg, Harry, *How You Can Learn to Live With Computers*. Lippincott, Philadelphia, 1977.

Kidder, Tracy, *Soul of a New Machine*. Little Brown, Boston, 1981.

Perry, Robert Louis, *Owning Your Home Computer*. Everest House, New York, 1980.

Teja, Edward, *Teaching Your Computer To Talk*. Tab Books, Blue Ridge Summit, PA, 1981.

Wanous, Samuel, *Introduction to Automated Data Processing*, 2nd ed. South Western, Cincinnati, 1979.

Willis, Jerry, *Computers for Everybody*, Tab Books, Blue Ridge Summit, PA, 1982.

Magazine articles on computers from NLS:

Boy's Life, "How Computers Help the Handicapped," Robert L. Perry. February 1983: 42.

Changing Times, "Home Computers: A Guide for Bewildered Buyers," vol 36. August 1982: 24-28.

Money, "Choosing the Best Computer For You," Augustin Hegberg. Vol 11, November 1982: 68-117. Compares 36 personal computers.

Playboy, "The Compleat Personal Computer," Danny Goodman. April 1982: 216, 218, 220. Software advances that permit computers to develop pseudo-intelligence.

Recording for the Blind
20 Roszel Rd
Princeton, NJ 08540
609-452-0606

60,000 titles on cassette, including computer books. Available to the legally certified blind at no charge since 1949. Application must be filed. 4-track tape recorder must be acquired elsewhere.

PERSONAL COMPUTERS AND THE DISABLED

VIII. STATES

At the state level, governments have a wide variety of agencies to serve the disabled community. Each state has anywhere from six to eight of these agencies, which are listed in the following order by state:

State Developmental Disabilities Council

Director of Special Education

Vocational Rehabilitation Agency

Vocational Rehabilitation Agency for the Blind

Governor's Committee on Handicapped Employment

Crippled Children's Services

Mental Retardation Program Director

Regional Library of the National Library System for the Blind & Handicapped

Strictly speaking, the Regional Libraries are not state agencies, but part of the Library of Congress National Library System.

PIC=Private Industry Councils

Nationwide government effort to employ the disabled. Each state is divided into geographic areas with one PIC each. California, for example, has 50 PIC's, including one for the city of San Francisco. A PIC is a Board of community leaders, more than half of whom must be prospective employers of the disabled. The local **Employment Development Dept (EDD)** will have information about the nearest PIC. At the state level, the **Governor's Committee on Employment of the Handicapped** provides information. Section VIIII will list the Governor's Committees by state. This decentralized structure, set up through the Job Training Partnership Act (JPTA), replaces CETA and makes Job placement more locally directed.

State Developmental Disabilities Councils

Decentralized planning agencies to administer funding from the Administration on Developmental Disabilities. These DD Councils are listed on the following pages by state. Here is a profile of one computer project recently begun by the Hawaii DD Council:

State Developmental Disabilities Council
Hawaii Dept. of Health
Box 3378
Honolulu, HI 96801
Lily Wang
808-548-8482

Program to train severely retarded students in data entry. Begun six months ago with five students and computers provided by Wang Labs. Seeking federal grants to expand and include other disabilities. Training manual in preparation.

Resources

ALABAMA

Dale W. Scott
Director
DD Planning Council
200 Interstate Park Dr.
P.O. Box 3710
Montgomery, AL 36193
205-271-9278

State Director of Special Education
Exceptional Children & Youth
State Department of Education
868 State Office Bldg.
Montgomery, AL 36104
205-832-3230

J.W. Cowen
Director
Division of Rehabilitation & Services
P.O. Box 11586
Montgomery, AL 36111
205-281-8780

Governor's Committee on
 Handicapped Employment
P. O. Box 11586
2129 E. South Blvd.
Montgomergy, AL 36111

Director
Crippled Children's Services
2129 E. South Blvd.
Montgomery, AL 36111
205-281-8780

Mental Retardation Program Director
Dept. of Mental Health
135 S. Union St.
Montgomery, AL 36130
205-834-4350

Library for the Blind &
 Physically Handicapped
Alabama Public Library Service
State of Alabama
Montgomery, AL 36130
205-277-7330

ALASKA

Dorothy J. Truran
Health Planner II
Governor's Council for the
 Handicapped & Gifted
600 University Ave., Suite C
Fairbanks, AK 99701
907-479-6507

State Director of Special Education
Exceptional Children & Youth
State Department of Education
Pouch F
Juneau, AK 99801
907-465-2970

Michael C. Morgan
Director
Division of Vocational Rehabilitation
Pouch F, MS 0581
Juneau, AK 99811
907-465-2814

Governor's Committee on
 Handicapped Employment
Hope Cottage
2805 Bering St., NO. 2-A
Anchorage, AK 99503

Director
State Department of Dept. Social Services
Family Health Section
Pouch H
Health and Welfare Bldg.
Juneau, AK 99801
907-465-3100

Mental Retardation Program Director
Dept. of Health and Social Services
Pouch H-04
Juneau, AK 99811
907-465-3372

Services for the Blind &
 Physically Handicapped
State Library
650 W. International Airport Road
Anchorage, AK 99502
907-274-6625

PERSONAL COMPUTERS AND THE DISABLED

ARIZONA

William C. Donovan
Executive Director
Governor's Council on DD
1717 W. Jefferson St. MS 0742
Phoenix, AZ 85007
602-255-4040

State Director of Special Education
State Department of Education
Division of Special Education
1535 W. Jefferson St.
Phoenix, AZ 85007
602-255-3183

Thomas G. Tyrrell
Adminstrator
Rehabilitation Services Administration
Dept. of Economic Security
1300 W. Washington St.
Phoenix, AZ 85007
602-255-3332

Governor's Committee on
  Handicapped Employment
2nd Floor, Education Bldg.
1535 W. Jefferson St.
Phoenix, AZ 85007

Director
State Crippled Children's Hospital
200 N. Curry Rd.
Tempe, AZ 85281
602-244-9471

Mental Retardation Program Director
Dept. of Economic Security
P.O. Box 6760
Phoenix, AZ 85005
602-255-5775

Library for the Blind &
  Physically Handicapped
3120 E. Roosevelt St.
Phoenix, AZ 85008
602-255-5578

ARKANSAS

Mary Eddy Thomas
Executive Director
Governor's DD Planning Council
4815 West Markham St.
Little Rock, AR 72201
501-661-2399

State Director of Special Education
Division of Institutional Services
State Department of Education
Arch Ford Educational Bldg.
Little Rock, AR 72201
501-371-2161

E. Russel Baxter
Commissioner
Rehabilitation Services Administration
Arkansas Department of Human Services
P.O. Box 37381
Little Rock, AR 72203
501-371-2571

Governor's Committee on
  Handicapped Employment
P.O. Box 2981
Little Rock, AR 72203

Director
Department of Social Services
Crippled Children's Section
Box 1437
Little Rock, AR 72203
501-371-2277

Mental Retardation Program Director
Mental Health/DD Services
Dept. of Human Services
Ste. 400, Waldon Bldg.
7th and Main
Little Rock, AR 72201
501-371-3419

Dick Seifert
Acting Commissioner
Division of Services for the Blind
Dept. of Human Services
P.O. Box 3237
Little Rock, AR 72203
501-371-2587

Library for the Blind &
  Physically Handicapped
MAC Bldg., One Capitol Mall
Little Rock, AR 72201
501-371-1155

Resources

CALIFORNIA

Jim Shorter
Executive Director
State Council on DD
1507 21st St.
Room 320
Sacramento, CA 95816
916-322-8481

State Director of Special Education
Special Education Division
Department of Public Instruction
721 Capitol Mall, Room 614
Sacramento, CA 95814
916-445-4036

P. Cecilio Fontanoza, Ph.D.
Director
Dept. Of Rehabilitation
830 K St. Mall
Sacramento, CA 95814
916-445-3971

Governor's Committee on
  Handicapped Employment
800 Capitol Mall, Room 5054
Sacramento, CA 95814

Director
State Department of Health
Crippled Children's Services Section
741-744 P St.
Sacramento, CA 95814
916-322-2090

Mental Retardation Program Director
Dept. of Developmental Services
714 P St. #650
Sacramento, CA 95814
916-323-3131

Library
Braille Institute of America, Inc.
741 N. Vermont Ave.
Los Angeles, CA 90029
213-663-1111

COLORADO

Merril Stern
Executive Director
Colorado DD Council
4126 S. Knox Court
Denver, CO 80236
303-761-0220

State Director of Special Education
Pupil Services Department
State Department of Education
State Office Bldg.
201 E. Colfax
Denver, CO 80203
303-839-2727

Mark E. Litvin, Ph.D.
Director
Division of Rehabilitation
Dept. of Social Services
1575 Sherman St.
Denver, CO 80203
303-866-2652

Governor's Committee on
  Handicapped Employment
1515 Sherman St., 5th Floor
Denver, CO 80203

Director
Department of Health
Handicapped Children's Program
4210 E. 11th Ave.
Denver, CO 80220
303-388-6111

Mental Retardation Program Directors
Division for Developmental Disabilities
4150 S. Lowell Blvd.
Denver, CO 80236
303-761-0220

Services for the Blind &
  Physically Handicapped
State Library
1313 Sherman St.
Denver, CO 80203
303-839-2081

PERSONAL COMPUTERS AND THE DISABLED

CONNECTICUT

Edward T. Preneta
Staff Director
DD Office—Dept. of Mental Retardation
342 N. Main St.
West Hartford, CT 06117
203-236-2531

State Director of Special Education
Bureau of Pupil Personnel
 & Special Education
State Dept. of Education
P.O. Box 2219
Hartford, CT 06115
203-566-4383

Joseph R. Galotti
Associate Commissioner
State Dept. of Education
Division of Vocational Rehabilitation
600 Asylum Ave.
Hartford, CT 06105
203-566-4440

Governor's Committee on
 Handicapped Employment
200 Folly Brook Blvd.
Wethersfield, CT 06109

Director
State Department of Health
Crippled Children's Section
79 Elm St.
Hartford, CT 06115
203-566-5425

Mental Retardation Program Director
Dept. of Mental Health
342 N. Main Street
West Hartford, CT 06117
203-236-2531

William E. Patton, ACSW
Director
Board of Education & Services for the Blind
170 Ridge Road
Wethersfield, CT 06109
203-566-5800

Library for the Blind &
 Physically Handicapped
State Library
90 Washington St.
Hartford, CT 06106
203-566-3028

DELAWARE

James F. Linehan
Administrator
DD Planning Council
Dept. of Community Affairs
P.O. Box 1401
156 S. State St. Priscilla Bldg.
Dover, DE 19901
302-736-4456

State Director of Special Education
Special Programs Division
Dept. of Public Instruction
Townsend Bldg.
Dover, DE 19901
302-678-5471

Tony Sokolowski
Director
Division of Vocational Rehabilitation
Dept. of Labor
State Office Bldg. 7th floor
820 N. French St.
Wilmington, DE 19801
302-571-2850

Governor's Committee on
 Handicapped Employment
1500 Shallcross Ave.
P.O. Box 1190
Wilmington, DE 19899

Director
Bureau of Personal Health Services
Division of Public Health
Jessee Cooper Memorial Bldg.
Capital Sq.
Dover, DE 19901
302-678-4768

Mental Retardation Program Director
Division of Mental Retardation
Route 1, Box 1000
Georgetown, DE 19947
302-934-8031

Norman Balot
Director
Division for the Visually Impaired
Dept. of Health and Social Services
305 W. 8th St.
Wilmington, DE 19801
302-571-3333

Division of Libraries
Special Services Group
215 Dover St.
Dover, DE 19901
302-678-4523

Resources

DISTRICT OF COLUMBIA

Katherine Williams
Executive Director
Randall School Room 306
1st & I Sts., SW
Washington, DC 20034
202-727-5905

State Director of Special Education
State Department of Education
Division of Special Education Programs
415 12th St., NW
Washington, DC 20004
202-724-4018

Vernon Hawkins
Administrator
D.C. Rehabilitation Services Administration
Dept. of Human Services
605 G St., NW
Room 1101
Washington, DC 20001
202-727-3227

Governor's Committee on
 Handicapped Employment
Room 200
122 C St., NW
Washington, DC 20001

Director
D.C. Department of Human Resources
Crippled Children's Services
1875 Connecticut Ave., NW
Washington, DC 20001
202-673-6670

Mental Retardation Program Director
Dept. of Human Services
Presidential Bldg.
Room 410
415 12th St., NW
Washington, DC 20004
202-673-6904

Library for the Blind &
 Physically Handicapped
901 G St., NW
Washington, DC 20001
202-727-2142

FLORIDA

Joe Krieger
Administrator
DD Dept. of Health &
 Rehabilitative Services
Florida DD Planning Council
1323 Winewood Blvd.
Bldg. 1, Room 308
Tallahassee, FL 32301
904-488-4180

State Director of Special Education
Bureau of Education for
 Exceptional Students
State Department of Education
319 Knott Bldg.
Tallahassee, FL 32304
904-488-1570

Ms. Lani Deauville
Director
Office of Vocational Rehabilitation
Dept. of Health & Rehabilitative
 Services
1317 Winewood Blvd.
Tallahassee, FL 32301
904-488-6210

Governor's Committee on
 Handicapped Employment
210 Caldwell Bldg.
Tallahassee, FL 32304

Director
Dept. of Health & Human Services
Children's Medical Services Program
1323 Winewood Blvd., Bldg. 5
Tallahassee, FL 32301
904-487-2690

Mental Retardation Program Director
Developmental Services Program
1311 Winewood Blvd.
Bldg. 5, Room 215
Tallahassee, FL 32301
904-488-4257

Donald H. Wedewer
Director
Division of Blind Services
Dept. of Education, W. Douglas Bldg.
2540 Executive Center Circle
Tallahassee, FL 32301
904-488-1330

Library for the Blind &
 Physically Handicapped
P.O. Box 2299
Daytona Beach, FL 32105
904-252-4722

PERSONAL COMPUTERS AND THE DISABLED

GEORGIA

Zebe Schmitt
Executive Director
Georgia Council on DD
878 Peachtree St., NE, Room 620
Atlanta, GA 30308
404-894-5790

State Director of Special Education
Department of Education
Program for Exceptional Children
State Office Bldg.
Atlanta, GA 30334
404-656-2678

Thomas R. Gaines
Director
Division of Rehabilitation Services
Dept. of Human Services
Floyd Memorial Veterans Bldg.
47 Trinity Ave., S.W., 10th Floor
Atlanta, GA 30334
404-656-2621

Governor's Committee on
 Handicapped Employment
1599 Memorial Dr., SE
Atlanta, GA 30317

Director
Department of Dept. of Human Resources
Crippled Children's Unit
618 Ponce de Leon Ave., NE
Atlanta, GA 30308
404-894-4081

Mental Retardation Program Director
Dept. of Mental Health Services
47 Trinity Ave., SW
Atlanta, GA 30334
404-656-6370

Library for the Blind &
 Physically Handicapped
1050 Murphy Ave., SW
Atlanta, GA 30310
404-656-2465

HAWAII

Lily I. Wang
Executive Secretary
State Council on DD
P.O. Box 3378
Honolulu, HI 96801
808-548-5994

State Director of Special Education
Special Needs Branch
State Department of Education
P.O. Box 2360
Honolulu, HI 96804
808-548-6923

Toshio Nishoika
Administrator
Vocational Rehabilitation &
 Services for Blind
Dept. of Social Services
P.O. Box 339
Honolulu, HI 96809
808-548-4769

Governor's Committee on
 Handicapped Employment
250 S. King St.
Room 603
Honolulu, HI 96813

Director
State Department of Health
P.O. Box 3378
Honolulu, HI 96801
808-548-5830

Mental Retardation Program Director
State Planning and Advisory Council
P.O. Box 3378
Honolulu, HI 96801
808-548-5994

Library for the Blind &
 Physically Handicapped
402 Hapahulu Ave.
Honolulu, HI 96815
808-732-7767

Resources

IDAHO

John Watts
Director
Idaho State Council of DD
Towers Bldg., 10th Floor
450 W. State St.
Boise, ID 83720
208-334-4408

State Director of Special Education
Special Education Division
State Department of Education
Len B. Jordan Bldg.
Boise, ID 83720
208-334-3940

George Pelletier
Administrator
Division of Vocational Rehabilitation
Len B. Jordan Bldg. Room 150
650 W. State St.
Boise, ID 83720
208-334-3390

Governor's Committee on
  Handicapped Employment
P.O. Box 35
Boise, ID 83707

Bureau of Child Health
State Department of Health & Welfare
Crippled Children's Services
State House
700 W. State St.
Boise, ID 83720
208-384-2136

Mental Retardation Program Director
Bureau of Adult and Child Development
State House
Boise, ID 83720
208-334-4181

Larry Selland
Acting Administrator
Commission for the Blind
State House
Boise, ID 83704
208-334-3220

Library for the Blind &
  Physically Handicapped
Idaho State Library
325 W. State St.
Boise, ID 83702
208-384-2150

ILLINOIS

Ann Kiley
Acting Director
Illinois Governor's Planning Council on DD
222 S. College
Springfield, IL 62706
217-782-9696

Director of Special Education
Dept. of Special Educational Services
State Department of Education
100 N. 1st St.
Springfield, IL 62777
217-782-6601

Robert Granzeier
Director
Dept. of Rehabilitation Services
623 E. Adams St.
Springfield, IL 62706
217-782-2093

Governor's Committee on
  Handicapped Employment
623 E. Monroe St., 1st Floor
Springfield, IL 62701

Director
Services for Crippled Children
540 Iles Park Pl.
Springfield, IL 62718
217-782-7001

Mental Retardation Program Director
Dept. of Mental Health
402 Stratton Office Bldg.
Springfield, IL 62706
217-782-7395

Library for the Blind &
  Physically Handicapped
Chicago Public Library
1055 W. Roosevelt Rd.
Chicago, IL 60608
312-738-9210

PERSONAL COMPUTERS AND THE DISABLED

INDIANA

Susan Jackson
Director
Indiana DD Advisory Council
429 N. Pennsylvania, Room 253
Indianapolis, IN 46204
317-232-7885

Director of Special Education
Division of Special Education
229 State House
Indianapolis, IN 46204
317-927-0216

Wendell J. Walls
Director
Rehabilitation Services
P.O. Box 7070
Indianapolis, IN 46204
317-232-1663

Commission for the Handicapped
1330 W. Michigan St.
Indianapolis, IN 46206

Director
Division of Services for
　Crippled Children
Department of Public Welfare
Room 701
100 N.Senate Ave
Indianapolis, IN 46204
317-232-4402

Mental Retardation Program Director
Dept. of Mental Health
5 Indiana Square
Indianapolis, IN 46204
317-232-7836

Indiana State Library
Blind & Physically
　Handicapped Division
140 N. Senate Ave.
Indianapolis, IN 46204
317-232-3684

IOWA

Joann Young
Council Coordinator
Governor's Planning Council for DD
Dept. of Human Services
5th Floor, Hoover State Office Bldg.
Des Moines, IA 50319
515-281-5646

Director of Special Education
Division of Special Education
Grimes State Office Bldg.
Des Moines, IA 50319
515-281-3176

Jerry L. Starkweather
Associate Superintendent
Rehabilitation Education & Services
Dept. of Public Instruction
510 E. 12th St.
Des Moines, IA 50319
515-281-4311

Governor's Committee on
　Handicapped Employment
Grimes State Office Bldg.
Des Moines, IA 50319

Director
Services for Crippled Children
University of Iowa
Iowa City, IA 52242
319-353-4431

Mental Retardation Program Director
Dept. of Social Services
Lucas State Office Bldg.
Des Moines, IA 50319
515-281-6003

Nancy A. Morman
Director
Commission for the Blind
4th and Keosauqua
Des Moines, IA 50309
515-283-2601

Resources

KANSAS

Janet Schalansky
Executive Director
Kansas Planning Council
  on DD Services
Dept. of Social and
  Rehabilitation Services
State Office Bldg., 5th Floor
Topeka, KS 66612
913-296-2608

Director of Special Education
Division of Special Education
120 E. 10th St.
Topeka, KS 66612
913-296-3866

Gabriel R. Faimon
Commissioner
Dept. of Social &
  Rehabilitative Services
2700 W. 6th,
Biddle Bldg., 2nd Floor
Topeka, KS 66606
913-296-3911

Governor's Committee on
  Handicapped Employment
126 S. 1st Floor
State Office Bldg.
Topeka, KS 66611

Director
Department of Health & Environment
Bureau of Maternal & Child Health
Topeka, KS 66620
913-862-9360

Mental Retardation Program Director
Dept. of Disabilities Services
State Office Bldg., 6th Floor
Topeka, KS 66612
913-296-3471

Richard A. Schuta, Ph.D.
Director
Division of Services for the Blind
State Dept. of Social &
  Rehabilitation Services
Biddle Bldg., 1st Floor
2700 W. 6th St.
Topeka, KS 66606
913-296-4454

Kansas State Library
Division for the Blind &
  Physically Handicapped
529 Kansas Ave.
Topeka, KS 66603
913-296-3642

KENTUCKY

Richard Eversman
Acting Director
DD Planning Council
275 E. Main St.
Frankfort, KY 40601
502-564-7841

Director of Special Education
Bureau of Education for
  Exceptional Children
Capitol Plaza Tower, 8th Floor
Frankfort, KY 40601
502-564-4970

Laurel True
Assistant Superintendent
Bureau of Rehabilitative Services
Dept. of Education
Capital Plaza Tower
Frankfort, KY 40601
502-564-4440

Governor's Committee on
  Handicapped Employment
600 W. Cedar St.
Louisville, KY 40203

Director
State Department of
  Human Resources
Bureau for Health Services
275 E. Main St.
Frankfort, KY 40601
502-564-4830

Mental Retardation Program Director
Community Services for the
  Mentally Retarded
Department of Human Resources
275 E. Main St.
Frankfort, KY 40601
502-564-3418

Charles W. McDowell
Director
Bureau of Blind Services
Education & Arts Cabinet
State Office Bldg., Annex
P.O. Box 758
Frankfort, KY 40601
502-564-4754

Library for the Blind &
  Physically Handicapped
Twilight Trail, Bldg. C
P.O. Box 818
Frankfort, KY 40602
502-564-5532

PERSONAL COMPUTERS AND THE DISABLED

LOUISIANA

Dr. Anne E. Farber
Executive Director
DD Planning Council
P.O. Box 44215
Baton Rouge, LA 70802
504-342-6804

Director of Special Education
Special Educational Services
Capitol Station
P.O. Box 44064
Baton Rouge, LA 70804
504-342-3631

Lester Soileau
Director
Division of Vocational Rehabilitation
Dept. of Health & Human Resources
P.O. Box 44371
Baton Rouge, LA 70804
504-342-2285

Governor's Committee on
  Handicapped Employment
530 Lakeland Dr.
Baton Rouge, LA 70802

Director
Department of Human Resources
P.O. Box 60630
New Orleans, LA 70160
504-568-5048

Mental Retardation Program Director
Dept. of Mental Health Services
721 Government St.
Room 308
Baton Rouge, LA 70802
504-342-6811

Jerry Swearingen
Director
Division of Blind Services
Dept. of Health &
  Human Development
1755 Florida St.
Baton Rouge, LA 70804
504-342-5284

Dept. for the Blind &
  Physically Handicapped
Louisiana State Library
P.O. Box 131
Baton Rouge, LA 70821
504-342-4943

MAINE

Peter Stowell
Executive Director
Dept. of Mental Health & Corrections
State Office Bldg., Room 411
Augusta, ME 04333

Division of Special Education
Director of Special Education,
State Department of
  Educational Services
State House Complex
Augusta, ME 04330
207-289-3451

C. Owen Pollard
Director
Bureau of Rehabilitation Services
Dept. of Health & Welfare
32 Winthrop St.
Augusta, ME 04330
207-289-2266

Governor's Committee on
  Handicapped Employment
32 Winthrop St.
Augusta, ME 04330

Director
Division of Child State Health
State House
Augusta, ME 04330
207-289-3311

Mental Retardation Program Director
Dept. of Mental Health Corrections
State House, Room 400
Augusta, ME 04330
207-289-3161

Library Services for the Handicapped
Maine State Library
State House Station 64
Augusta, ME 04333
207-289-3950

Resources

MARYLAND

Catherine Raggio
Acting Director
Developmental Disabilities Council
Dept. of Health and Mental Hygiene
O'Conner Bldg., 4th Floor
201 W. Preston St.
Baltimore, MD 21201
301-383-3358

Director of Special Education
Division of Special Education
200 W. Baltimore St.
Baltimore, MD 21021
301-659-2000

Richard Batterton
Assistant Superintendent
Division of Vocational Rehabilitation
State Dept. of Education
200 W. Baltimore St.
Baltimore, MD 21201
301-659-2294

Governor's Committee on
 Handicapped Employment
2100 Guilford
Room 201
Baltimore, MD 21218

Director
Dept. of Health and Mental Hygiene
Preventative Medicine Administration
201 W. Preston St.
Baltimore, MD 21201
301-383-2821

Mental Retardation Program Director
Dept. of Health and Mental Hygiene
201 W. Preston Street
Baltimore, MD 21201
301-383-3354

Library for the Blind &
 Physically Handicapped
1715 N. Charles St.
Baltimore, MD 21201
301-383-3111

MASSACHUSETTS

Steve Rosner
Director
DD Planning Council
One Ashburton Place, Room 1319
Boston, MA 02108
617-727-6374

Director of Special Education
Division of Special Education
31 St. James Ave.
Boston, MA 02116
617-727-6217

Elmer C. Bartels
Commissioner
Rehabilitation Commission
Statler Office Bldg., 11 Floor
20 Providence St.
Boston, MA 02116
617-727-2172

Governor's Committee on
 Handicapped Employment
C. F. Hurley Employment
Security Bldg.
Government Center
Boston, MA 02114

Director
State Department of Public Health
Division of Family Health
39 Boylston St.
Boston, MA 02116
617-737-3372

Mental Retardation Program Director
Dept. of Mental Health
160 N. Washington St.
Boston, MA 02114
617-727-5608

Edward J. McHugh
Commissioner
Commission for the Blind
110 Tremont St., 6th Floor
Boston, MA 02108
617-727-5550

Library for the Blind &
 Physically Handicapped
Perkins School for the Blind
175 N. Beacon St.
Watertown, MA 02172
617-924-3434

PERSONAL COMPUTERS AND THE DISABLED

MICHIGAN

Beth Ferguson
Acting Director
DD Planning Council
Lewis Cass Bldg., 6th Floor
Lansing, MI 48926
517-373-6443

Director of Special Education
Special Educational Services
P.O. Box 420
Lansing, MI 48902
517-373-1695

Peter Griswold
Director
Michigan Bureau of
  Vocational Rehabilitation
Dept. of Education
P.O. Box 30010
Lansing, MI 48909
517-373-0683

Governor's Committee on
  Handicapped Employment
7150 Harris Drive
Lansing, MI 48929

Director
Department of Public Health
Bureau of Maternal and
  Child Health
3500 N. Logan St.
Lansing, MI 48914
517-373-3650

Mental Retardation Program Director
Dept. of Mental Health
Lewis Cass Bldg., 6th Floor
Lansing, MI 48926
517-373-2900

Philip E. Peterson
Director
Commission for the Blind
Dept. of Labor
309 N. Washington Square
Lansing, MI 48909
517-373-2062

Library for the Blind &
  Physically Handicapped
33030 Van Born Rd.
Wayne, MI 48184
313-274-2600

MINNESOTA

Colleen Wieck, Ph.D
Director
DD Planning Council
200 Capitol Square Bldg.
550 Cedar St.
St. Paul, MN 55101
612-296-4018

Director of Special Education
Special Educational Section
Capitol Sq., 550 Cedar St.
St. Paul, MN 55101
612-296-4163

Edward O. Opheim
Assistant Commissioner
Vocational Rehabilitation
Department of Economic Security
Space Center, 3rd Floor
444 Lafayette Rd.
St. Paul, MN 55101
612-296-1822

Council for the Handicapped
Metro Square, 7th and Roberts Sts.
Suite 208
St. Paul, MN 55101

Director
Department of Health
Crippled Children's Services
717 Delaware St.
Minneapolis, MN 55440
612-296-5372

Mental Retardation Program Director
Dept. of Public Welfare
Centennial Office Bldg.
5th Floor
St. Paul, MN 55155
612-296-2160

C. Stanley Potter
Director
State Services for the Blind
Division of Rehabilitation Services
Dept. of Minnesota Public Welfare
1745 University Ave., 1st Floor
St. Paul, MN 55104
612-296-6080

Library for the Blind &
  Physically Handicapped
Braille & Sight Saving School
Faribault, MN 55021
507-332-3279

Resources

MISSISSIPPI

Ed Bell
Planning Coordinator
DD Planning Council
Dept. of Mental Health
1102 Robert E. Lee Bldg.
Jackson, MS 39201
601-359-1290

Director of Special Education
Division of Special Education
P.O. Box 771
Jackson, MS 39205
601-354-6950

Bradley Sanders
Director
Vocational Rehabilitation
P.O. Box 1698
Jackson, MS 39205
601-354-6825

Governor's Committee on
   Handicapped Employment
Box 1698
Jackson, MS 39205

Director
State Board of Health
Bureau of Family Health Services
Crippled Children's Services
P.O. Box 1700
Jackson, MS 39205
601-354-6680

Mental Retardation Program Director
Dept. of Mental Health
1100 Robert E. Lee Bldg.
Jackson, MS 39210
601-354-6692

J. Elton Moore, Ph.D.
Director
Vocational Rehabilitation
   for the Blind
P.O. Box 4872
Jackson, MS 39216
601-354-6412

Services for the Handicapped
Mississippi Library Commission
P.O. Box 3260
Jackson, MS 39207
601-354-7208

MISSOURI

Ken Dowden
Coordinator
DD Planning Council
Division of MR/DD
Dept. of Mental Health
2002 Missouri Blvd.
Jefferson City, MO 65102
314-751-4054

Director of Special Education
Division of Special Education
P.O. Box 480
Jefferson City, MO 65101
314-751-2965

Don Gann, Ph.D.
Assistant Commissioner
Division of Vocational Rehabilitation
State Department of Education
2401 E. McCarty
Jefferson City, MO 65101
314-751-3251

Governor's Committee on
   Handicapped Employment
P.O. Box 59
421 E. Dunklin
Jefferson City, MO 65101

Director
Department of Social Services
Division of Health
Crippled Children's Services
Broadway State Office Building
Jefferson City, MO 65101
314-751-4667

Mental Retardation Program Director
Dept. of Mental Health
2002 Missouri Blvd.
P.O. Box 687
Jefferson City, MO 65101
314-751-4054

Gary Stangler
Interum Deputy Director
Bureau for the Blind
Division of Family Services
619 E. Capitol
Jefferson City, MO 65101
314-751-4249

Wolfner Memorial Library for the
   Blind & Physically Handicapped
1808 Washington Ave.
St. Louis, MO 63103
314-241-4227

PERSONAL COMPUTERS AND THE DISABLED

MONTANA

Clyde Muirheid
Staff Director
DD Planning Council
P. O. Box 4210
Helena, MT 59601
406-444-3878

Director of Special Education
Division of Special Education
State Capitol
Helena, MT 59601
406-449-5660

W.R. Donaldson
Administrator
Rehabilitative Services
Dept. of Social &
 Rehabilitation Services
P.O. Box 4210
Helena, MT 59601
406-444-3434

Governor's Committee on
 Handicapped Employment
P.O. Box 1723
Helena, MT 59601

Director
Department of Health &
 Environmental Sciences
Health Services Division
Maternal and Child Health
Cogswell Bldg.
Helena, MT 59601
406-449-2554

Mental Retardation Program Director
Developmental Disabilities Division
P.O. Box 4210
Helena, MT 59601
406-449-2995

Montana State Library
Division for the Blind &
 Physically Handicapped
930 E. Lyndale Ave.
Helena, MT 59601
406-449-3004

NEBRASKA

Eric Evans
Acting Staff Director
DD Planning Council
P. O. Box 95007
Lincoln, NE 68509
402-471-2981

Director of Special Education
Division of Special Education
State Department of Education
223 S. 10th St.
Lincoln, NE 68508
402-471-2471

Jason D. Andrew, Ph.D.
Assistant Commissioner
Division of Rehabilitation Services
State Dept. of Rehabilitative
 Services
301 Centennial Mall, 6th Floor
Lincoln, NE 68509
402-471-2961

Governor's Committee on
 Handicapped Employment
550 S 16th
P.O. Box 949600
State House Station
Lincoln, NE 68509

Director
Department of Public Welfare
Services for Crippled Children
301 Centennial Mall, Fifth Floor
Lincoln, NE 68509
402-471-3121

Mental Retardation Program Director
Office of Mental Health
State House
Box 94738
Lincoln, NE 68508
402-471-2165

James S. Nyman, Ph.D.
Director
Services for the Visually Impared
Dept. of Public Institutions
1047 S. St.
Lincoln, NE 68502
402-471-2891

Library for the Blind &
 Physically Handicapped
Nebraska Library Commission
1420 P St.
Lincoln, NE 68508
402-471-2045

Resources

NEVADA

Michael A. Becker
Planner
DD Planning Council
Rehab Div. Dept. of Human Resources
505 E. King St., Room 502
Carson City, NV 89710
702-885-4440

Director of Special Education
Division of Special Education
State Department of Education
440 W. King St.
Capitol Complex
Carson City, NV 89101
702-885-5700

Del Frost
Administrator
Rehabilitation Division
Dept. of Human Resources
Kinkead Bldg., 5th Floor
505 E. King St.
Carson City, NV 89710
702-885-4440

Governor's Committee on
  Handicapped Employment
505 E. King St.
State Capitol Complex
Carson City, NV 98710

Director
Division of Public Health
State Department of Human Resources
505 E. King St.
Room 205, Capitol Complex
Carson City, NV 89701
702-885-4885

Mental Retardation Program Director
Dept. of Mental Health
1937 N. Carson St., Ste. 244
Capitol Mall Complex
Carson City, NV 89710
702-885-5943

Special Services Division
Nevada State Library
Capitol Complex
Carson City, NV 89710
702-885-5155

NEW HAMPSHIRE

Susan P. Parker
Executive Director
DD Planning Council
1 Eagle Square, Suite 510
Concord, NH 03301
603-271-4709

Director of Special Education
Division of Special Education
State Department of Education
105 Loudon Rd., Bldg. #3
Concord, NH 03301
603-271-3741

Bruce A. Archambault
Chief
Division of Vocational Rehabilitation
State Dept. of Rehabilitation
101 Pleasant St. State Office Park So.
Concord, NH 03301
603-271-3121

Governor's Committee on
  Handicapped Employment
6 Loudon Rd.
Concord, NH 03301

Director
State Department of Health/Welfare
Division of Public Health
16 S. Spring St.
Concord, NH 03301
603-842-2681

Mental Retardation Program Director
Comm. Developmental Services/
  Health & Welfare
Hazen Drive
Concord, NH 03301
603-271-4711

Library Services for the Handicapped
17 Fruit St.
Concord, NH 03301
603-271-3429

PERSONAL COMPUTERS AND THE DISABLED

NEW JERSEY

Catherine Rowan
Executive Director
DD Planning Council
108-110 N. Broad St., CN 700
Trenton, NJ 08625
609-292-3745

Director of Special Education
Division of Special Education
State Department of Education
225 W. State St.
Trenton, NJ 08625
609-984-4955

George R. Chizmadia
Director
Division of Vocational
  Rehabilitation Services
Labor and Industry Bldg., Room 1005
John Fitch Plaza
Trenton, NJ 08625
609-292-5987

Governor's Committee on
  Handicapped Employment
Labor and Industry Bldg.
Room 1005
Trenton, NJ 08625

Director
Crippled Children's Program
State Department of Health
Health/Agricultural Bldg.
Trenton, NJ 08625
609-292-5676

Mental Retardation
  Program Director
Dept. of Human Services
222 S. Warren St.
Capitol Place One
Trenton, NJ 08625
609-292-3742

Norma Farrar Krajczar
Executive Director
Commission for the Blind
1100 Raymond Blvd.
Newark, NJ 07102
201-648-2324

Library for the
  Blind & Handicapped
1676 N. Olden Ave. Ext.
Trenton, NJ 08638
609-292-6450

NEW MEXICO

Marie Fritz
Director
DD Planning Council
Dept. of Finance and Administration
440B Cerrillos Road
Maya Bldg., Suite B
Santa Fe, NM 87503
505-827-7371

Director of Special Education
Division of Special Section
State Department of Education
300 Don Gaspar Ave
Sante Fe, NM 87503
505-827-2793

Orlando Giron
Dept. of Education
Division of Vocational
  Rehabilitation
604 W. San Mateo
Santa Fe, NM 87503
505-476-5581

Governor's Committee on
  Handicapped Employment
401 Broadway, NE
Albuquerque, NM 87103

Director
Health and Social Services
  Department
Office of Family Services
P.O. Box 2348
Santa Fe, NM 87501
505-827-3201

Mental Retardation Program Director
HED-Behavioral Health Services
P.O. Box 968
Santa Fe, NM 87501
505-827-5271

New Mexico State Library
Library for the Blind &
  Physically Handicapped
P.O. Box 1629
Santa Fe, NM 87503
505-827-2033

Resources

NEW YORK

Louis Grumet
Executive Secretary
DD Planning Council
Empire State Plaza
Agency Building #1, 10th Floor
Albany, NY 12223
518-474-3655

Director of Special Education
Office for Education of
 Handicapped Children
State Department of Education
55 Elk St.
Albany, NY 12234
518-474-5548

Richard M. Switzer
Acting Commissioner
Office of Vocational
 Rehabilitation
The University of the
 State of N.Y.
99 Washington Ave., Room 1910
Albany, NY 12230
518-473-4595

Governor's Committee on
 Handicapped Employment
Human Resources Center
Albertson, NY 11507

Director
State Department of Health
Bureau of Medical Rehabilitation
Empire State Plaza
Tower Bldg.
Albany, NY 12237
518-474-1911

Mental Retardation
 Program Director
Mental Health/
 Develop. Disabilities Offices
44 Holland Ave.
Albany, NY 12229
518-474-3231

Jack L. Ryan, Jr.
Director
Commission for the
 Blind & Visually Handicapped
10 Eyck Office Bldg.
40 North Pearl St.
Albany, NY 12243
518-473-1801

Library for the Blind
 & Physically Handicapped
Cultural Education Center
Empire State Plaza
Albany, NY 12230
518-474-5935

NORTH CAROLINA

Director of Special Education
Division of Exceptional Children
State Department of
 Public Instruction
Raleigh, NC 27611
919-733-3921

Claude A. Myer
Director
Vocational Rehabilitation Services
Dept. of Human Resources
State Office
P.O. Box 26053
Raleigh, NC 27611
919-733-3364

Governor's Committee on
 Handicapped Employment
306 N. Wilmington St.
Raleigh, NC 27611

Director
State Department of
 Human Resources
Crippled Children's Section
Division of Health Services
P.O. Box 2091
Raleigh, NC 27602
919-733-7437

Mental Retardation
 Program Director
Mental Health Services
Albemarle Bldg.
325 N. Salisbury St.
Raleigh, NC 27611
919-733-3654

Herman O. Gruber
Director
Division of Services for the Blind
N.C. Dept. of Human Resources
309 Ashe Ave.
Raleigh, NC 27606
919-733-9822

Dept. of Cultural Resources
Library for the Blind &
 Physically Handicapped
1811 N. Blvd.
Raleigh, NC 27635
919-733-4376

PERSONAL COMPUTERS AND THE DISABLED

NORTH DAKOTA

Darvin Hirsch
Director
DD Planning Council
State Capitol Annex
Bismarck, ND 58505
701-224-2769

Director of Special Education
Special Education Division
Department of Public Instruction
State Capitol
Bismarck, ND 58501
701-224-2277

James O. Fine
Director
Division of Vocational Rehabilitation
State Capitol Bldg.
Bismarck, ND 58505
701-224-2907

Governor's Committee on
  Handicapped Employment
State Capitol, 13th Floor
Bismarck, ND 58505

Director
State Department Social Services Board
State Capitol Bldg.
Bismarck, ND 58501
701-224-2436

Mental Retardation Program Director
Community Mental Health Programs
Dept. of Health
909 Basic Ave.
Bismarck, ND 58505
701-224-2769

OHIO

Denis W. Stoddard, Ph.D.
Executive Director
Ohio DD Planning Council
145 High Street
Columbus, OH 43215
614-466-5205

Director of Special Education
Division of Special Education
933 High Street
Worthington, OH 43085
614-466-2650

Robert L. Rabe
Administrator
Rehabilitation Services Commission
4656 Heaton Road
Columbus, OH 43229
614-438-1210

Governor's Committee on
  Handicapped Employment
4656 Heaton Road
Columbus, OH 43229

Director
State Department of Health
P.O. Box 118
450 E. Town St.
Columbus, OH 43215
614-466-3263

Mental Retardation
  Program Director
Dept. Mental Health/
  Develop. Disabilities
State Office Tower
30 E. Broad St.
Room 1284
Columbus, OH 43215
614-466-5214

Braille and Talking Book Dept.
Cleveland Public Library
325 Superior Ave.
Cleveland, OH 44114
216-623-2911

Library for the Blind &
  Physically Handicapped
444 W. 3rd St.
Cincinnati, OH 45202
513-369-6074

Resources

OKLAHOMA

Ray Ashworth
Council Coordinator
DD Planning Council
P.O. Box 25352
Oklahoma City, OK 73125
405-521-2989

Director of Special Education
Division of Special Education
State Department of Education
2500 N. Lincoln, Suite 263
Oklahoma City, OK 73105
405-521-3351

James A. West, Ph.D.
Director
Division of Rehabilitative
  & Visual Services
Dept. of Human Services
P.O. Box 25352
Oklahoma City, OK 73125
405-521-3646

Governor's Committee on
  Handicapped Employment
301 Will Rogers Bldg.
Oklahoma City, OK 73105

Director
Department of Rehabilitative Services
Crippled Children's Unit
P.O. Box 25352
Oklahoma City, OK 73125
405-271-3902

Mental Retardation Program Director
Dept. of Human Services
P.O. Box 25325
Oklahoma City, OK 73125
405-521-3646

Library for the Blind &
  Physically Handicapped
1108 NE 36th St.
3Oklahoma City, OK 73111
405-521-3514

OREGON

Jack Horner
Council Coordinator
DD Planning Council
800 Public Service Bldg.
Salem, OR 97310
503-378-2314

Director of Special Education
Division of Special Education
State Department of Education
942 Lancaster Dr. NE
Salem, OR 97310
503-378-3598

Joil Southwell
Administrator
Division of Vocational Rehabilitation
Dept. of Human Resources
2045 Silverton Road, NE
Salem, OR 97310
503-378-3850

Governor's Committee on
  Handicapped Employment
Oregon State Employment Division
875 Union St., NE
Salem, OR 97310

Director
Crippled Children's Division
3181 Southwest Sam Jackson
  Park Rd.
Portland, OR 97201
503-225-8362

Mental Retardation Program Director
Program for Mental Health/
  Develop. Disabilities
Mental Health Division
2570 Center St., NE
Salem, OR 97310
503-378-2429

Charles Young
Administrator
Commission for the Blind
535 S.E. 12th Ave.
Portland, OR 97214
503-238-8380

Oregon State Library
Services for the Blind & Handicapped
555 13th St., NE
Salem, OR 97301
503-378-3849

PERSONAL COMPUTERS AND THE DISABLED

PENNSYLVANIA

David Schwartz
Executive Director
DD Planning Council
Room 569, Forum Bldg.
Commonwealth Ave.
Harrisburg, PA 17120
717-787-6057

Director of Special Education
Bureau of Special Education
State Department of Education
P.O. Box 911
Harrisburg, PA 17126
717-783-1264

George Lowe, Jr.
Executive Director
Office of Vocational Rehabilitation
Labor & Industry Bldg.
7th and Forster Sts.
Harrisburg, PA 17120
717-787-5244

Governor's Committee on
  Handicapped Employment
Bureau of Employment Security
Rm. E-161
Seventh and Forster Sts.
Harrisburg, PA 17121

Director
State Department of Health
Bureau of Children's Services
407 S. Cameron St.
Harrisburg, PA 17120
717-783-5436

Joseph A. Snyder
Commissioner
Bureau of Blindness &
  Visual Services
Dept. of Public Welfare
Capital Association Bldg., Room 300
P.O. Box 2675
Harrisburg, PA 17120
717-787-6176

Library for the Blind &
  Physically Handicapped
Free Library of Philadelphia
919 Walnut St.
Philadelphia, PA 19107
215-925-3213

Library for the Blind &
  Physically Handicapped
Carnegie Library of Pittsburgh
4724 Baum Blvd.
Pittsburgh, PA 15213
412-687-2440

RHODE ISLAND

Michael Slachek
Director
DD Planning Council
600 New London Ave.
Cranston, RI 02920
401-464-3191

Director of Special Education
Division of Special Education
State Department of Education
235 Promenade St.
Providence, RI 02908
401-277-3505

Edward Carley
Administrator
Vocational Rehabilitation Services
Division of Community Services
40 Fountain St.
Providence, RI 02903
401-421-7005

Governor's Committee on
  Handicapped Employment
Bureau of Employment Security
24 Mason St.
Providence, RI 02903

Director
Department of Health
Division of Child Health
75 Davis St.
Room 302
Providence, RI 02908
401-277-2312

Mental Retardation
  Program Director
Division of Retardation
Dept. of Mental Health
Aime J. Forand Bldg.
600 New London Ave.
Cranston, RI 02920
401-464-3234

E. Lyman D'Andrea
Administrator
Services for the Blind
  & Visually Impaired
Dept. of Social &
  Rehabilitational Services
46 Abord St.
Providence, RI 02903
401-277-2300

Library for the Blind &
  Physically Handicapped
Rhode Island Dept. of Library Services
95 Davis St.
Providence, RI 02908
401-277-2726

Resources

SOUTH CAROLINA

Mary Barnett
Director
DD Planning Council
1205 Pendleton St., Room 408
Edgar Brown Bldg.
Columbia, SC 29201
803-758-8016

Director of Special Education
Office of Program for Handicapped
State Department of Education
Room 309, Rutledge Bldg.
Columbia, SC 29201
803-758-7432

Joseph S. Dunesbury
Commissioner
Vocational Rehabilitation Dept.
P.O. Box 4945
Columbia, SC 29240
803-758-3237

Governor's Committee on
　Handicapped Employment
Bureau of Employment Security
P.O. Box 1406
1550 Gadsen St.
Columbia, SC 29202

Director
Department of Health &
　Environmental Control
Children's Services
J. Marion Sims Bldg.
Columbia, SC 29201
803-758-5594

Mental Retardation Program Director
Dept. of Mental Health
2712 Middleburg Dr.
P.O. Box 4706
Columbia, SC 29240
803-758-3671

Maxine R. Bowles
Commissioner
Commission for the Blind
1430 Confederate Ave.
Columbia, SC 29201
803-758-2595

Library for the Blind &
　Physically Handicapped
Regional Library
700 Knox Abbott Drive
Cayce, SC 29033
803-758-2726

SOUTH DAKOTA

Thomas E. Scheinost
Program Administrator
Office of DD
State Office
Richard F. Kneip Bldg.
Pierre, SD 57501
605-773-3438

Director of Special Education
Section for Special Education
Division of Elementary &
　Secondary Education
New State Office Bldg.
Pierre, SD 57501
605-773-3678

John E. Madigan
Secretary
Division of Rehabilitative Services
Dept. of Rehabilitation
State Office Bldg. Illinois St.
Pierre, SD 57501
605-773-3195

Governor's Committee on
　Handicapped Employment
State Office Bldg., 2nd Floor
Illinois St.
Pierre, SD 57501

Director
State Department of Health
Division of Health Services
Foss Bldg.
Pierre, SD 57501
605-224-3141

Mental Retardation Program Director
Div. of Mental Health
Dept. of Social Services
State Office Bldg., 3rd Floor
Pierre, SD 57501
605-773-3438

State Library for the Handicapped
State Library Bldg.
Pierre, SD 57501
605-773-3514

PERSONAL COMPUTERS AND THE DISABLED

TENNESSEE

Pat Oates
Director
DD Planning Council
505 Deaderick St.
James K. Polk Bldg., 4th Floor
Nashville, TN 37219
615-741-6433

Director of Special Education
Education for the Handicapped
State Department of Education
103 Cordell Hull Bldg.
Nashville, TN 37219
615-741-2851

William M. Jenkins, Ed.D.
Assistant Commissioner
Division of Rehabilitation Services
1808 West End Bldg., Room 900
Nashville, TN 37203
615-741-2095

Governor's Committee on
   Handicapped Employment
Room 424
1808 West End Bldg.
Nashville, TN 37203

Director
State Department of Public Health
Crippled Children's Services
347 Cordell Hull Bldg.
Nashville, TN 37219
615-741-7335

Mental Retardation Program Director
Dept. of Mental Health
501 Union Bldg.
Nashville, TN 37219
615-741-3803

Library for the Blind &
   Physically Handicapped
729 Church St.
Nashville, TN 37203
615-741-3915

TEXAS

Joellen Flores-Simmons
Director
DD Planning Council
118 E. Riverside Dr.
Austin, TX 78704
512-445-8867

Director of Special Education
Division of Special Education
Texas Education Agency
201 E. 11th St.
Austin, TX 78701
512-475-3501

Vernon M. Arrell
Commissioner
Rehabilitation Commission
118 E. Riverside Dr.
Austin, TX 78704
512-445-8100

Governor's Committee on
   Handicapped Employment
Texas Employment Commission
15th and Congress
TEC Bldg.
Austin, TX 78778

Director
Department of Health
Crippled Children's Program
1100 W. 49th St.
Austin, TX 78576
512-458-7700

Mental Retardation Program Director
Dept. of Mental Health
P.O. Box 12668, Capitol Station
Austin, TX 78711
512-454-3761

John C. Wilson
Executive Director
State Commission for the Blind
P.O. Box 12866, Capitol Station
Austin, TX 78711
512-475-6810

Library for the Blind &
   Physically Handicapped
P.O. Box 12927, Capitol Station
Austin, TX 78711
512-475-4758

Resources

UTAH

Ineda Roe
Director
Council for Handicapped
 and DD Persons
P. O. Box 11356
Salt Lake City, UT 84147
801-533-6770

Director of Special Education
Pupil Services Coordinator
State Department of Education
250 E. 5th St.
Salt Lake City, UT 84111
801-533-5982

Judy Buffmire, Ph.D.
Administrator
Division of Rehabilitation Services
Utah State Office of Education
250 E. 5th St.
Salt Lake City, UT 84111
801-533-5991

Governor's Committee on
 Handicapped Employment
250 E. 500 St.
Salt Lake City, UT 84111

Director
State Division of Health
Crippled Children's Services
44 Medical Dr.
Salt Lake City, UT 84113
801-533-4390

Mental Retardation Program Director
Dept. of Social Services
150 West N. Temple, Ste. 370
P.O. Box 2500
Salt Lake City, UT 84110
801-533-7146

Warren Thompson
Director
Services for the Visually Handicapped
Utah State Office of Education
309 E. First St.
Salt Lake City, UT 84111
801-533-9393

Library for the Blind &
 Physically Handicapped
State Library Commission
2150 S. 300 W., Ste. 16
Salt Lake City, UT 84115
801-533-5855

VERMONT

Thomas Pomdar
Executive Secretary
DD Planning Council
Waterbury Office Complex
103 S. Main St.
Waterbury, VT 05676
802-241-2612

Director of Special Education
Special Education and
 Pupil Personnel Services
State Department of Education
Montpelier, VT 05602
802-828-3141

Richard W. Hill
Director
Vocational Rehabilitation Division
Osgood Bldg., Waterbury Complex
103 S. Main St.
Waterbury, VT 05676
802-241-2189

Governor's Committee on
 Handicapped Employment
81 River St.
Montpelier, VT 05602

Director
Department of Health
Child Health Services
115 Colchester Ave.
Burlington, VT 05402
802-862-5701

Mental Retardation Program Director
Dept. of Mental Health
State Office Bldg.
Montpelier, VT 05602
802-241-2636

David Mentasti
Director
Division for the Blind &
 Visually Handicapped
Osgood Bldg., Waterbury Complex
103 S. Main St.
Waterbury, VT 05676
802-241-2211

Library for the Blind &
 Physically Handicapped
Dept. of Libraries
Montpelier, VT 05602
802-828-3273

PERSONAL COMPUTERS AND THE DISABLED

VIRGINIA

Linda Veldheen
Director
DD Planning Council
P.O. Box 1797
Richmond, VA 23214
804-786-1331

Director of Special Education
Division of Special Education
State Department of Education
322 E. Grace
Richmond, VA 23216
804-786-2673

Altamont Dickerson, Jr.
Commissioner
Dept. of Rehabilitative Services
Commonwealth of Virginia
4901 Fitzhugh Ave.
P.O. Box 11045
Richmond, VA 23230
804-257-0316

Governor's Committee on
 Handicapped Employment
P.O. Box 1358
Richmond, VA 23211

Director
State Department of Health
Division of Hospital Medical Services
Bureau of Crippled Children's Services
109 Covernor St.
Richmond, VA 23219
804-770-3691

Mental Retardation Program Director
Dept. of Mental Health
P.O. Box 1797
Richmond, VA 23214
804-786-4982

William T. Coppage
Commissioner
Dept. for the Visually Handicapped
397 Azalea Ave.
Richmond, VA 23227
804-264-3140

Library for the Blind &
 Physically Handicapped
1901 Roane St.
Richmond, VA 23222
804-786-8016

WASHINGTON

Sharon M. Hansen
Director
DD Planning Council
Mail Stop 41-P
Olympia, WA 98504
206-753-3908

Director of Special Education
Department of Public Instruction
Special Services Section
Old Capitol Bldg.
Olympia, WA 98504
206-753-2563

Leslie James
Director
Division of Rehabilitation
State Office Bldg., No. 2
Dept. of Social and Health Services
P.O. Box 1788 (MS21-c)
Olympia, WA 98504
206-753-0293

Governor's Committee on
 Handicapped Employment
212 Maple Park
Olympia, WA 98504

Director
State Department of Social
 & Health Services
Division of Health Services
Child Health Section
MS: LC-12-A
Olympia, WA 98504
206-753-2571

Mental Retardation
 Program Director
Div. of Developmental
 Disabilities/Dept. of Health
Box 1788, OB-42C
Olympia, WA 98532
206-753-3900

Paul Dziedzic
Director
Dept. of Services for the Blind
921 Lakeridge Dr., 2nd Floor
Mail Stop SW-21
Olympia, WA 98502
206-754-1224

Library for the Blind &
 Physically Handicapped
811 Harrison St.
Seattle, WA 98129
206-464-6930

Resources

WEST VIRGINIA

Richard Kelly
Staff director
DD Planning Council
C/o Dept. of Mental Health
State Capitol
Charleston, WV 25305
304-348-2276

Director of Special Education
Division of Special Education
State Department of Education
Capitol Complex
Room B-057
Charleston, WV 25305
304-348-2034

Earl W. Wolfe
Director
Division of Vocational
  Rehabilitation
State Board of
  Vocational Education
State Capitol Complex
Charleston, WV 25305
304-348-2375

Governor's Committee on
  Handicapped Employment
4407 MacCorkle Ave., SE
Charleston, WV 25304

Director
State Department of Welfare
Division of Crippled
  Children's Services
1212 Lewis St., Morris Sq.
Charleston, WV 25301
304-348-3071

Mental Retardation
  Program Director
Develop. Disabilities Services/
  Health Dept.
State Capitol Bldg.
Charleston, WV 25305
304-348-2276

Library for the Blind &
  Physically Handicapped
Science and Culture Center
Greenbrier and Washington Sts.
Charleston, WV 25305
304-348-4061

WISCONSIN

Jayn Wittenmyer
Director
DD Planning Council
P.O. Box 7851
Madison, WI 53702
608-266-7826

Director of Special Education
Division for Handicapped Children
GEF III, 4th Floor, B 93
125 S. Webster
Madison, WI 53702
608-266-1649

Patricia Kallesen
Administrator
Division of Vocational
  Rehabilitation
Dept. of Health & Social Services
131 W. Wilson St., 7th Floor
P.O. Box 7852
Madison, WI 53702
608-266-5466

Governor's Committee on
  Handicapped Employment
Park Regent Bldg., 4th floor
1 S. Park St.
Madison, WI 53715

Director
State Department of
  Public Instruction
Bureau for Crippled Children
126 Langdon St.
Madison, WI 53702
608-266-3886

Mental Retardation
  Program Director
Bureau of Mental Health/
  Health Dept.
1 W. Wilson Street
Madison, WI 53702
608-267-7921

Library for the Blind &
  Physically Handicapped
814 W. Wisconsin Ave.
Milwaukee, WI 53233
414-278-3045

PERSONAL COMPUTERS AND THE DISABLED

WYOMING

Sharron Kelsey
Director
DD Planning Council
P.O. Box 1205
Cheyenne, WY 82001
307-632-7105

Director of Special Education
Office of Exceptional Children
State Department of Education
Cheyenne, WY 82002
307-777-7416

Robert D. Dingwall, Ed.D.
Administrator
Division of Vocational
 Rehabilitation
Dept. of Health & Social Services
326 Hathaway Bldg.
Cheyenne, WY 82002
307-777-7385

Governor's Committee on
 Handicapped Employment
611 E. 16th St.
Cheyenne, WY 82001

Director
State Department of Health/
 Social Services
Hathaway Office Bldg.
Cheyenne, WY 82002
307-777-7121

Mental Retardation Program Director
Coordinator for Human Resources
Board of Charities and Reform
State Capitol Bldg.
Cheyenne, WY 82001
307-777-7407

For information about **The McWilliams Letter** ("Some's News, Some's Not"), an informal ten-times-per-year update on the world of personal computers, please write to:

>Prelude Press
>Box 69773
>Los Angeles, CA 90069

We'll send you a "descriptive brochure" (as they say in the travel industry).

Addresses

Here are the addresses of the manufacturers mentioned in the text and the Buying Guide. There are also others here who were not mentioned.

Acorn Computer
400 Unicorn Park Drive
Woburn, MA 01801
(617) 935-1190

Advanced Software Interface
2655 Campus Drive
Suite 260
San Mateo, CA 94403
(415) 572-1347
(Keynote software for IBM)

Advent Products
965 North Main Street
Orange, CA 92667
(714) 997-0800
(Anti-glare screens)

Alfred Glossbrenner
St. Martin's Press
175 Fifth Avenue
New York, NY 10010
(Personal Computer
Communications Book)

American Training International
3770 Highland Avenue
Suite 201
Manhattan Beach, CA 90266
(213) 546-4725
(Teach Yourself Software)

Anchor Automation
6624 Valjean Avenue
Van Nuys, CA 91406
(818) 997-6493
(Signalman modems)

Apple Computer
10260 Bandley Drive
Cupertino, CA 95014
(408) 996-1010

Artificial Intelligence
Research Group
921 N. La Jolla
Los Angeles, CA 90046
(213) 656-7368
(Eliza)

Ashton-Tate
9929 West Jefferson Boulevard
Culver City, CA 90230
(213) 204-5570
(dBase II)

Atari, Inc.
1265 Borregas Avenue
Sunnyvale, CA 94086
(408) 745-2000

Axel Johnson Corp.
666 Howard Street
San Francisco, CA 94105
(415) 777-3800
(Autocode software)

Brother International
20 Goodyear
Irvine, CA 92714
(714) 859-9700

BRS
1200 Route 7
Latham, NY 12110
(800) 833-4707
(BRS After Dark database)

Bruce & James Publishers
The Wharfside Building
680 Beach Street—Suite 357
San Francisco, CA 94109
(415) 775-8400
(WordVision for IBM)

Business Computer Network
P.O. Box 36
1000 College View Drive
Riverton, WY 82501
(800) 446-6255
(BCN Communications Network)

Businessoft
24 Jean Lane
Monsey, NY 10952
(201) 783-6888
(Wondertype)

BYTE
70 Main Street
Peterborough, NH 03458
(603) 924-9281
(Magazine)

Bytewriter
125 Northview Road
Ithaca, NY 14850
(607) 272-1132

Centram Systems, Inc.
P.O. Box 511
Camp Hill, PA 17011
(717) 763-1198
(Networking Kaypros)

Chuck Atkinson Programs
Rt. 5, Box 277-C
Benbrook, TX 76126
(817) 249-0166
(Pro Bookkeeper, Quick Check, RIP programs)

Coleco Industries
999 Quaker Lane South
West Hartford, CT 06110
(203) 725-6000
(Coleco Adam)

Columbia Data Products, Inc.
8990 Route 108
Columbia, MD 21045
(301) 992-3400
(Columbia MPC)

Commodore Computer Systems
1200 Wilson Drive
West Chester, PA 19380
(215) 431-9100

Compal Computer Center
8500 Wilshire Boulevard
Suite 103
Beverly Hills, CA 90211
(213) 652-2263
(Wordpal)

Compaq Computer Corp.
12330 Perry Road
Houston, TX 77070
(713) 370-7040
(Compaq computers)

CompuServe Information Service
5000 Arlington Centre Boulevard
P.O. Box 20212
Columbus, OH 43220
(800) 848-8199
(Database)

Computers International
3540 Wilshire Boulevard
Los Angeles, CA 90010
(213) 386-3111
(Daisywriter printer)

Comrex
3701 Skypark Drive
Suite #120
Torrance, CA 90505
(213) 373-0280
(Letter quality printers)

Continental Software
11223 South Hindry Avenue
Los Angeles, CA 90045
(213) 410-3977
(The Home Accountant)

Cord Ltd.
2815 Junipero Avenue
Building #102
Signal Hill, CA 90806
(213) 595-4446
(Supercord)

Corona Data Systems
313 Via Colinas
Westlake Village, CA 91362
(818) 991-8120

Creative Computing
Box 789-M
Morristown, NJ 07960
(Magazine)

Cromemco
280 Bernardo Avenue
Mountain View, CA 94043
(415) 964-7400
(C-10 computer)

Cuadra Associates, Inc.
2001 Wilshire Boulevard
Suite 305
Santa Monica, CA 90403
(213) 829-9972
(Directory of Online Databases)

Cuesta Systems, Inc.
3440 Roberto Court
San Luis Obispo, CA 93401
(805) 541-4160
(DataSaver line conditioner)

Data Base Research Corp.
66 South Van Gordon, Suite 155
Lakewood, CO 80228
(303) 987-2588
(Champion business accounting software)

Datatran
1195 South Huron Street
Denver, CO 80223
(303) 778-0870
(Datatracker breakout box)

DIALOG Information Services, Inc.
3460 Hillview Avenue
Palo Alto, CA 94304
(415) 852-3901
(DIALOG and Knowledge Index databases)

Digisoft Computers
1501 Third Avenue
New York, NY 10028
(212) 734-3875
(Mail-Com)

Digital Equipment Corporation (DEC)
2 Mount Royal Avenue
Marlboro, MA 01752
(617) 264-1669
(DEC Rainbow and DECmate II)

Digital Marketing
2670 Cherry Lane
Walnut Creek, CA 94596
(415) 938-2880
(Micro Link II)

Dover Publications
180 Varick Street
New York, NY 10014
(Publishers of Dover
Archive Series)

Dow Jones News/Retrieval
Service
P.O. Box 300
Princeton, NJ 08540
(800) 257-5114
(Database)

Dvorak International
Federation
11 Pearl Street
Brandon, VT 05733
(802) 247-6020
(Dvorak Keyboard group)

DynaType
740 East Wilson Avenue
Glendale, CA 91206
(213) 243-1114
(Typesetting using modems)

Dynax
5698 Bandini Boulevard
Bell, CA 90201
(213) 260-7121
(Distributor of the Brother
printers)

Eagle Business Systems
983 University Avenue
Los Gatos, CA 95030
(408) 395-5005
(Eagle Computer)

Epson America, Inc.
3415 Kashiwa Street
Torrance, CA 90505
(213) 539-9140
(QX-10 computer and
FX-80 printer)

Franklin Computer
7030 Colonial Highway
Pennsauken, NJ 08109
(609) 482-5900
(Franklin Ace 1000 and 1200)

FYI
P.O. Box 26481
Austin, TX 78755
(512) 346-0133
(SuperFile and FYI 3000)

Grid Systems Corp.
2535 Garcia Drive
Mountain View, CA 94043
(415) 961-4800
(Compass Computer)

Hayes Microcomputer Products, Inc.
5923 Peachtree
Industrial Boulevard
Norcross, GA 30092
(404) 449-8791
(Hayes SmartModem)

Head Computer Products
18533 Burbank Boulevard
Tarzana, CA 91356
(818) 342-9600
(Head Head Cleaner)

Heathkit Electronics Corporation
P.O. Box 167
St. Joseph, MI 49805
(616) 982-3285
(Heath H-89)

Heritage Software, Inc.
2130 South Vermont Avenue
Los Angeles, CA 90007
(213) 737-7252
(SmartKey)

Hewlett-Packard
974 East Arques Street
Sunnyvale, CA 94086
(408) 720-3367

IBM
Information Systems Division
P.O. Box 1328
Boca Raton, FL 33432
(305) 241-6007

IJG Inc.
1953 West 11th Street
Upland, CA 91786
(714) 946-5805
(Electric Pencil)

Information Unlimited Software
281 Arlington Avenue
Berkeley, CA 94707
(415) 331-6700
(Easy Writer II)

InfoWorld
1060 Marsh Road
Suite C-200
Menlo Park, CA 94025
(415) 328-4602
(Magazine)

Interactive Structures, Inc.
146 Montgomery Avenue
Bala Cynwyd, PA 19004
(215) 667-1713
(ShuffleBuffer)

Interface Age
P.O. Box 1234
Cerritos, NJ 90701
(Magazine)

IQ Technologies, Inc.
11811 N.E. First Street
Bellevue, WA 98005
(206) 451-0232
(Smart Cable)

ITT Dialcom
1109 Spring Street
Silver Spring, MD 20910
(301) 588-1572
(Dialcom database)

John-Roger
Baraka Books
3500 West Adams Boulevard
Los Angeles, CA 90018
(Author of *Consciousness of Wealth*)

Jonos Ltd.
1835 Dawns Way
Fullerton, CA 92631
(714) 999-6661
(Jonos Computers)

Kaypro Corporation
533 Stevens Avenue
Solana Beach, CA 92075
(619) 481-3424
(Kaypro II, 4, 10)

Keytronics
P.O. Box 14687
Spokane, WA 99214
(509) 928-8000
(Keyboard for IBM-PC)

KREPEC Software, Inc.
5460 Royalmount
Suite 208
Montreal, Quebec
CANADA H4P 1H8
(514) 735-4749
(Reportmaker)

Langley-St. Clair
132 West 24th Street
New York, NY 10011
(212) 989-6876
(Eye-Guard radiation shield)

Lanier Business Products
1700 Chantilly Drive Northeast
Atlanta, GA 30324
(800) 241-1706

Lassen Software, Inc.
P.O. Box 1190
Chico, CA 95927
(916) 891-6957
(Diskette Manager)

Leading Edge Products, Inc.
21 Highland Circle
Needham Heights, MA 02194
(617) 449-4655
(Leading Edge PC)

Lexisoft
Box 267
Davis, CA 95617
(916) 758-3630
(Spellbinder)

Lexocorp
7100 Havenhurst Avenue
Van Nuys, CA 91406
(213) 786-1600
(Lexorbiter Series III)

Lifeboat Associates
1651 Third Avenue
New York, NY 10028
(Software distributors)

Lifetree Software
177 Webster Street
Suite 342
Monterey, CA 93940
(408) 373-4718
(VolksWriter for IBM)

Lotus Development Corporation
161 First Street
Cambridge, MA 02138
(617) 492-7171
(123 software)

Mannesmann Tally
8301 South 180th Street
Kent, WA 98032
(206) 251-5500
(Mannesmann Tally 160L)

MCI Mail
2000 M Street, NW
Washington, DC 20036
(202) 293-4255
(Electronic Mail)

Micro Solutions
125 South Fourth Street
DeKalb, IL 60115
(815) 756-3421
(UniForm Disk Formatting Program)

MicroPro International
1229 Fourth Street
San Rafael, CA 94901
(415) 499-1200
(WordStar and other software)

Morrow Designs
600 McCormick Street
San Leandro, CA 94577
(415) 430-1970
(Morrow Micro Decision)

Muse Software
347 North Charles Street
Baltimore, MD 21201
(301) 659-7212
(Word processing for Apples)

NEC Information Systems, Inc.
5 Militia Drive
Lexington, MA 02173
(617) 862-3120
(Spinwriter letter quality
printer)

NewsNet
945 Haverford Road
Bryn Mawr, PA 19010
(215) 527-8030
(Database)

NorthStar Computers, Inc.
14440 Catalina Street
San Leandro, CA 94577
(415) 357-8500

Norton-Lambert Corp.
P.O. Box 4085
Santa Barbara, CA 93103
(805) 687-8896
(LYNC communications
software)

Novation
20409 Prairie Street
Chatsworth, CA 91311
(818) 996-5060
(D-Cat and AutoCat modems)

Oasis Systems
3692 Midway Drive
San Diego, CA 92110
(619) 222-1153
(The WORD Plus, Punctuation
and Style)

Official Airline Guides, Inc.
2000 Clearwater Drive
Oak Brook, IL 60521
(Database)

Okidata Corporation
3300 Keller Street
Suite #201
Santa Clara, CA 95050
(408) 986-1890
(Dot matrix printers)

Otrona Corporation
4725 Walnut Street
Boulder, CO 80301
(800) 525-7550
(Otrona 2001)

Palantir, Inc.
3400 Montrose Boulevard
Suite #718
Houston, TX 77006
(713) 520-8221

Peachtree Software
3 Corporate Square
Suite 700
Atlanta, GA 30329
(404) 325-8533
(PeachText and other software)

Pearlsoft
25195 Southwest Parkway
P.O. Box 638
Wilsonville, OR 97070
(503) 682-3636
(Personal Pearl data base manager)

Peggy Glenn
924 Main Street
Huntington Beach, CA 92648
(714) 536-4926
(Home Word Processing Service Book)

Perfect Software, Inc.
702 Harrison Street
Berkeley, CA 94710
(415) 524-1926

Personal Computing
4 Disk Drive (cute, huh?)
Box 1408
Riverton, NJ 08077
(Magazine)

Pion, Inc.
101R Walnut Street
Watertown, MA 02172
(617) 923-8009
(Interstellar drive)

Plu*Perfect Systems
P.O. Box 1494
Idyllwild, CA 92349
(714) 659-4432
(CP/M 2.2E and Plu*Perfect Writer)

Popular Computing
P.O. Box 307
Martinsville, NJ 08836
(Magazine)

Printek, Inc.
1737 North First Street
Suite 510
San Jose, CA 95112
(408) 275-1905
(Dot matrix printers)

Profile Computer Systems, Inc.
2509 South West 59th Street
Oklahoma City, OK 73119
(405) 682-3606
(speed-up and co-processor boards)

PSC Computers, Inc.
2934 Wilshire Boulevard
Santa Monica, CA 90403
(213) 826-3128
(Epson QX-10 book)

R.J. Brady Company
Routes 197 and 450
Bowie, MD 20715
(301) 262-6300
(Publishers of Z-100 users guide)

Radio Shack/Tandy
1800 One Tandy Center
Fort Worth, TX 76102
(817) 390-3011

Ring King Visibles, Inc.
215 West Second Street
Muscatine, IA 52761
(800) 553-9647
(Makers of disk storage files)

Rising Star Industries
24050 Madison Street
Suite #113
Torrance, CA 90505
(213) 378-9861
(Valdocs software for QX-10)

Rocky Mountain Software
Systems
P.O. Box 3282
Walnut Creek, CA 94598
(415) 680-8378
(NewWord Software)

Samna
2700 N.E. Expressway
Suite #C-1200
Atlanta, GA 30345
(800) 241-2065
(Samna Word II)

Sanyo
51 Joseph Street
Moonachie, NJ 07074
(201) 440-9300

Screenplay Systems
211 East Olive Avenue
Suite 203
Burbank, CA 91502
(818) 843-6557
(Scriptor)

Seequa Computer Corp.
8305 Telegraph Road
Odenton, MD 21113
(301) 672-3600

Select Information Systems
919 Sir Francis Drake Boulevard
Kentfield, CA 94904
(415) 459-4003

Sheepshead Software
P.O. Box 486
Boonville, CA 95415
(Drive Diagnostic Kit)

Silver-Reed America, Inc.
19600 South Vermont Avenue
Torrance, CA 90502
(213) 516-7008
(Letter-quality Printers)

Sinclair Research
50 Staniford Street
Suite 800
Boston, MA 02114
(617) 742-4826
(Sinclair QL)

Small Systems Engineering
1056 Elwell Court
Palo Alto, CA 94303
(415) 964-8201
(CP/M card for Victor 9000)

Smith-Corona
65 Locust Avenue
New Canaan, CT 06840
(203) 972-1471
(L-1000 printer)

SoftCraft, Inc.
8726 South Sepulveda Boulevard
Suite 1641
Los Angeles, CA 90045
(213) 821-8476
(Fancy Font)

Software Products International
10343 Roselle Street
Suite A
San Diego, CA 92121
(619) 450-1526
(LogiQuest III)

Solution Technology, Inc.
1499 Palmetto Park Road
Suite 218
Boca Raton, FL 33432
(305) 368-6226
(Compare Software)

SOS Computers
362 South La Brea Avenue
Los Angeles, CA 90036
(213) 857-0317
(Porta-Micro Mate
computer stand)

South Bay Word Processing
P.O. Box 331
Nestor, CA 92053
(619) 575-8381
(Word Processing Service
Start-Up Kit)

Star Micronics, Inc.
3 Oldfield Drive
Irvine, CA 92714
(714) 768-4340
(Printers)

Supersoft
P.O. Box 1628
Champaign, IL 61820
(217) 359-2112
(Disk Doctor)

Telehance Industries
28631 Canwood Street
Unit M
Agoura, CA 91301
(818) 706-1557
(Hard disks for TeleVideo)

Teleram
2 Corporate Park Drive
White Plains, NY 10604
(914) 694-9270
(Teleram T-3000)

TeleVideo
1170 Morse Avenue
Sunnyvale, CA 94086
(408) 745-7760

Texas Instruments, Inc.
P.O. Box 1444, MS 7896
Houston, TX 77001
(713) 895-3000

The Source
1616 Anderson Road
McLean, VA 22102
(703) 734-7500
(Databank)

The Systems House
Village Center
Box 617
Great Falls, VA 22066
(703) 759-6800
(Free Flier)

Thunderhawk Corporation
485 Antelope Boulevard
Suite 3
Red Bluff, CA 96080
(916) 529-3000
(Thunder 'Tector Power Saver)

Toshiba America
Information Systems Division
2441 Michelle Drive
Tustin, CA 92680
(714) 730-5000
(T-300 computer)

Transtar
P.O. Box C-96975
Bellevue, WA 98009
(206) 454-9250
(Letter quality printers)

U.S. Robotics
1123 West Washington
Chicago, IL 60607
(312) 733-0497
(Password modem)

Victor, United
13477 Prospect Road
Strongville, OH 44136
(216) 238-8448

VisiCorp
2895 Zanker Road
San Jose, CA 95134
(408) 946-9000
(VisiCalc and other software)

Wang Electronic Publishing
1 World Trade Center
Room 3271
New York, NY 10048
(212) 432-2131
(Random House Thesaurus and Strunk & White)

Wang Laboratories
6059 Bristol Parkway
Culver City, CA 90230
(213) 642-7433
(Wang Personal Computer)

Western Telematic Inc.
2435 South Anne Street
Santa Ana, CA 92704
(714) 979-0363
(Smart Switch)

Western Union
One Lake Street
Upper Saddle River, NJ 07458
(201) 825-5000
(EasyLink Electronic Mail)

Westnofa USA, Inc.
7618 North Rogers Avenue
Chicago, IL 60626
(312) 761-4610
(Balans Chairs)

WP News
211 East Olive Street
Suite 210
Burbank, CA 91501
(818) 845-7809
(A word processing newsletter)

Wyndham Group, Ltd., The
125 Mirona Road
Portsmouth, NH 03801
(603) 431-4800
(Letterbank Software)

Xedex Corporation
1345 Avenue of the Americas
New York, NY 10105
(Baby Blue Board for IBM)

Xerox Corporation
Stamford, CT 06904
(203) 329-8700
(Xerox 820-II)

Zenith Data Systems
1000 Milwaukee Avenue
Glenview, IL 60025
(312) 391-8744
(Z-100 computer)